"*In the Realm of Hungry Ghosts* is a survey of scientific evidence on addiction. . . . Drug-addled, yes—but Maté's patients are often perceptive, sensitive and struggling to keep whatever dignity society has left them. . . . That the well-off and the destitute are considered together in this book reminds us that addiction transcends class. . . . Maté is obviously an effective communicator on medical issues."

The Gazette

"A nuanced and complex meditation on what opium-eater Thomas de Quincy called the 'abiding darkness'. . . . A powerful and compassionate work."

NOW

"Excellent. . . . One of the book's strengths is Maté's detailed and compassionate characterization of the afflicted addicts he treats, but this is not just a memoir. Rather, using his own experience as well as the most advanced recent research, he attempts to delineate the closely interrelated psychological, social, and neurological dimensions of addiction. . . . A calm, unjudging, compassionate attentiveness to what is happening within."

The Walrus

"Powerful. . . . Maté wades through the vast learning behind the root causes of addiction, applying a clinical and psychological view to the physical manifestation and unearthing some surprising (to the layman anyway) answers for why people do such frightening and destructive things to themselves. . . . *In the Realm of Hungry Ghosts* is enormously compelling and Maté, as noted, is admirably, sometimes inexplicably, empathetic to all who cross his path."

Toronto Star

"Maté presents a well-reasoned critique of the so-called war on drugs and offers suggestions for how we might respond more effectively to chronic addiction."

The Vancouver Sun

"Dr. Maté's latest book [is] a moving, debate-provoking and multi-layered look at how addiction arises, the people afflicted with it and why he supports decriminalization of all drugs, including crystal meth. . . . [*In the Realm of Hungry Ghosts*] reads not only as a lively textbook analysis of the physiological and psychological causes of drug addiction, but also as an investigation into his heart and mind."

The Globe and Mail

"Gabor Maté's connections—between the intensely personal and the global, the spiritual and the medical, the psychological and the political—are bold, wise and deeply moral. He is a healer to be cherished and this exciting book arrives at just the right time."

Naomi Klein, author of *No Logo* and *The Shock Doctrine*

"It seems odd to use the word 'beautiful' to describe a book that focuses frequently, in graphic, unrelenting detail, on the lives of some of the most hopeless outcasts of our society: the hard-core street addicts with whom Dr. Gabor Maté works. Yet that's the word that came repeatedly to mind as I read *In the Realm of Hungry Ghosts*. It's not only the grace of Maté's writing, though that's certainly a great part of it. It's the sense of compassion that infuses the entire book. . . . Maté offers no easy fixes (pun intended), but does offer hope and understanding."

The Record

"With superb descriptive talents, Gabor Maté takes us into the lives of the emotionally destitute and drug addicted human beings who are his patients. In this highly readable and penetrating book, he gives us the disturbing truths about the nature of addiction and its roots in people's early years—truths that are usually concealed by time and protected by shame, secrecy and social taboo."

Vincent Felitti, M.D., Clinical Professor of Medicine,
University of California, and Co-Principal Investigator,
Adverse Childhood Experiences Study

GABOR MATÉ, M.D.

In the Realm of
Hungry Ghosts

Close Encounters with Addiction

VINTAGE CANADA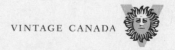

VINTAGE CANADA EDITION, 2009

Published in Canada by Vintage Canada, a division of Random House of Canada Limited, Toronto, in 2009. Originally published in hardcover in Canada by Alfred A. Knopf Canada, a division of Random House of Canada Limited, Toronto, in 2008. Distributed by Random House of Canada Limited, Toronto.

Vintage Canada and colophon are registered trademarks of Random House of Canada Limited.

www.randomhouse.ca

LIBRARY AND ARCHIVES CANADA CATALOGUING IN PUBLICATION

Maté, Gabor
In the realm of hungry ghosts : close encounters with addiction / Gabor Maté.

Includes bibliographical references and index.

ISBN 978-0-676-97741-7

1. Compulsive behavior. 2. Substance abuse. 3. Maté, Gabor—
Mental health. I. Title.

RC533.M38 2009   616.85'84   C2008-903680-8

Book design by CS Richardson

Printed and bound in the United States of America

2 4 6 8 9 7 5 3 1

To beloved Rae, my wife and dearest friend, who has lived these pages with me for forty years through thick and thin, for better or worse, and always for the best.

The persons, quotes, case examples and life histories in this book are all authentic; no embellishing details have been added and no "composite" characters have been created. To protect privacy, pseudonyms are used for All my patients, except for two people who directly requested to be named. In two other cases I have provided disguised physical descriptions, again in the interests of privacy.

Permission has been received from the persons whose lives are laid bare here. they have in all cases read the material pertinent to them. Similarly, prior permission and final approval was granted by the subjects whose photographs appear in these pages.

All scientific research quoted is fully referenced for each chapter in the Endnote section, but there was no space to list all the other journal articles that were consulted in the preparation of this manuscript. Professionals—indeed, any readers—are welcome to contact me for further information. I may be reached through my website: www.drgabormate.com. I welcome all comments but cannot respond to requests for specific medical advice.

Finally, a note regarding the photo portraits that accompany the text. Humbling as it is for a writer to accept that a picture is worth a thousand words, there may be no better proof of that dictum than the remarkable photographs contributed to this volume by Rod Preston. Having worked in the Downtown Eastside, Rod knows the people I've written about well and his camera has captured their experience with accuracy and feeling. His website is www.rodpreston.com.

What is addiction, really? It is a sign, a signal, a symptom of
distress. It is a language that tells us about a plight
that must be understood.

ALICE MILLER
Breaking Down the Wall of Silence

In the search for truth human beings take two steps forward and one
step back. Suffering, mistakes and weariness of life thrust them
back, but the thirst for truth and stubborn will drive them forward.
And who knows? Perhaps they will reach the real truth at last.

ANTON CHEKHOV
The Duel

CONTENTS

PART VII: THE ECOLOGY OF HEALING

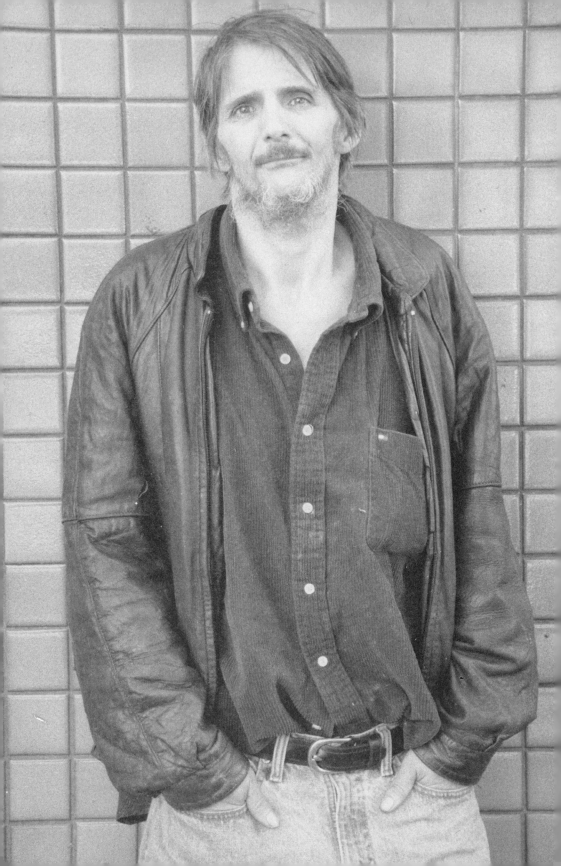

Hungry Ghosts: The Realm of Addiction

—

Yon Cassius has a lean and hungry look.

WILLIAM SHAKESPEARE

Julius Caesar

The *mandala,* the Buddhist Wheel of Life, revolves through six realms. Each realm is populated by characters representing aspects of human existence—our various ways of being. In the Beast Realm we are driven by basic survival instincts and appetites such as physical hunger and sexuality, what Freud called the id. The denizens of the Hell Realm are trapped in states of unbearable rage and anxiety. In the God Realm we transcend our troubles and our egos through sensual, aesthetic or religious experience, but only temporarily and in ignorance of spiritual truth. Even this enviable state is tinged with loss and suffering.

The inhabitants of the Hungry Ghost Realm are depicted as creatures with scrawny necks, small mouths, emaciated limbs and large, bloated, empty bellies. This is the domain of addiction, where we constantly seek something outside ourselves to curb an insatiable yearning for relief or fulfillment. The aching emptiness is perpetual because the substances, objects or pursuits we hope will soothe it are not what we really need. We don't know what we need, and so long as we stay in the hungry ghost mode, we'll never know. We haunt our lives without being fully present.

Some people dwell much of their lives in one realm or another. Many of us move back and forth between them, perhaps through all of them in the course of a single day.

My medical work with drug addicts in Vancouver's Downtown Eastside has given me a unique opportunity to know human beings who spend almost all their time as hungry ghosts. It's their attempt, I believe, to escape the Hell Realm of overwhelming fear, rage and despair. The painful longing in their hearts reflects something of the emptiness that may also be experienced by people with apparently happier lives. Those whom we dismiss as "junkies" are not creatures from a different world, only men and women mired at the extreme end of a continuum on which, here or there, all of us might well locate ourselves. I can personally attest to that. "You slink around your life with a hungry look," someone close once said to me. Facing the harmful compulsions of my patients, I have had to encounter my own.

No society can understand itself without looking at its shadow side. I believe there is one addiction process, whether it is manifested in the lethal substance dependencies of my Downtown Eastside patients; the frantic self-soothing of overeaters or shopaholics; the obsessions of gamblers, sexaholics and compulsive Internet users; or the socially acceptable and even admired behaviours of the workaholic. Drug addicts are often dismissed and discounted as unworthy of empathy and respect. In telling their stories my intent is twofold: to help their voices to be heard and to shed light on the origins and nature of their ill-fated struggle to overcome suffering through substance abuse. They have much in common with the society that ostracizes them. If they seem to have chosen a path to nowhere, they still have much to teach the rest of us. In the dark mirror of their lives, we can trace outlines of our own.

There is a host of questions to be considered. Among them:

- What are the causes of addictions?
- What is the nature of the addiction-prone personality?
- What happens physiologically in the brains of addicted people?
- How much choice does the addict really have?

- Why is the "War on Drugs" a failure and what might be a humane, evidence-based approach to the treatment of severe drug addiction?
- What are some of the paths for redeeming addicted minds *not* dependent on powerful substances—that is, how do we approach the healing of the many behaviour addictions fostered by our culture?

The narrative passages in this book are based on my experience as a medical doctor in Vancouver's drug ghetto and on extensive interviews with my patients—more than I could cite. Many of them volunteered in the generous hope that their life histories might be of assistance to others who struggle with addiction problems or that they could help enlighten society regarding the experience of addiction. I also present information, reflections and insights distilled from many other sources, including my own addictive patterns. And finally, I provide a synthesis of what we can learn from the research literature on addiction and the development of the human brain and personality.

Although the closing chapters offer thoughts and suggestions concerning the healing of the addicted mind, this book is not a prescription. I can say only what I have learned as a person and describe what I have seen and understood as a physician. Not every story has a happy ending, as the reader will find out, but the discoveries of science, the teachings of the heart and the revelations of the soul all assure us that no human being is ever beyond redemption. The possibility of renewal exists so long as life exists. How to support that possibility in others and in ourselves is the ultimate question.

I dedicate this work to all my fellow hungry ghosts, be they inner-city street dwellers with HIV, inmates of prisons or their more fortunate counterparts with homes, families, jobs and successful careers. May we all find peace.

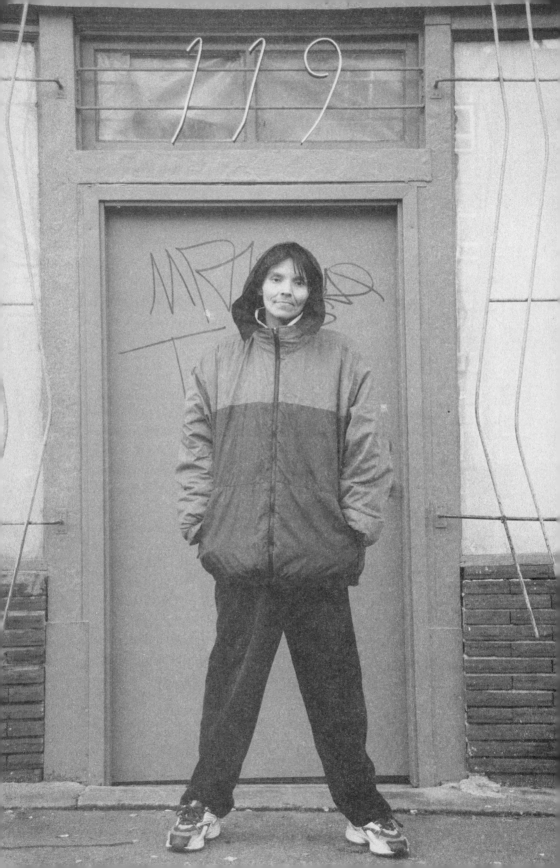

PART I

Hellbound Train

What was it that did in reality make me an opium eater?
Misery, blank desolation, abiding darkness.
THOMAS DE QUINCEY
Confessions of an English Opium Eater

CHAPTER I

The Only Home He's Ever Had

As I pass through the grated metal door into the sunshine, a setting from a Fellini film reveals itself. It is a scene both familiar and outlandish, dreamlike and authentic.

On the Hastings Street sidewalk Eva, in her thirties but still waif-like, with dark hair and olive complexion, taps out a bizarre cocaine flamenco. Jutting her hips, torso and pelvis this way and that, bending now at the waist and thrusting one or both arms in the air, she shifts her feet about in a clumsy but concerted pirouette. All the while she tracks me with her large, black eyes.

In the Downtown Eastside this piece of crack-driven improvisational ballet is known as "the Hastings shuffle," and it's a familiar sight. During my medical rounds in the neighbourhood one day, I saw a young woman perform it high above the Hastings traffic. She was balanced on the narrow edge of a neon sign two storeys up. A crowd had gathered to watch, the users among them more amused than horrified. The ballerina would turn about, her arms horizontal like a tightrope walker's, or do deep knee bends—an aerial Cossack dancer, one leg kicked in front. Before the top of the firemen's ladder could reach her cruising altitude, the stoned acrobat had ducked back inside her window.

Eva weaves her way among her companions, who crowd around me. Sometimes she disappears behind Randall—a wheelchair-bound, heavy-set, serious-looking fellow, whose unorthodox thought patterns do not mask a profound intelligence. He recites an ode of autistic praise to his indispensable motorized chariot. "Isn't it amazing, Doc, isn't it, that Napoleon's cannon was pulled by horses and oxen in the Russian mud and snow. And now I have this!" With an innocent smile and earnest expression, Randall pours out a recursive stream of facts, historical data, memories, interpretations, loose associations, imaginings, and paranoia that almost sound sane— almost. "That's the Napoleonic Code, Doc, which altered the transportational mediums of the lower rank and file, you know, in those days when such pleasant smorgasboredom was still well fathomed." Poking her head above Randall's left shoulder, Eva plays peek-a-boo.

Beside Randall stands Arlene, her hands on her hips and a reproachful look on her face, clad in skimpy jean shorts and blouse—a sign, down here, of a mode of earning drug money and, more often than not, of having been sexually exploited early in life by male predators. Over the steady murmur of Randall's oration comes her complaint: "You shouldn't have reduced my pills." Arlene's arms bear dozens of horizontal scars, parallel, like railway ties. The older ones white, the more recent red, each mark a souvenir of a razor slash she has inflicted on herself. The pain of self-laceration obliterates, if only momentarily, the pain of a larger hurt deep in the psyche. One of Arlene's medications controls this compulsive self-wounding, and she's always afraid I'm reducing her dose. I never do.

Close to us, in the shadow of the Portland Hotel, two cops have Jenkins in handcuffs. Jenkins, a lanky Native man with black, scraggly hair falling to below his shoulders, is quiet and compliant as one of the officers empties his pockets. He arches his back against the wall, not a hint of protest on his face. "They should leave him alone," Arlene opines loudly. "That guy doesn't deal. They keep grabbing him and never find a thing." At least in the broad daylight of Hastings Street, the cops go about their search with exemplary politeness—not, according to my patients, a consistent police attitude. After a minute or two Jenkins is set free and lopes silently into the hotel with his long stride.

Meanwhile, within the span of a few minutes, the resident poet laureate of absurdity has reviewed European history from the Hundred Years' War to Bosnia and has pronounced on religion from

Moses to Mohammed. "Doc," Randall goes on, "the First World War was supposed to end all wars. If that was true, how come we have the war on cancer or the war on drugs? The Germans had this gun Big Bertha that spoke to the Allies but not in a language the French or the Brits liked. Guns get a bad rap, a bad reputation—a bad *raputation,* Doc—but they move history forward, if we can speak of history moving forward or moving at all. Do you think history moves, Doc?"

Leaning on his crutches, paunchy, one-legged, smiling Matthew—bald, and irrepressibly jovial—interrupts Randall's discourse. "Poor Dr. Maté is trying to get home," he says in his characteristic tone: at once sarcastic and sweetly genuine. Matthew grins at us as if the joke is on everyone but himself. The chain of rings piercing his left ear glimmers in the bronzed gold of the late afternoon sun.

Eva prances out from behind Randall's back. I turn away. I've had enough street theatre and now I want to escape. The good doctor no longer wants to be good.

We congregate, these Fellini figures and I—or I should say we, this cast of Fellini characters—outside the Portland Hotel, where they live and I work. My clinic is on the first floor of this cement-and-glass building designed by Canadian architect Arthur Erickson, a spacious, modern, utilitarian structure. It's an impressive facility that serves its residents well, replacing the formerly luxurious turn-of-the-century establishment around the corner that was the first Portland Hotel. The old place, with its wooden balustrades, wide and winding staircases, musty landings and bay windows, had a character and history the new fortress lacks. Although I miss its Old World aura, the atmosphere of faded wealth and decay, the dark and blistered windowsills varnished with memories of elegance, I doubt the residents have any nostalgia for the cramped rooms, the corroded plumbing or the armies of cockroaches. In 1994 there was a fire on the roof of the old hotel. A local newspaper ran a story and a photograph featuring a female resident and her cat. The headline proclaimed, "Hero Cop Saves Fluffy." Someone phoned the Portland to complain that animals should not be allowed to live in such conditions.

The nonprofit Portland Hotel Society, for whom I am the staff physician, turned the building into housing for the nonhousable. My patients are mostly addicts, although some, like Randall, have enough derangement of their brain chemicals to put them out of touch with reality even without the use of drugs. Many, like Arlene, suffer from both mental illness and addiction. The PHS administers several similar facilities within a radius of a few blocks: the Stanley, Washington, Regal and Sunrise hotels. I am the house doctor for them all.

The new Portland faces the Army and Navy department store across the street, where my parents, as new immigrants in the late 1950s, bought most of our clothing. Back then, the Army and Navy was a popular shopping destination for working people—and for middle-class kids looking for funky military coats or sailor jackets. On the sidewalks outside, university students seeking some slumming fun mixed with alcoholics, pickpockets, shoppers and Friday night Bible preachers.

No longer. The crowds stopped coming many years ago. Now these streets and their back alleys serve as the centre of Canada's drug capital. One block away stood the abandoned Woodward's department store, its giant, lighted "W" sign on the roof a long-time Vancouver landmark. For a while squatters and antipoverty activists occupied the building, but it has recently been demolished; the site is to be converted into a mix of chic apartments and social housing. The Winter Olympics are coming to Vancouver in 2010 and with it the likelihood of gentrification in this neighbourhood. The process has already begun. There's a fear that the politicians, eager to impress the world, will try to displace the addict population.

Eva intertwines her arms, stretches them behind her back and leans forward to examine her shadow on the sidewalk. Matthew chuckles at her crackhead yoga routine. Randall rambles on. I glance out eagerly at the rush-hour traffic flowing by. Finally, rescue arrives. My son Daniel drives up and opens the car door. "Sometimes I don't believe my life," I tell him, easing into the passenger's seat. "Sometimes I don't believe your life either," he nods. "It can get pretty intense down here." We pull away. In the rearview mirror the receding figure of Eva gesticulates, legs splayed, head tilted to the side.

—

The Portland and the other buildings of the Portland Hotel Society represent a pioneering social model. The purpose of the PHS is to provide a system of safety and caring to marginalized and stigmatized people—the ones who are "the insulted and the injured," to borrow from Dostoevsky. The PHS attempts to rescue such people from what a local poet has called the "streets of displacement and the buildings of exclusion."

"People just need a space to be," says Liz Evans, a former community nurse, whose upper-tier social background might seem incongruous with her present role as a founder and director of the PHS. "They need a space where they can exist without being judged and hounded and harassed. These are people who are frequently viewed as liabilities, blamed for crime and social ills, and . . . seen as a waste of time and energy. They are regarded harshly even by people who make compassion their careers."

From very modest beginnings in 1991, the Portland Hotel Society has grown to participate in activities such as a neighbourhood bank; an art gallery for Downtown Eastside artists; North America's first supervised injection site; a community hospital ward, where deep-tissue infections are treated with intravenous antibiotics; a free dental clinic; and the Portland Clinic, where I have worked for the past eight years. The core mandate of the PHS is to provide domiciles for people who would otherwise be homeless.

The statistics are stark. A review done shortly after the Portland was established revealed that among the residents three-quarters had over five addresses in the year before they were housed, and 90 per cent had been charged or convicted of crimes, often many times over, usually for petty theft. Currently 36 per cent are HIV positive or have frank AIDS, and most are addicted to alcohol or other substances—anything from rice wine or mouthwash, cocaine or heroin. Over half have been diagnosed with mental illness. The proportion of Native Canadians among

Portland residents is five times their ratio in the general population.

For Liz and the others who developed the PHS, it was endlessly frustrating to watch people go from crisis to crisis, with no consistent support. "The system had abandoned them," she says, "so we've tried to set up the hotels as a base for other services and programs. It took eight years of fundraising and four provincial government ministries and four private foundations to make the new Portland a reality. Now people finally have their own bathrooms, laundry facilities and a decent place to eat food."

What makes the Portland model unique and controversial among addiction services is the core intention to accept people as they are—no matter how dysfunctional, troubled and troubling they may be. Our clients are not the "deserving poor"; they are just poor—undeserving in their own eyes and in those of society. At the Portland Hotel there is no chimera of redemption nor any expectation of socially respectable outcomes, only an unsentimental recognition of the real needs of real human beings in the dingy present, based on a uniformly tragic past. We may (and do) hope that people can be liberated from the demons that haunt them and work to encourage them in that direction, but we don't fantasize that such psychological exorcism can be forced on anyone. The uncomfortable truth is that most of our clients will remain addicts, on the wrong side of the law as it now stands. Kerstin Stuerzbecher, a former nurse with two liberal arts degrees, is another Portland Society director. "We don't have all the answers," she says, "and we cannot necessarily provide the care people may need in order to make dramatic changes in their lives. At the end of the day it's never up to us—it's within them or not."

Residents are offered as much assistance as the Portland's financially stretched resources permit. Home support staff clean rooms and assist with personal hygiene for the most helpless. Food is prepared and distributed. When possible, patients are accompanied to specialists' appointments or for X-rays or other medical investigations. Methadone, psychiatric medications and HIV drugs are dispensed by the staff. A laboratory comes to the Portland every few months to screen for HIV and hepatitis and for follow-up blood tests. There is a writing and poetry group, an art group—a quilt based on residents' drawings hangs on the wall of my office. There are visits from an acupuncturist, hairdressing, movie nights, and while we still had the funds people were taken away from the grimy confines of the Downtown Eastside for an annual camping outing. My son Daniel, a sometime employee at the Portland, has led a monthly music group.

"We had this talent evening at the Portland a few years ago," says Kerstin, "with the art group and the writing group, and there was also a cabaret show. There was art on the wall and people read their poetry. A long-time resident came up to the microphone. He said he didn't have a poem to recite or anything else creative. . . . What he shared was that the Portland was his first home. That this is the only home he's ever had and how grateful he was for the community he was part of. And how proud he was to be part of it, and he wished his mom and dad could see him now."

"The only home he's ever had"—a phrase that sums up the histories of many people in the Downtown Eastside of "one of the world's most livable cities."*

The work can be intensely satisfying or deeply frustrating, depending on my own state of mind. Often I face the refractory nature of people who value their health and well-being less than the immediate, drug-driven needs of the moment. I also have to confront my own resistance to them as people. Much as I want to accept them, at least in principle, some days I find myself full of disapproval and judgment, rejecting them and wanting them to be other than who they are. That contradiction originates with me, not with my patients. It's my problem—except that, given the obvious power imbalance between us, it's all too easy for me to make it their problem.

* As Vancouver is often described internationally, most recently in the *New York Times*, 8 July 2007.

My patients' addictions make every medical treatment encounter a challenge. Where else do you find people in such poor health and yet so averse to taking care of themselves or even to allowing others to take care of them? At times, one literally has to coax them into hospital. Take Kai, who has an immobilizing infection of his hip that could leave him crippled, or Hobo, whose breastbone osteomyelitis could penetrate into his lungs. Both men are so focused on their next hit of cocaine or heroin or "jib"—crystal meth—that self-preservation pales into insignificance. Many also have an ingrained fear of authority figures and distrust institutions, for reasons no one could begrudge them.

"The reason I do drugs is so I don't feel the fucking feelings I feel when I don't do drugs," Nick, a forty-year-old heroin and crystal meth addict once told me, weeping as he spoke. "When I don't feel the drugs in me, I get depressed." His father drilled into his twin sons the notion that they were nothing but "pieces of shit." Nick's brother committed suicide as a teenager; Nick became a lifelong addict.

The Hell Realm of painful emotions frightens most of us; drug addicts fear they would be trapped there forever but for their substances. This urge to escape exacts a fearful price.

The cement hallways and the elevator at the Portland Hotel are washed clean frequently, sometimes several times a day. Punctured by needle marks, some residents have chronic draining wounds. Blood also seeps from blows and cuts inflicted by their fellow addicts or from pits patients have scratched in their skin during fits of cocaine-induced paranoia. One man picks at himself incessantly to get rid of imaginary insects.

Not that we lack *real* infestation in the Downtown Eastside. Rodents thrive between hotel walls and in the garbage-strewn back alleys. Vermin populate many of my patients' beds, clothes and bodies: bedbugs, lice, scabies. Cockroaches occasionally drop out from shaken skirts and pant legs in my office and scurry for cover under my desk. "I like having one or two mice around," one young man told me. "They eat the cockroaches and bedbugs. But I can't stand a whole nest of them in my mattress."

Vermin, boils, blood and death: the plagues of Egypt.

In the Downtown Eastside the angel of death slays with shocking alacrity. Marcia, a thirty-five-year-old heroin addict, had moved out of her PHS residence and was living in a tenement half a block away. One morning, I received a frantic phone call about a suspected overdose. I found Marcia in bed, her eyes wide open, lying on her back and already in rigor mortis. Her arms were extended, palms outward in a gesture of alarmed protest as if to say: "No, you've come to take me too soon, much too soon!" Plastic syringes cracked under my shoes as I approached her body. Marcia's dilated pupils and some other physical cues told the story—she died not of overdose but of heroin withdrawal. I stood for a few moments by her bedside, trying to see in her body the charming, if always absent-minded, human being I had known. As I turned to leave, wailing sirens signalled the arrival of emergency vehicles outside.

Marcia had been in my office just the week before, in good cheer, asking for help with some medical forms she needed to fill out, to get back on welfare. It was the first time I'd seen her in six months. During that period, as she explained with nonchalant resignation, she had helped her boyfriend, Kyle, blow through a hundred-and-thirty-thousand-dollar inheritance—a process selflessly aided by many other user friends and hangers-on. For all that popularity, she was alone when death caught her.

Another casualty was Frank, a reclusive heroin addict who would grudgingly let you into his cramped quarters at the Regal Hotel only when he was very ill. "No fucking way I'm dying in hospital," he declared, once it became clear that the grim reaper AIDS was knocking at his door. There was no arguing with Frank about that or anything else. He died in his own ragged bed, but *his* bed, in 2002.

Frank had a sweet soul that his curmudgeonly abrasiveness could not hide. Although he never talked to me about his life experience, he expressed the gist of it in "Downtown Hellbound Train," a poem he wrote a few months before his death. It is a requiem for himself and for the dozens of women—drug users, sex trade workers—said to have been murdered at the infamous Pickton pig farm outside Vancouver.

Went downtown—Hastings and Main
Looking for relief from the pain
All I did was find
A one-way ticket on a Hellbound Train

On a farm not far away
Several friends were taken away
Rest their souls from the pain
End their ride on the Hellbound Train

Give me peace before I die
The track is laid out so well
We all live our private hell
Just more tickets on the Hellbound Train

Hellbound Train
Hellbound Train
One-way ticket on a Hellbound Train

Having worked in palliative medicine, care of the terminally ill, I have encountered death often. In a real sense, addiction medicine with this population is also palliative work. We do not expect to cure anyone, only to ameliorate the effects of drug addiction and its attendant ailments and to soften the impact of the legal and social torments our culture uses to punish the drug addict. Except for the rare fortunate ones who escape the Downtown Eastside drug colony, very few of my patients will live to old age. Most will die of some complication of their HIV or hepatitis C or of meningitis or a massive septicemia contracted through multiple self-injections during a prolonged cocaine run. Some will succumb to cancer at a relatively young age, their stressed and debilitated immune systems unable to keep malignancy in check. That's how Stevie died, of liver cancer, the sweet-sardonic expression that always played on her face obscured by deep jaundice. Or they'll do a bad fix one night and die of an overdose, like Angel at the Sunrise Hotel or like Trevor, one floor above, who always smiled as if nothing ever bothered him.

One darkening February evening, Leona, a patient who lives in a nearby hotel, awoke on the cot in her room to find her eighteen-year-old son, Joey, lifeless and rigid in her bed. She had taken him in from the street and was keeping watch to save him from self-harm. Mid-morning, after an all-night vigil, she fell asleep; he overdosed in the afternoon. "When I woke up," she recalled, "Joey was lying motionless. Nobody had to tell me. The ambulance and fire guys came, but there was nothing anybody could do. My baby was dead." Her grief is oceanic, her sense of guilt fathomless.

One constant at the Portland Clinic is pain. Medical school teaches the three signs of inflammation, in Latin: *calor, rubror, dolor*—heat, redness and pain. The skin, limbs or organs of my patients are often inflamed, and for that my ministrations can be at least temporarily adequate. But how to soothe souls inflamed by the intense torment imposed first by childhood experiences almost too sordid to believe and then, with mechanical repetition, by the sufferers themselves? And how to offer them comfort when their sufferings are made worse every day by social ostracism—by what the scholar and writer Elliot Leyton has described as "the bland, racist, sexist and 'classist' prejudices buried in Canadian society: an institutionalized contempt for the poor, for sex trade workers, for drug addicts and alcoholics, for aboriginal people." The pain here in the Downtown Eastside reaches out with hands begging for drug money. It stares from eyes cold and hard or downcast with submission and shame. It speaks in cajoling tones or screams aggressively. Behind every look, every word, each violent act or disenchanted gesture is a history of anguish and degradation, a self-writ tale with new chapters added each day and scarcely a happy end.

—

As Daniel drives me home, we're listening to CBC on the car radio, broadcasting its whimsical afternoon cocktail of lighthearted patter, classics and jazz. Jolted by the disharmony between the urbane radio space and the troubled world I've just left, I recall my first patient of the day.

Madeleine sits hunched, elbows resting on her thighs, her gaunt, wiry body convulsed by sobbing. She clutches her head in her hands, periodically clenching her fists and beating rhythmically at her temples. Straight brown hair, fallen forward, veils her eyes and cheeks. Her lower lip is swollen and bruised, and blood trickles from a small cut. Her thick, boyish voice is hoarse with rage and pain. "I've been fucked over again," she cries. "It's always me, the sucker for everyone else's bullshit. How do they know they can do it to me every time?" She coughs as the tears trickle down her windpipe. She's like a child telling her story, asking for sympathy, pleading for help.

The tale she tells is a variation on a theme familiar in the Downtown Eastside: drug addicts exploiting each other. Three women Madeleine knows well give her a hundred-dollar bill. The deal is, she buys twelve "rocks" of crack from the person she calls the "Spic." She gets one; they'll keep some for themselves and resell the rest. "We can't let the cops see us buy that much," they tell her. The transaction is completed, money and rocks are exchanged. Ten minutes later the "great big Spic" catches up with Madeleine, "grabs me by the hair, throws me on the ground, gives me a punch in the face." The hundred-dollar bill is counterfeit. "They set me up. 'Oh, Maddie, you're my buddy, you're my friend.' I had no idea it was a bogus hundred."

My clients often speak about the "Spic," but he's an unseen presence, a mythical figure I only hear about. On the street corners near the Portland Hotel, young, olive-hued Central Americans congregate, black baseball caps over their eyes. As I walk by, they call out to me in a low whisper, even with my signal stethoscope around my neck: "up, down" or "good rock." (Up and down are junkie slang for cocaine—an upper, a stimulant—and for heroin—a downer, a sedative. Rock is crack cocaine.) "Hey, can't you see that's the doctor?" someone occasionally hisses. The Spic may well be amongst that group or perhaps the epithet is a generic term that refers to any of them.

I don't know who he is or the path that led him to Vancouver's Skid Row, where he pushes cocaine and slaps around the emaciated women who steal, deal, cheat or sell cheap oral sex to pay him.

Where was he born? What war, what deprivation forced his parents out of their slum or their mountain village to seek a life so far north of the Equator? Poverty in Honduras, paramilitaries in Guatemala, death squads in El Salvador? How did he become the Spic, a villain in a story told by the rake-thin, distraught woman in my office who, choking on her tears, explains her bruises and asks that I don't hold it against her that she failed to show for last week's methadone visit.

"I haven't had juice for seven days," Madeleine says. ("Juice" is slang for methadone: the methadone powder is dissolved in orange-flavoured Tang.) "And I won't ask anybody for help on the street because if they help you, you owe them your goddamn life. Even if you pay them back, they still think you owe them. 'There's Maddie, we can hustle her for it. She'll give it to us.' They know I won't fight. 'Cause if I ever fight I'm going to fucking kill one of these bitches down here. I don't want spend the rest of my life in jail because of some goddamn cunt I never should've got involved with in the first place. That's what's going to happen. I can only take so much."

I hand her the methadone prescription and invite her back to talk after she's had her dose at the pharmacy. Although Madeleine agrees, I won't see her again today. As always, the need for the next fix beckons.

Another visitor that morning was Stan, a forty-five-year-old Native man just out of jail, also here for his methadone script. In his eighteen months of incarceration he has become pudgy, and this has softened the menacing air bestowed by his height, muscular build, glowering dark eyes, Apache hair and Fu Manchu moustache. Or perhaps he's mellowed, since he's been off cocaine all this time. He peers out the window at the sidewalk across the street, where a few of his fellow addicts are involved in a scene outside the Army and Navy store. There is much gesticulation and apparently aimless striding back and forth. "Look at them," he says. "They're stuck here. You know, Doc, their life stretches from here to maybe Victory Square to the left and Fraser Street to the right. They never get out. I want to move away, don't want to waste myself down here anymore.

"Ah, what's the use. Look at me, I don't even have socks." Stan points at his worn-out running shoes and baggy, red-cotton jogging pants with the elastic bunched a few inches above his ankles. "When I get on the bus in this outfit, people just know. They move away from me. Some stare; most don't even look in my direction. You know what that feels like? Like I'm an alien. I don't feel right till I'm back here; no wonder nobody ever leaves."

When he returns for a methadone script ten days later, Stan is still living on the street. It's a March day in Vancouver: grey, wet and unseasonably cold. "You don't want to know where I slept last night, Doc," he says.

For many of Vancouver's chronic, hard-core addicts, it's as if an invisible barbed-wire barrier surrounds the area extending a few blocks from Main and Hastings in all directions. There is a world beyond, but to them it's largely inaccessible. It fears and rejects them and they, in turn, do not understand its rules and cannot survive in it.

I am reminded of an escapee from a Soviet Gulag camp who, after starving on the outside, voluntarily turned himself back in. "Freedom isn't for us," he told his fellow prisoners. "We're chained to this place for the rest of our lives, even though we aren't wearing chains. We can escape, we can wander about, but in the end we'll come back."[2]

———

People like Stan are among the sickest, the neediest and the most neglected of any population anwhere. All their lives they've been ignored, abandoned and, in turn, self-abandoned time and again. Where does a commitment to serve such a community originate? In my case, I know it is rooted in my beginnings as a Jewish infant in Nazi-occupied Budapest in 1944. I've grown up with the awareness of how terrible and difficult life can be for some people—through no fault of their own.

But if the empathy I feel for my patients can be traced to my childhood, so can the reactively intense scorn, disdain and judgment that sometimes erupt from me, often towards these same pain-driven individuals. Later on, I'll discuss how my own addictive tendencies stem from my early childhood experiences. At heart,

I am not that different from my patients—and sometimes I cannot stand seeing how little psychological space, how little heaven-granted grace separates me from them.

My first full-time medical position was at a clinic in the Downtown Eastside. It was a brief, six-month stint but it left its mark, and I knew that someday I'd come back. When, twenty years later, I was presented with the opportunity to become the clinic physician at the old Portland, I seized it because it felt right: just the combination of challenge and meaning I was seeking at that time in my life. With hardly a moment's thought I left my family practice for a cockroach-infested downtown hotel.

What draws me here? All of us who are called to this work are responding to an inner pull that resonates with the same frequencies that vibrate in the lives of the haunted, drained, dysfunctional human beings in our care. But of course, we return daily to our homes, outside interests and relationships while our addict clients are trapped in their downtown gulag.

Some people are attracted to painful places because they hope to resolve their own pain there. Others offer themselves because their compassionate hearts know that here is where love is most needed. Yet others come out of professional interest: this work is ever challenging. Those with low self-esteem may be attracted because it feeds their egos to work with such powerless individuals. Some are lured by the magnetic force of addictions because they haven't resolved, or even recognized, their own addictive tendencies. My guess is that most of us physicians, nurses and other professional helpers who work in the Downtown Eastside are impelled by some mixture of these motives.

Liz Evans began working in the area at the age of twenty-six. "I was overwhelmed," she recalls. "As a nurse, I thought I had some expertise to share. While that was true, I soon discovered that, in fact, I had very little to give—I could not rescue people from their pain and sadness. All I could offer was to walk beside them as a fellow human being, a kindred spirit.

"A woman I'll call Julie was locked in her room and force-fed a liquid diet and beaten by her foster family from age seven on—she has a scar across her neck from where she slashed herself when she was only sixteen. She's used a cocktail of painkillers, alcohol, cocaine and heroin ever since and works the streets. One night she came home after she'd been raped and crawled into my lap, sobbing. She told me repeatedly that it was her fault, that she was a bad person and deserved nothing. She could barely breathe. I longed to give her anything that would ease her pain as I sat and rocked her. It was too intense for me to bear." As Liz discovered, something in Julie's pain triggered her own. "This experience showed me that we have to keep our own issues from turning into barriers."

"What keeps me here?" muses Kerstin Stuerzbecher. "In the beginning I wanted to help. And now . . . I still want to help, but it's changed. Now I know my limits. I know what I can and cannot do. What I can do is to be here and advocate for people at various stages in their lives, and to allow them to be who they are. We have an obligation as a society to . . . support people for who they are, and to give them respect. That's what keeps me here."

There's another factor in the equation. Many people who've worked in the Downtown Eastside have noticed it: a sense of authenticity, a loss of the usual social games, the surrender of pretence—the reality of people who cannot declare themselves to be anything other than what they are.

Yes, they lie, cheat and manipulate—but don't we all, in our own way? Unlike the rest of us, they can't pretend not to be cheaters and manipulators. They're straight-up about their refusal to take responsibility, their rejection of social expectation, their acceptance of having lost everything for the sake of their addiction. That isn't much by the straight world's standards, but there's a paradoxical core of honesty wrapped in the compulsive deceit any addiction imposes. "What do you expect, Doc? After all, I'm an addict," a small, skinny forty-seven-year-old man once said to me with a wry and disarming smile, having failed to wheedle a morphine prescription. Perhaps there's a fascination in that element of outrageous, unapologetic pseudo-authenticity. In our secret fantasies who among us wouldn't like to be as carelessly brazen about our flaws?

"Down here you have honest interactions with people," says Kim Markel, the nurse at the Portland Clinic. "I can come here and actually be who I am. I find that rewarding. Working in the hospitals or in different community settings, there's always pressure to toe the line. Because our work here is so diverse and because we're among people whose needs are so raw and who have nothing left to hide, it helps me maintain honesty in what I do. There's not that big shift between who I am at work and who I am outside of work."

Amidst the unrest of irritable drug seekers hustling and scamming for their next high, there also occur frequent moments of humanity and mutual support. "There are amazing displays of warmth all the time," Kim says. "Although there's a lot of violence, I see many people caring for each other," adds Bethany Jeal, a nurse at Insite, North America's first supervised injection site, located on Hastings, two blocks from the Portland. "They share food, clothing and makeup—anything they have." People tend to each other through illness, report with concern and compassion on a friend's condition and often display more kindness to someone else than they usually give themselves.

"Where I live," Kerstin says, "I don't know the person two houses down from me. I vaguely know what they look like, but I certainly don't know their name. Not down here. Here people know each other, and that has its pros and its cons. It means that people rail at each other and rage at each other, and it also means that people will share their last five pennies with each other.

"People here are very raw, so what comes out is the violence and ugliness that often gets highlighted in the media. But that rawness also brings out raw feelings of joy and tears of joy—looking at a flower I hadn't noticed but someone living in a one-room at the Washington Hotel has noticed because he's down here every day. This is his world and he pays attention to different details than I do. . . ."

Nor is humour absent. As I walk my Hastings rounds from one hotel to another, I witness much back-slapping banter and raucous laughter. "Doctor, doctor, gimme the news," comes a jazzy sing-song from under the archway of the Washington. "Hey, you need a shot of rhythm an' blues," I chant back over my shoulder. No need to look around. My partner in this well-rehearsed musical routine is Wayne, a sunburned man with long, dirty blond curls and Schwarzenegger arms tattooed from wrist to biceps.

I wait to cross an intersection with Laura, a Native woman in her forties, whose daunting life history, drug dependence, alcoholism and HIV have not extinguished her impish wit. As the red hand on the pedestrian traffic light yields to the little walking figure, Laura chimes up, her tone a shade sardonic: "White man says go." Our paths coincide for the next half-block, and all the while Laura chuckles loudly at her joke. So do I.

The witticisms are often fearlessly self-mocking. "Used to bench press two hundred pounds, Doc," Tony, emaciated, shrivelled and dying of AIDS, cracked during one of his last office visits. "Now I can't even bench press my own dick."

When my addict patients look at me, they are seeking the real me. Like children, they are unimpressed with titles, achievements, worldly credentials. Their concerns are too immediate, too urgent. If they come to like me or to appreciate my work with them, they will spontaneously express pride in having a doctor who is occasionally interviewed on television and is an author. But only then. What they care about is my presence or absence as a human being. They gauge with unerring eye whether I am grounded enough on any given day to co-exist with them, to listen to them as persons with feelings, hopes and aspirations as valid as mine. They can tell instantly whether I'm genuinely committed to their well-being or just trying to get them out of my way. Chronically unable to offer such caring to themselves, they are all the more sensitive to its presence or absence in those charged with caring for them.

It is invigorating to operate in an atmosphere so far removed from the regular workaday world, an atmosphere that insists on authenticity. Whether we know it or not, most of us crave authenticity, the reality beyond roles, labels and carefully honed personae. With all its festering problems, dysfunctions, diseases and crime, the Downtown Eastside offers the fresh air of truth, even if it's the stripped, frayed truth of desperation. It holds up a mirror in which we all, as individual human beings and collectively as a society, may recognize ourselves. The fear, pain and longing we see are our own fear, pain and longing. Ours, too, are the beauty and compassion we witness here, the courage and the sheer determination to surmount suffering.

—

CHAPTER 2

The Lethal Hold of Drugs

—

Nothing records the effects of a sad life so
graphically as the human body.

NAGUIB MAHFOUZ
Palace of Desire

From behind his lectern at an East Hastings funeral chapel,
the elderly priest proclaims the world's farewell to Sharon.
"How exuberant and joyful she was. 'Here I am, Sha-na-na!'
she announced as she burst into a room. On seeing her, who could
not feel glad to be alive?"

Behind the family the mourners are dispersed through the
sparsely filled chapel. A group of Portland staffers are present, along
with five or six residents and a few people I don't recognize.

The young Sharon, I've been told, was model beautiful. Hints of
that beauty still remained when I met her six years ago, traces gradually erased by her increasingly pallid complexion, sunken cheeks
and decaying teeth. In her last years Sharon was often in pain. Two
large patches on her left shin were denuded of skin by injection-
induced bacterial infections. Reinfection caused repeated skin grafts
to slough off, leaving the flesh continually exposed. The exasperated
plastic surgeons at St. Paul's Hospital considered further intervention futile. In her chronically swollen left knee a bone abscess
lurked, flaring up every so often and then subsiding. That
osteomyelitis was never fully treated because Sharon couldn't

endure the six to eight weeks of hospitalization required to complete the intravenous antibiotic regimen—not even when it appeared that amputation might be the only alternative. Unable to weight-bear owing to her inflamed knee joint, Sharon became hostage to a wheelchair in her early thirties. She'd propel it along the Hastings sidewalk at astonishing speed, employing her strong arms and her right leg to boost herself along.

The priest tactfully avoids evoking the pain-haunted Sharon, whose drug obsession drove her back to the Downtown Eastside, but honours her vital essence.

"Forgive us, Lord, for we do not know how to cherish . . . Life is eternal, love is immortal . . . For every joy that passes, something beautiful is created . . . ," intones the priest. At first all I hear is a litany of funerary clichés and I am annoyed. Soon, however, I find myself comforted. In the face of untimely death, it occurs to me, there are no clichés. "For always Sharon, that voice, that spirit . . . For the peace of eternity, immortal peace . . ."

The quiet sobbing of women vibrates in counterpoint to the priest's consoling words. Closing the book on the lectern, he looks solemnly around the room. As he steps off the podium, music is piped in: Andrea Bocelli crooning a sentimental Italian aria. Mourners are invited to pay their last respects to Sharon, who rests in an open coffin below the stage. One by one they walk up, bow their heads and step back to honour the family. Beverly, cocaine-induced pick marks disfiguring her face, approaches the coffin. She supports Penny, who is bent over her walker. The two were close friends of Sharon. Tom, whose hoarse, alcohol-fuelled evening bellowing resounds up and down Hastings, is dressed in his finest. Stone sober and sombre in white shirt and tie, he bows in prayerful silence over the flower-decorated bier and crosses himself.

Sharon's white-powdered face wears a naïve, uncertain expression, rouged lips closed and slightly awry. It occurs to me that this faintly befuddled, childlike look probably reflects the inner world of the live Sharon more accurately than the raucous character she often presented in my office.

Sharon's body was found in her bed one April morning. She lay there on her side as if in dreamy repose, her features undistorted by pain or distress. We could only guess at the cause of death, but over-dose was the best surmise. Despite her long-standing HIV infection and her low immune counts, she had not been ill, but we knew she was heavily into heroin use since she'd left the recovery home. There was no drug paraphernalia in her room. It seems she'd injected what-ever killed her in a neighbour's apartment before returning to her own.

The failed attempt at rehabilitation saddened everyone who cared for her. By all accounts she'd appeared to be doing well. "Another four weeks without injection, Maté," she'd proudly report during her monthly telephone calls. "Send in my methadone script, would you? I don't want to come there to pick it up—I'll just be pulled into using again." Staff visiting the recovery shelter reported that she was vibrant, in good colour, cheerful and optimistic. Despite her heroin relapse, her death was a shock, and even now, with her body laid out in the chapel, hard to accept. Her vivacity, cheer and irrepressible energy had been so much a part of our lives. After the priest's kind and celebratory words, Sharon should have stood up and walked out with the rest of us.

Service over, the mourners mingle in the parking lot for a while before going their separate ways. It's a bright, dazzling day, the first time this year the spring sun has shown its face in the Vancouver sky. I say hello to Gail, a Native woman who's bravely approaching the end of her third month without cocaine. "Eighty-seven days," she beams at me. "I can't believe it." It's no mere exercise in willpower. Gail was hospitalized for a fulminant abdominal infection two years ago and had a colostomy to rest her inflamed intestines. The severed segments of bowel should have been surgically rejoined long before now, but the procedure was always cancelled because Gail's intra-venous cocaine use jeopardized the chances of healing. The origi-nal surgeon has declined to see her again. "I booked the OR for nothing at least three times," he told me. "I won't take another chance." I couldn't argue with his logic. A new specialist has reluctantly agreed to proceed with the operation, but only under the strictest understanding that Gail will stay off the cocaine. Failing this last opportunity, she may, for the rest of her life, dis-charge her feces into the plastic receptacle taped to her belly. She hates having to change the bag, sometimes several times a day.

"How ya doin,' Doc," says the ever-affable Tom, lightly kneading my shoulder. "Good ta see ya. You're a good man." "Thanks," I say. "So are you." Still supported by her hefty friend Beverly, skinny little Penny shuffles up. She leans on her walker with her right hand, shading her eyes against the noonday sun with the left. Penny has only recently finished a six-month course of IV antibiotics for a spinal infection that has left her hunch-backed and weak-legged. "I never expected to see Sharon die before me," she says. "I really thought in hospital last summer I was a goner." "You were close enough to scare even me," I reply. We both laugh.

I look at this small cluster of human beings gathered at the funeral of a comrade who met her death in her mid-thirties. How powerful the addiction, I think, that not all the physical disease and pain and psychological torment can shake loose its lethal hold on their souls. "In the Nazi *Arbeit* [work] camps back in '44 when a man was caught smoking one cigarette, the whole barracks would die," a patient, Ralph, once told me. "For one cigarette! Yet even so, the men did not give up their inspiration, their will to live and to enjoy what they got out of life from certain substances, like liquor or tobacco or what-ever the case may be." I don't know how accurate his account was as history, but as a chronicler of his own drug urges and those of his fellow Hastings Street addicts, Ralph spoke the bare truth: people jeopardize their lives for the sake of making the moment livable. Nothing sways them from the habit—not illness, not the sacrifice of love and relationship, not the loss of all earthly goods, not the crushing of their dignity, not the fear of dying. The drive is that relentless.

How to understand the death grip of drug addiction? What keeps Penny injecting after the spinal suppuration that nearly made her paraplegic? Why can't Beverly give up shooting cocaine despite the HIV, the recurring abscesses I've had to drain on her body and the joint infections that repeatedly put her in hospital? What could have drawn Sharon back to the Downtown Eastside and her suici-dal habit after her six-month getaway? How did she shrug off the deterrents of HIV and hepatitis, a crippling bone infection and the chronic burning, piercing pain of exposed nerve endings?

What a wonderful world it would be if the simplistic view were accurate: that human beings need only negative consequences to teach them hard lessons. Then any number of fast-food franchises would be tickets to bankruptcy, the TV room would be a deserted spot in our homes, and the Portland Hotel could reinvent itself as something more lucrative: perhaps a luxury housing unit with Mediterranean pretensions for downtown yuppies, similar to the sold-out "Firenze" and "España" condo developments still under construction around the corner.

—

On the physiological level drug addiction is a matter of brain chemistry gone askew under the influence of a substance and, as we will see, even before the use of mind-altering substances begins. But we cannot reduce human beings to their neurochemistry; and even if we could, people's brain physiology doesn't develop separately from their life events and their emotions. The addicts sense this. Easy as it would be to pin responsibility for their self-destructive habits on a chemical phenomenon, few of them do so. Few of them accept a narrow medical model of addiction as illness, for all the genuine value of that model.

What is the truly fatal attraction of the drug experience? That's a question I've put to many of my clients at the Portland Clinic. "You've got this miserable, swollen, ulcerated leg and foot—red, hot and painful," I say to Hal, a friendly, jocular man in his forties, one of my few male patients without a criminal record. "You have to drag yourself to the emergency every day for IV antibiotics. You have HIV. And you won't give up injecting speed. What do you suppose is behind that for you?"

"I don't know," Hal mutters, his toothless gums smothering his words. "You ask anybody . . . anybody, including myself, why should you put something into your body that in the next five minutes makes you drool, look gooey, you know, distort your brainwave patterns to the point where you can't think reasonably, inhibits your speech pattern—and then want to do it again." "And gives you an abscessed leg," I add helpfully. "Yes, an abscessed leg. Why? I really don't know."

In March 2005, I had a similar discussion with Allan. Also in his forties, also with HIV, Allan had been to Vancouver Hospital with sharp chest pains a few days earlier. He was told he'd probably suffered a flare-up of endocarditis, an infection of the heart valves. Declining to be admitted to hospital, Allan presented himself instead for a second opinion at the emergency ward of St. Paul's, where he was assured that everything was fine. Now he was in my office for a third assessment.

On examination I can see he isn't acutely ill but is nevertheless in terrible shape. "What should I do, Doc?" he asks, raising his shoulders and spreading his arms out in helpless consternation. "Okay," I say, reviewing his chart. "Your father died of heart disease. Your brother died of heart disease. You're a heavy smoker. You have a history of endocarditis from IV drug use. I'm treating you for cardiac failure and even now your legs are swollen because your heart isn't pumping efficiently. Your HIV is controlled by strong medications and, with your Hep C, your liver is just hanging in there. But you still keep injecting. And you're asking me what you should do. What's wrong with this picture?"

"I was hoping you'd say that," Allan replies. "You need to tell me I'm a fucking retard. It's the only way I learn."

"Okay," I oblige. "You're a fucking retard."

"Thanks, Doc."

"The trouble is, you're not a fucking retard; you're addicted. And how are we to understand that?"

Allan died four months later, cold and blue at midnight on the floor of his room in a nearby hotel. He was injecting, rumour had it, from a bad lot of methadone heisted in a break-in at a local pharmacy and subsequently adulterated with crystal meth or who knows what. According to the coroner's office, that little enterprise in independent drug marketing caused the death of at least eight people

"I'm not afraid of dying," a client told me. "Sometimes I'm more afraid of living."

That fear of life as they have experienced it underlies my patients' continued drug use. "Nothing bothers me when I'm high. There's no stress in my life," one person said—a sentiment echoed by many addicted people. "Makes me just forget," said Dora, an inveterate cocaine user. "I forget about my problems. Nothing ever seems quite as bad as it really is, until you wake up the next morning, and then it's worse. . . ." In the summer of 2006 Dora left the Portland and moved back to the streets, hustling for dope. In January she died of multiple brain abscesses in the intensive care unit of St. Paul's Hospital.*

Alvin is in his fifties, a portly, thick-armed, former long-distance trucker. On methadone to control his heroin addiction, he has recently been increasing his crystal meth use. "The first part of the day it makes me feel like I want to puke," he says, "but then, after eight or nine hoots on the pipe . . . How does it make me feel? Like a fool first of all, but I dunno, it's a ritual, I guess."

"Here's what I'm hearing," I counter. "For the privilege of being nauseated and feeling like a fool, you spend a thousand dollars a month. Is this what you're telling me?" Alvin laughs. "I only puke on the first one of the day, though. I get a high of some sort, which lasts about three to five minutes, and then . . . you say to yourself, Why did I do that? But then it's too late. Something makes you keep doing it, and that's what's called addiction. And I don't know how to curb that. Honest to God, I hate the shit, I honestly hate that shit." "But you still get something out of it." "Well, yeah, or I wouldn't be doing it, obviously—sort of like having an orgasm, I guess."

Beyond the addict's immediate orgasmic release of the moment, drugs have the power to make the painful tolerable and the humdrum worth living for. "There is a memory so fixed and so perfect that on certain days my brain listens to no other," writes Stephen Reid—author, incarcerated bank robber and self-described junkie—of his first hit of narcotics, at age eleven. "I am in profound awe of the ordinary—the pale sky, the blue spruce tree, the rusty barbed-wire fence, those dying yellow leaves. I am high. I am eleven years old and in communion with this world. Wholly innocent, I enter into the heart of unknowing."[1] In a similar vein, Leonard Cohen has written about "the promise, the beauty, the salvation of cigarettes. . . ."

Like patterns in a tapestry, recurring themes emerge in my interviews with addicts: the drug as emotional anaesthetic; as an antidote to a frightful feeling of emptiness; as a tonic against fatigue,

* Infections fester from bacteria injected into the tissues during drug injection and are carried by blood circulation to internal organs like the lungs, liver, heart, spine and brain.

boredom, alienation and a sense of personal inadequacy; as stress reliever and social lubricant. And, as in Stephen Reid's description, the drug may—if only for a brief instant—open the portals of spiritual transcendence. In places high and low these themes blight the lives of hungry ghosts everywhere. They act with lethal force on the cocaine-, heroin- and crystal-meth-wired addicts of the Downtown Eastside. We will return to them in the next chapter.

—

In a photo we have at the Portland, Sharon, in a black bathing suit, sits on a sun-dappled deck, her legs immersed in the shimmering, clear water of a blue-tiled pool. Relaxed and composed, she smiles directly at the photographer's lens. This is the young woman of joy and possibility memorialized by the priest, captured here by the camera a few months before her death, revelling in the warmth of a late fall afternoon at the home of her Twelve-Step sponsor.

In the twelve years Sharon spent in the Downtown Eastside, she could not complete those twelve steps. She'd been so dysfunctional and cocaine aggressive that until the day she was accepted as a resident at the Portland, she'd been barred from even visiting the hotel. "That's how it works," Portland Society director Kerstin Stuerzbecher told me in the foyer of the chapel after Sharon's funeral. "There are only two choices: either you're too much trouble to be allowed to live here or you're so much trouble you can live only here.

"And die only here," Kerstin added as we stepped out into the sunlight.

CHAPTER 3

—

The Keys of Paradise:
Addiction as a Flight from Distress

—

*Dismissing addictions as "bad habits" or "self-destructive
behaviour" comfortably hides their functionality in the life
of the addict.*[1]

VINCENT FELITTI, M.D., PHYSICIAN AND RESEARCHER

I t is impossible to understand addiction without asking what
relief the addict finds, or hopes to find, in the drug or the
addictive behaviour.

The early-nineteenth-century literary figure Thomas De Quincey
was an opium user. "The subtle powers lodged in this mighty drug,"
he rhapsodized, "tranquilize all irritations of the nervous system . . .
sustain through twenty-four hours the else drooping animal energies
. . . O just, subtle and all-conquering opium . . . Thou only givest
these gifts to man; and thou hast the keys of Paradise." De Quincey's
words encapsulate the blessings of all drugs as the addict experiences
them—indeed, as we shall see later, the appeal of all addictive
obsessions, with or without drugs.

Far more than a quest for pleasure, chronic substance use is the
addict's attempt to escape distress. From a medical point of view,
addicts are self-medicating conditions like depression, anxiety,
post-traumatic stress or even ADHD (attention deficit hyperactivity disorder).

Addictions always originate in pain, whether felt openly or hidden in the unconscious. They are emotional anaesthetics. Heroin and cocaine, both powerful physical painkillers, also ease psychological discomfort. Infant animals separated from their mothers can be soothed readily by low doses of narcotics, just as if it was actual physical pain they were enduring.*[2]

The pain pathways in humans are no different. The very same brain centres that interpret and "feel" physical pain also become activated during the experience of emotional rejection: on brain scans they "light up" in response to social ostracism just as they would when triggered by physically harmful stimuli.[3] When people speak of feeling "hurt" or of having emotional "pain," they are not being abstract or poetic but scientifically quite precise.

The hard-drug addict's life has been marked by a surfeit of pain. No wonder she desperately craves relief. "In moments I go from complete misery and vulnerability to total invulnerability," says Judy, a thirty-six-year-old heroin and cocaine addict who is now trying to kick her two-decade habit. "I have a lot of issues. A lot of the reason why I use is to get rid of those thoughts and emotions and cover them up."

The question is never "Why the addiction?" but "Why the pain?"

The research literature is unequivocal: most hard-core substance abusers come from abusive homes.[4] The majority of my Skid Row patients suffered severe neglect and maltreatment early in life. Almost all the addicted women inhabiting the Downtown Eastside were sexually assaulted in childhood, as were many of the men. The autobiographical accounts and case files of Portland residents tell stories of pain upon pain: rape, beatings, humiliation, rejection, abandonment, relentless character assassination. As children they were obliged to witness the violent relationships, self-harming life patterns or suicidal addictions of their parents— and often had to take care of them. Or they had to look after younger siblings and defend them from being abused even as they

* In popular usage "narcotic" may refer loosely to any illicit drug. In this book, as
  in medical language, narcotics is a term only for opioid drugs either derived
  from the Asian poppy, like heroin and morphine, or synthetic, like oxycodone.

themselves endured the daily violation of their own bodies and souls. One man grew up in a hotel room where his prostitute mother hosted a nightly procession of men as her child slept, or tried to, on his cot on the floor.

Carl, a thirty-six-year-old Native man, was banished from one foster home after another, had dishwashing liquid poured down his throat at age five for using foul language and was tied to a chair in a dark room in attempts to control his hyperactivity. When he's angry at himself—as he was one day for having used cocaine—he gouges his foot with a knife as punishment. He confessed his "sin" to me with the look of a terrorized urchin who'd just smashed some family heirloom and dreaded the harshest retribution.

Another man described the way his mother used a mechanical babysitter when he was three years old. "She went to the bar to drink and pick up men. Her idea of keeping me safe and from getting into trouble was to stick me in the dryer. She put a heavy box on top so I couldn't get out." The air vent ensured that the little boy wouldn't suffocate.

My prose is unequal to the task of depicting such nearly inconceivable trauma. "Our difficulty or inability to perceive the experience of others . . . is all the more pronounced the more distant these experiences are from ours in time, space, or quality," wrote the Auschwitz survivor Primo Levi.[5] We can be moved by the tragedy of mass starvation on a far continent; after all, we have all known physical hunger, if only temporarily. But it takes a greater effort of emotional imagination to empathize with the addict. We readily feel for a suffering child, but cannot see the child in the adult who, his soul fragmented and isolated, hustles for survival a few blocks away from where we shop or work.

Levi quotes Jean Améry, a Jewish-Austrian philosopher and resistance fighter who fell into the grasp of the Gestapo. "Anyone who was tortured remains tortured . . . Anyone who has suffered torture never again will be able to be at ease in the world . . . Faith in humanity, already cracked by the first slap in the face, then demolished by torture, is never acquired again."[6] Améry was a full-grown adult when he was traumatized, an accomplished intellectual captured by the foe in the course of a war of liberation. We may then imagine the shock, loss of faith and unfathomable despair of the child who is traumatized not by hated enemies but by loved ones.

Not all addictions are rooted in abuse or trauma, but I do believe they can all be traced to painful experience. A hurt is at the centre of *all* addictive behaviours. It is present in the gambler, the Internet addict, the compulsive shopper and the workaholic. The wound may not be as deep and the ache not as excruciating, and it may even be entirely hidden—but it's there. As we'll see, the effects of early stress or adverse experiences directly shape both the psychology and the neurobiology of addiction in the brain.

—

I asked fifty-seven-year-old Richard, an addict since his teens, why he kept using. "I don't know, I'm just trying to fill a void," he replied. "Emptiness in my life. Boredom. Lack of direction." I knew all too well what he meant. "Here I am, in my late fifties," he said. "I have no wife, no children. I appear to be a failure. Society says you should be married and have children, a job, that kind of stuff. This way, with the cocaine, I can sit there and do some little thing like rewire the toaster that wasn't working, and not feel like I've lost out on life." He died a few months after our interview, succumbing to a combination of lung disease, kidney cancer and overdose.

"I didn't use for six years," says Cathy, forty-two-year-old heroin and cocaine user, back in a grubby Downtown Eastside hotel after a long absence. She's contracted HIV since her return. "The whole six years I craved. It was the lifestyle. I thought I was missing something. And now I look around myself and I think, What the hell was I missing?" Cathy reveals that when she wasn't using, she missed not only the effect of the drugs but also the excitement of drug seeking and the rituals the drug habit entails. "I just didn't know what to do with myself. It felt empty."

A sense of deficient emptiness pervades our entire culture. The drug addict is more painfully conscious of this void than most people and has limited means of escaping it. The rest of us find other ways of suppressing our fear of emptiness or of distracting ourselves from it. When we have nothing to occupy our minds, bad memories, troubling anxieties, unease or the nagging mental stupor we call boredom can arise. At all costs, drug addicts want to escape spending "alone time" with their minds. To a lesser degree, behavioural addictions are also responses to this terror of the void.

—

Opium, wrote Thomas De Quincey, is a powerful "counter agent . . . to the formidable curse of *taedium vitae*"—the tedium of life.

Human beings want not only to survive, but also to live. We long to experience life in all its vividness, with full, untrammelled emotion. Adults envy the open-hearted and open-minded explorations of children; seeing their joy and curiosity, we pine for our own lost capacity for wide-eyed wonder. Boredom, rooted in a fundamental discomfort with the self, is one of the least tolerable mental states.

For the addict the drug provides a route to feeling alive again, if only temporarily. "I am in profound awe of the ordinary," recalls author and bank robber Stephen Reid of his first hit of morphine. Thomas De Quincey extols opium's power "to stimulate the capacities of enjoyment."

Carol is a twenty-three-year-old resident of the Portland Hotel Society's Stanley Hotel. Her nose and lips are pierced with rings. Around her neck she wears a chain with a black metal cross. Her hairdo is a pink-dyed Mohawk that tapers to blond locks cascading at the back to her shoulders. A bright, mentally agile young woman, Carol has been an injection crystal meth user and heroin addict since she ran away from home at age fifteen. The Stanley is her first stable domicile after five years on the streets. These days she is active in promoting harm reduction and in supporting fellow addicts. She has attended international conferences, and her writings have been quoted by addiction experts.

During a methadone appointment, she explains what she cherishes about the crystal meth experience. She speaks nervously and rapidly and fidgets incessantly, effects that result from her long-standing stimulant habit and likely from the early-onset hyperactivity disorder she had before she ever used drugs. As befits a street-educated child of her generation, Carol's every second word seems to be "like" or "whatever."

"When you do, like, a good hit or whatever you get like a cough or whatever, like a warm feeling, you really feel a hit, start breathing hard or whatever," she says. "Kind of like a good orgasm if you are a more sexual person—I never really thought of it that way, but my body still experiences the same physical sensations. I just don't associate it with sex.

"I get all excited, whatever you're into . . . I like playing with clothes, or I like going out at night in the West End when there's not a whole lot of people, walking down back alleys, singing to myself. People leave stuff out, I look for what I can find, scavenging, and it's all so interesting."

The addict's reliance on the drug to reawaken her dulled feelings is no adolescent caprice. The dullness is itself a consequence of an emotional malfunction not of her making: the internal shutdown of vulnerability.

From the Latin word *vulnerare*, "to wound," vulnerability is our susceptibility to be wounded. This fragility is part of our nature and cannot be escaped. The best the brain can do is to shut down conscious awareness of it when pain becomes so vast or unbearable that it threatens to overwhelm our capacity to function. The automatic repression of painful emotion is a helpless child's prime defence mechanism and can enable the child to endure trauma that would otherwise be catastrophic. The unfortunate consequence is a wholesale dulling of emotional awareness. "Everybody knows there is no fineness or accuracy of suppression," wrote the American novelist Saul Bellow in *The Adventures of Augie March*; "if you hold down one thing you hold down the adjoining."[7]

Intuitively, we all know that it's better to feel than not to feel. Beyond their energizing subjective charge, emotions have crucial survival value. They orient us, interpret the world for us and offer us vital information. They tell us what is dangerous and what is benign, what threatens our existence and what will nurture our growth. Imagine how disabled we would be if we could not see or hear or taste or sense heat or cold or physical pain. Emotional shutdown is similar. Our emotions are an indispensable part of our sensory apparatus and an essential part of who we are. They make life worthwhile, exciting, challenging, beautiful and meaningful.

When we flee our vulnerability, we lose our full capacity for feeling emotion. We may even become emotional amnesiacs, not remembering ever having felt truly elated or truly sad. A nagging void opens, and we experience it as alienation, as profound *ennui*, as the sense of deficient emptiness described above.

The wondrous power of a drug is to offer the addict protection from pain while at the same time enabling her to engage the world with excitement and meaning. "It's not that my senses are dulled— no, they open, expanded," explained a young woman whose substances of choice are cocaine and marijuana. "But the anxiety is removed, and the nagging guilt and—yeah!" The drug restores to the addict the childhood vivacity she suppressed long ago.

———

Emotionally drained people often lack physical energy, as anyone who has experienced depression knows, and this is a prime cause of the bodily weariness that beleaguers many addicts. There are many more: dismal nutrition; a debilitating lifestyle; diseases like HIV, hepatitis C and their complications; disturbed sleep patterns that date back, in many cases, to childhood—another consequence of abuse or neglect. "I just couldn't go to sleep, ever," says Maureen, a sex-trade worker and heroin addict. "I never even knew there was such a thing as a good sleep until I was twenty-nine years old." Like Thomas De Quincey, who used opium to "sustain through twenty-four hours the else drooping animal energies," present-day addicts turn to drugs for a reliable energy boost.

"I can't give up cocaine," a pregnant patient named Celia once told me. "With my HIV, I have no energy. The rock gives me strength." Her phrasing sounded like a morbid reconfiguration of the psalmist's words: *"He only is my rock and my salvation; he is my defence. I shall not be moved."*

"I enjoy the rush, the smell and the taste," says Charlotte, long-time cocaine and heroin user, pot smoker and self-confessed speed freak. "I guess I've been smoking or doing some form of drugs for so long,

I don't know . . . I think, What if I stopped? Then what? That's where I get my energy from."

"Man, I can't face the day without the rock," says Greg, a multi-drug addict in his early forties. "I'm dying for one right now."

"You're not dying *for* it," I venture. "You're dying *because* of it." Greg is tickled. "Nah, not me. I'm Irish and half Indian."

"Right. There are no dead Irish or dead Indians around."

From Greg, more jollity. "Everybody has to go sometime. When your number comes up, that's it."

These four don't know it, but beyond illness or the inertia of emotional and physical exhaustion, they are also up against the brain physiology of addiction.

Cocaine, as we shall see, exerts its euphoric effect by increasing the availability of the reward chemical dopamine in key brain circuits, and this is necessary for motivation and for mental and physical energy. Flooded with artificially high levels of dopamine triggered by external substances, the brain's own mechanisms of dopamine secretion become lazy. They stop functioning at anywhere near full capacity, relying on the artificial boosters instead. Only long months of abstinence allow the intrinsic machinery of dopamine production to regenerate, and in the meantime, the addict will experience extremes of physical and emotional exhaustion.

—

Aubrey, a tall, rangy, solitary man now approaching middle age, is also hooked on cocaine. His face is permanently lined by sadness, and his customary tone is one of resignation and regret. He feels incomplete and incompetent as a person without the drug, a self-concept that has nothing to do with his real abilities and everything to do with his formative experiences as a child. By his own assessment, inadequacy and the sense that he was a failed human being were part and parcel of his personality before he ever touched drugs.

"After Grade Eight I grew up on drugs," Aubrey says. "When I turned to drugs, I found that I fit in with other kids . . . Yeah, it was a big important thing, to fit in. See, as a kid when you picked somebody for a soccer game, I was always the last guy to be picked.

"See," he continues, "I've been in institutions a lot, I've spent a long time in a four-by-eight cell. So I've been by myself a lot. And before then, too. See, I had a rough childhood, going from foster home to foster home. I was shipped off quite a bit, eh."

"At what age were you sent to foster homes?" I ask.

"About eleven. My father was killed, hit by a truck. My mother couldn't take care of all of us kids, and so Children's Aid stepped in. Me being the oldest, they took me out. I got two brothers. They were younger. They stayed home."

Aubrey believes he was chosen for foster care because he was "so hyper as a kid" that his mother couldn't handle him.

"I was there for five years. Well, not in one place. No. I got shipped around. They'd keep me for maybe a year and then they couldn't . . . and I had to go to another one."

"How did it feel to be shunted about like that?"

"It hurt me. I was feeling like I wasn't wanted. I was just a kid . . . It's like, I'm a kid and nobody wants me. Even in school. The nuns taught me, but I never learned to read or write or nothing. They just pushed me from one class to another . . . I was always disciplined for something, and they'd take me out of that class and put me in a class for four- or five-year-old kids . . . so I felt so uncomfortable. It was hard for me. I felt stupid. I'm sitting there with all these little kids around me, looking at me. The teacher is teaching spelling . . . And they're doing it and I can't do it . . . I kept it all to myself. I didn't want to talk for the longest time . . . I couldn't even talk to people. I stuttered; I had a hard time explaining myself. I kept it all inside me for so long. When I get hyper I can't talk proper . . .

"Strange, the cocaine calms me down.* And the pot. I smoke five or six joints a day. That relaxes me, too. It takes the edge off. At the end of the day I just lay back with it. That's just what happens, that's my life. I smoke a joint and I go to sleep."

Shirley, in her forties, addicted to both opiates and stimulants and stricken with the usual roster of diseases, also confesses to a

---

* A patient's report that a stimulant drug like cocaine or crystal meth has a calming effect is virtual confirmation that he or she has ADHD (Attention Deficit Hyperactivity Disorder). See Appendix II.

sense of inadequacy without her drugs and sees cocaine as a life necessity. "I was thirteen when I first used. It took most of my inhibitions away, and my uneasiness, my inadequacies—how we feel about ourselves I guess is a better way to put it."

"When you say inhibitions, what do you mean?" I ask.

"Inhibitions . . . it's like the awkwardness a man and a woman feel when you first meet, and you don't know whether to kiss each other, except I always felt that way. It makes everything go easier . . . your movements are more relaxed, so you're not awkward anymore."

No less a figure than the young Dr. Sigmund Freud was enthralled with cocaine for a while, relying on it "to control his intermittent depressed moods, improve his general sense of well-being, help him relax in tense social encounters, and *just make him feel more like a man*."[*][8] Freud was slow to accept that cocaine could creat a dependence problem.

Enhancing the personality, the drug also eases social interactions, as Aubrey and Shirley both testify. "Usually, I'm feeling down," says Aubrey. "I do coke, I'm totally a different person. I could talk to you a lot better now if I was high on cocaine. I don't slur my words. It wakes me. It makes it easier to see people. I'll want to start a conversation with somebody. I'm usually not very interesting to talk to . . . That's why most of the time I don't want to be with other people. I don't have that drive. I stay in my room by myself."

Many addicts report similar improvements in their social abilities under the influence, in contrast to the intolerable aloneness they experience when sober. "It makes me talk, it opens me up; I can be friendly," says one young man wired on crystal meth. "I'm never like this normally." We shouldn't underestimate how desperate a chronically lonely person is to escape the prison of solitude. It's not a matter here of common shyness but of a deep psychological sense of isolation experienced from early childhood by people who felt rejected by everyone, beginning with their caregivers.

Nicole is in her early fifties. After five years as my patient she revealed that, as a teenager, she'd been repeatedly raped by her father. She, too, has HIV, and the ravages of an old hip infection

* Italics mine throughout unless otherwise noted.

have left her hobbling around with a cane. "I'm more social with the drug," she says. "I get talkative and confident. Usually I'm shy and withdrawn and not very impressive. I let people walk all over me."

———

Another powerful dynamic perpetuates addiction despite the abundance of disastrous consequences: the addict sees no other possible existence for himself. His outlook on the future is restricted by his entrenched self-image as addict. No matter how much he may acknowledge the costs of his addiction, he fears a loss of self if it were absent from his life. In his own mind, he would cease to exist as he knows himself.

Carol says she was able to experience herself in a completely new and positive way under the influence of crystal meth. "I felt like I was smarter, like a floodgate of information or whatever just opened in my head . . . It opened my creativity. . . ." Asked if she has any regrets about her eight years of amphetamine addiction, she is quick to respond: "Not really, 'cause it helped bring me to who I am today." That may sound bizarre, but Carol's perspective is that drug use helped her escape an abusive family home, survive years of street living and connect her with a community of people with shared experiences. As many crystal meth users see it, this drug offers benefits to young street dwellers. Strange to say, it makes their lives more livable in the short term. It's hard to get a good night's sleep on the street: crystal meth keeps you awake and alert. No money for food? No need for hunger: crystal meth is an appetite suppressant. Tired, lacking energy? Crystal meth gives a user boundless energy.

Chris, a personable man with a mischievous sense of humour, whose well-muscled arms sport a kaleidoscope of tattoos, completed a year-long prison term a few months ago and is now back on the methadone program. In the Downtown Eastside he's known by the strange sobriquet "Toecutter," which he earned, legend has it, when he dropped a sharp, heavy industrial blade on someone's foot. He continues to inject crystal meth with dogged determination. "Helps me concentrate," he says. There's no doubt he's had

Attention Deficit Disorder all his life and he accepts the diagnosis, but he declines treatment. "This smart doctor once told me I'm self-medicating," he smirks, recalling a conversation we had years ago.

Chris recently came into the clinic with a fracture of his facial bones, sustained in a street brawl over a "paper" of heroin. Had the blow struck an inch higher, his left eye would have been destroyed. "I don't want to give up being an addict," he says when I ask him if it's all worth it. "I know this sounds pretty fucked up, but I like who I am."

"You're sitting here with your face smashed in by a metal pipe, and you're telling me you like who you are?"

"Yes, but I like who *I* am. I'm Toecutter, I'm an addict and I'm a nice guy."

—

Jake, methadone-treated opiate addict and heavy cocaine user, is in his mid-thirties. With his wispy blond facial stubble and lively body movements and a black baseball cap pulled rakishly low over his eyes, he could pass for ten years younger. "You've been injecting a lot of cocaine recently," I remark to him one day.

"It's hard to get away from it," he replies with his gap-toothed grin.

"You make coke sound like it's some wild animal, stalking you. Yet you're the one who's chasing it. What does it do for you?"

"It cuts the edge off everyday life down here, of dealing with everything."

"What is everything?"

"Responsibilities. I guess you could call it that—responsibilities. So long as I'm using, I don't care about responsibilities . . . When I'm older, I'll worry about pension plans and stuff like that. But right now, I don't care about nothin' except my old lady."

"Your old lady . . ."

"Yeah, I look upon the coke as my old lady, my family. It's my partner. I don't see my own family for a year, and I don't care, 'cause I've got my partner."

"So the coke is your life."

"Yeah, the coke's my life . . . I care more about the dope than my loved ones or anything else. For the past fifteen years . . . it's part of me now. It's part of my every day . . . I don't know how to be without it. I don't know how to live everyday life without it. You take it away, I don't know what I'm going to do . . . If you were to change me and put me in a regular-style life, I wouldn't know how to retain it. I was there once in my life, but it feels like I don't know how to go back. I don't have the . . . It's not the will I don't have; I just don't know how."

"What about the desire? Do you even want that regular life?"

"No, not really," Jake says quietly and sadly.

I don't believe that's true. I think deep in his heart there must live a desire for a life of wholeness and integrity that may be too painful to acknowledge—painful because, in his eyes, it's unattainable. Jake is so identified with his addiction that he doesn't dare imagine himself sober. "It feels like everyday life for me," he says. "It doesn't seem any different from anyone else's life. It's normal for me."

That reminds me of the frog, I tell Jake. "They say that if you take a frog and drop him in hot water, he'll jump out. But if you take the same frog, put him in water at room temperature and then slowly heat up the water, he'll boil to death because gradually, degree by degree, he becomes used to it. He perceives it as normal.

"If you had a regular life and somebody said to you, 'Hey, you could be in the Downtown Eastside hustling all day and blowing three or four hundred dollars a day on rock,' you'd say, 'What? Are you crazy? That's not for me!' But you've been doing it for so long, it's become normal for you."

Jake then shows me his hands and arms, covered with patches of silvery scales on a red, inflamed field of skin. On top of everything else, his psoriasis is acting up. "Do you think you could send me to a skin specialist?" he asks.

"I could," I reply, "but the last time I did, you didn't show for the appointment. If you miss this one, I won't refer you again."

"I'll go, Doc. Don't worry, I'll go."

I write out the prescriptions for methadone and for the dermatological creams Jake needs. We chat a little more, and then he leaves. He's my last patient of the day.

A few minutes later, as I'm about to check my voicemail messages, there's a knock. I pull the door ajar. It's Jake, who made it to the front gate of the Portland but has returned to tell me something. "You were right, you know," he says, grinning again.

"Right about what?"

"That frog you're talking about. That's me."

CHAPTER 4

You Wouldn't Believe My Life Story

M até, you wouldn't believe my life story. Everything I'm
saying to you is true."

"You think I wouldn't believe it?"

Serena gives me a look that's resigned and challenging at the
same time. A tall Native woman with long, black hair, she has a per-
petually world-weary expression on her thin face. Although she's
also capable of sudden mirth, even in laughter her eyes retain their
sadness. Just over thirty years old, Serena has spent almost half her
life here in the Downtown Eastside, wired on drugs.

What can you tell me, I think, that I haven't heard down here
before? Later, after I hear her out, I feel humbled.

Serena doesn't readily share anything about her inner life. She
comes for regular methadone appointments and every once in a
while attempts to scam me for some other narcotic prescription,
under the pretence of having a headache or back pain. When I
refuse, she's never argumentative. "Okay," she says quietly, shrug-
ging her shoulders. One day, two years ago, she appeared in my
office, asking for methadone to "carry"—that is, rather than having
to drink in front of the pharmacist every morning, she wanted several days' doses in advance. "My grandmother died in Kelowna," she
told me in a flat monotone. "I have to go home for the burial."

Downtown Eastside addicts often ask for methadone carries for
illicit purposes, such as selling the substance or injecting it to get a

bigger rush. Others go to the pharmacy, but instead of swallowing their whole dose, they hold some in their mouth and later spit it into a coffee cup. The expectorated methadone then becomes merchandise. Despite the risk of transmittable disease, buyers don't hesitate to drink a drug mixed with someone else's saliva. Pharmacists are expected to observe complete ingestion of the methadone they dispense, but the rule is often broken, so juice is always up for sale on the streets.

"I have to verify this before I can give you the carry," I replied to Serena. "Who's your grandmother's doctor?" Nonchalantly, she gave me the name. As she sat in my office and waited calmly, I dialled the physician's office in Kelowna. "Mrs. B . . . ," my colleague said on the speaker phone. "Oh, no, it so happens she was very much alive when I saw her this morning."

"You heard that," I said to Serena. No flicker of movement, not the barest sign of embarrassment, registered on her face. "Well," she shrugged, getting up to leave, "they told me she was dead." I've often been struck by the childlike insouciance of my addicted patients when they lie to me. A naïve manipulation like the one Serena attempted is simply part of the game, and being caught is no more shameful than being found while playing hide-and-seek.

Her HIV care has been a source of struggle between us, since she habitually refuses to have her blood counts done. "I can't know what treatment you need," I explain, "if I don't know the state of your immune system." Once, in utter frustration, I tried to coerce her into having the blood tests by threatening to withhold her methadone. A week later I recanted. "It's not my right to force you into anything," I said by way of apology. "The methadone has nothing to do with HIV. Whether you get yourself tested or not is entirely up to you. I can only offer you my best advice. I'm sorry." "Thank you, Maté," Serena said. "I just don't want anybody controlling me." Soon afterwards she did undergo the required tests voluntarily. And so far her immune counts have been high enough that antiviral medications haven't been needed.

The question of control is a touchy one. No segment of the population feels powerlessness more acutely than Downtown Eastside drug addicts. Even the average citizen finds it difficult to question medical authority, for a host of cultural and psychological reasons.

As an authority figure, the doctor triggers deeply ingrained feelings of childhood powerlessness in many of us—I had that experience even years after completing medical training when I needed care for myself. But in the case of the drug addict, the disempowerment is real, palpable and quite in the present. Engaged in illegal activities to support her habit—her very habit being illegal—she is on all sides hemmed in by laws, rules and regulations. It occurs to me at times that, in the view of my addicted patients, the roles of detective, prosecutor and judge are grafted onto my duties as physician. I am there not only as a healer, but also as an enforcer.

Coming most commonly from a socially deprived background and having passed through courts and prisons repeatedly, the Downtown Eastside addict is unaccustomed to challenging authority directly. Dependent on the physician for her lifeline methadone prescription, she is in no position to assert herself. If she doesn't like her doctor, she has little latitude to seek care elsewhere: downtown clinics are not eager to accept each other's "problem" clients. Many addicts speak bitterly about medical personnel who, they find, impose their "my-way-or-the-highway" authority with arrogance and insensitivity. In any confrontation with authority, be it nurse, doctor, police officer or hospital security guard, the addict is virtually helpless. No one will accept her side of the story—or act on it even if they do.

Power comes with the territory and it corrupts. At the Portland I've caught myself in behaviours that I would never permit myself in any other context. Not long ago another young Native woman was in my office, also methadone dependent and also with HIV. I'll call her Cindy. At the end of the visit I opened the door and called to Kim, the nurse whose office is directly next to mine: "Please draw blood for Cindy's HIV indices, and we'll need a urinalysis as well." Several clients were sitting in chairs in the waiting area, and my words were clearly audible to all. Cindy, looking hurt, reproached me quietly. "You shouldn't say that so loud." I was aghast. Back in the "respectable" family practice I ran for twenty years before coming to work in the Downtown Eastside, it would have been unthinkable for me to commit such a callous breach of confidentiality, to injure someone's dignity so brazenly. I closed the door and offered my regrets. "I was loud," I agreed. "Very stupid of me." "Yes, it was," Cindy shot back, but somewhat mollified. I thanked her for being forthright. "I'm tired of everyone pushing me around," she said as she stood up to leave.

There's also a deeper source of the exaggerated power imbalance that besets doctor–patient relationships in the Downtown Eastside—not unique to this neighbourhood, but here it's almost universal. Imprinted in the developing brain circuitry of the child subjected to abuse or neglect is fear and distrust of powerful people, especially of caregivers. In time this ingrained wariness is reinforced by negative experiences with authority figures such as teachers, foster parents and members of the legal system or the medical profession. Whenever I adopt a sharp tone with one of my clients or display indifference or attempt some well-meant coercion for her benefit, I unwittingly take on the features of the powerful ones who first wounded and frightened her decades ago. Whatever my intentions, I end up evoking pain and fear.

For all these reasons, and more, Serena's instinct is to guard her inner world from me. Her asking for help today owes something to the trust established between us but even more to her present despair.

"Is there anything you can give me for depression?" she begins. "My grandmother in Kelowna died three months ago. I've been thinking of going away to be with her."

"Killing yourself?"

"Not killing myself, just taking some pills so . . ."

"That's killing yourself."

"I don't call it that. Just going to sleep . . . Not waking up again." Serena looks crushed and disconsolate. This time the loss of her grandmother is real.

"Please tell me about her," I say.

"She was sixty-five. She raised me, from when my mother delivered me and left the hospital right away. The social worker had to phone my grandmother and tell her that if she didn't come and sign papers, I'd be put into a foster home." Throughout the entire discussion that follows Serena's voice is grief-stricken, choked and weepy. Her tears stop flowing only intermittently.

"Then she raised my daughter from a year old." Serena has a child, now fourteen years old, born to her when she herself was fifteen. Serena's mother, in her forties and also a patient of mine, was sixteen when she abandoned her newborn. She has a room with her boyfriend in the same Hastings hotel where Serena lives.

"Where's your daughter now?"

"With my Aunt Gladys. I guess she's doing all right. After my grand-mother died, she started getting into speed and everything like that . . .

"She raised me; she raised my brother Caleb and my sister Devona—my first cousins, actually, but we grew up like brother and sisters."

"What kind of a home did she give you?"

"She gave me a perfect home—until I left to find my mother. That's how I came down here, to look for my mom." What this poor woman calls a "perfect home" becomes devastatingly clear as she continues her narrative.

"Had you not met your mother before?"

"Never."

"Had you used before?"

"Not till I got down here to find my mother."

Apart from the movement of her right hand as she dabs her eyes, Serena sits motionless. The sunlight streaming into the office through the window behind her leaves her face in merciful obscurity.

"I had my daughter when I was fifteen. He was my auntie's boyfriend, whatever. He was molesting me and if I said anything, he vowed to beat my auntie."

"I see."

"Mate, you would not believe my life story. Everything I'm saying to you is true."

"You think I would not believe it?"

In the brief silence that follows, I recollect how ever since that fictitious report of her grandmother's death two years ago, I have dis-missed Serena as a manipulator, a drug seeker. I am prone to that human—but inhumane—failing of defining and categorizing people according to our interpretation of their behaviours. Our ideas and feelings about a person congeal around our limited experience of them, and around our judgments. In my eyes, Serena was reduced to an addict who inconvenienced me by wanting more drugs. I didn't perceive that she was a human being suffering unimaginable pain, soothing it, easing it in the only way she knew how.

I'm not always stuck in that blind mode. I move in and out of it, depending on how I am doing in my own life. I'm more subject to deadening judgments and definitions that restrict my view of the other when I'm tired or stressed and most especially when, in some way, I'm not conducting myself with integrity. At such times my addict clients experience the power imbalance between us most acutely.

"I was fifteen years old when I came down here to Hastings," Serena goes on. "I had five hundred dollars in my pocket I'd saved for food until I caught up with my mom. It took me a week to find her. I had about four hundred bucks left. When she found that out, she stuck a needle in my arm. The four hundred dollars was gone in four hours."

"And that was your first experience with heroin?"

"Yes." A long silence ensues, broken only by the throaty, weeping sounds Serena is trying to suppress.

"And then she sold me to a fucking big fat huge motherfucker while I was sleeping." These words are uttered with the helpless, plaintive rage of a child. "She's my mom. I love her, but we're not close. The one I call Mom is my grandmother. And now she's gone. She was the only one who cared whether I lived or died. If I died today, nobody would give a damn . . .

"I need to let her go. I'm holding her back."

Serena can see by my look that I don't follow. "I am not letting her go," she explains. "In our tradition, we have to let the spirits go. If not, they're still with us, stuck."

I suggest that it's almost impossible for her to find release, since she felt her grandmother was the only one who'd ever loved, accepted and supported her. "But what if you found someone else who really loved you and cared for you?"

"There is no one else. There is none."

"Are you sure of that?"

"Who? Myself? God?"

"I don't know. Both, perhaps."

Serena's voice breaks with grief. "You know what I think about God? Who is this God that keeps the bad people behind and takes away the good people?"

"How about yourself? How about you?"

"If I was strong enough for that, I'd let her go. I have a drug problem and it's hard for me to help myself. I've tried so many times, Maté. Tried and tried. I've quit for four, five, six months, a year, but I always end up coming back. This is the only place I know where I feel safe." Here in Canada, "our home and native land," the reality is that the Downtown Eastside, afflicted by addiction, illness, violence, poverty and sexual exploitation, is the only spot where Serena has any sense of security.

Serena has known two homes in her life: her grandmother's house in Kelowna and one or another ramshackle hotel on East Hastings. "I'm not safe in Kelowna," she says. "I was molested by my uncle and my grandfather, and the drug is keeping me from thinking about what happened. And my grandfather was telling my grandmother to tell me to come back and to forgive and forget. 'If you want to come back to Kelowna and talk about it in front of the whole family, you can.' Talk about fucking what? What? Everything is over and done with already. There is no turning back. He can't forget and change what he did to me. My uncle can't change what he did to me."

The sexual abuse began when Serena was seven years old and persisted until she gave birth to her child, at fifteen. All the while, she was looking after her younger siblings.

"I had to protect my brother and sister, too. I'd hide them in the basement with four or five bottles of baby food. They were still in diapers. When I was eleven years old, I tried to refuse my grandfather, but he said that if I didn't do exactly what he told me, he was going to do it to Caleb, too. Caleb was only eight then."

"Oh, Jesus," escapes from my lips. It's a blessing, I suppose, that after all these years working in the Downtown Eastside, I'm still capable of being shocked.

"And your grandmother didn't protect you."

"She couldn't. She was drinking so much until she quit. She began drinking every morning. She was drinking until my daughter was born."

Years later, Caleb was killed—beaten and drowned by three cousins after a drinking bout. "I still have trouble believing my brother is dead, too," Serena says. "We were so close when we were kids."

So this was the perfect home Serena grew up in, under the care of a grandmother who, no doubt, loved her grandchild but was utterly unable to defend her from the predatory males in the household or from her own alcoholism. And that grandmother, now deceased, was Serena's sole connection to the possibility of sustaining, consoling love in this world.

"Have you ever talked with anyone about this?" In the Downtown Eastside this is almost always a rhetorical question.

"No. Can't trust anybody . . . Can't talk to my mom. Me and my mom don't have a mother and daughter life. We live in the same building; we don't even see each other. She walks right by me. That hurts me large.

"I've tried everything. There's no point. I've tried so many years to see if my mom would get close to me. And the only time she gets close to me is if I have some dope or money in my pocket. It's the only time she'll say, 'Daughter, I love you.'"

I wince.

"The only time, Maté. The only time."

I have no doubt that if Serena's mother spoke about her life, an equally painful narrative would emerge. The suffering down here is multigenerational. Almost uniformly, the greatest anguish confessed by my patients, male or female, concerns not the abuse they suffered but their own abandonment of their children. They can never forgive themselves for it. The very mention of it draws out bitter tears, and much of their continued drug use is intended to dull the impact of such memories. Serena herself, speaking here as the wounded child, is silent about her own guilt feelings regarding her neglected daughter, now a crystal meth user. Pain begets pain. Let those who would judge either of these women look to themselves.

As always when I spend an unexpectedly long time with a patient, the waiting-room crowd erupts in noisy protest. "Hurry up," someone shouts coarsely. "We need our juice, too!" All of Serena's hurt and rage now explode out of her in a full-throated "Shut the fuck up!" I poke my head out the door to calm the anxious multitude.

I agree to prescribe Serena an antidepressant, explaining that it may or may not work and may or may not cause side effects, depending on a person's particular physiology. And I tell her we can try another one if this one doesn't work. I hand her the prescription and search in my heart to find compassionate words, words that may help soothe the anguish Serena bears in hers. And the words come, haltingly at first.

"What happened to you is truly horrible. There is no other word for it and there is nothing I can say that comes even close to acknowledging just how terrible, how unfair it is for any being, any child to be forced to endure all that. But no matter what, I still don't accept that things are hopeless for any human being. I believe there is a natural strength and innate perfection in everyone. Even though it's covered up by all kinds of terrors and all kinds of scars, it's there."

"I wish I could find it," Serena says in a voice so choked and quiet, I am reading her lips to make out the words.

"It's in you. I see it. I can't prove it to you, but I see it."

"I've tried to prove it to myself, and I failed."

"I know. You've tried and it didn't work and you're back here. It's very difficult. There ought to be a lot more support."

Finally, I tell Serena that to the depressed person, everything looks absolutely hopeless. "That's what it means to be depressed. We'll see how you'll do with the medication. Let's talk again in two weeks."

And here is where I'm humbled. I'm humbled by my feebleness in helping this person. Humbled that I had the arrogance to believe I'd seen and heard it all. You can never see and hear it all because, for all their sordid similarities, each story in the Downtown Eastside unfolded in the particular existence of a unique human being. Each one needs to be heard, witnessed and acknowledged anew, every time it's told. And I'm especially humbled because I dared to imagine that Serena was less than the complex and luminous person she is. Who am I to judge her for being driven to the belief that only through drugs will she find respite from her torments?

Spiritual teachings of all traditions enjoin us to see the divine in each other. "*Namaste*," the Sanskrit holy greeting, means: "The divine in me salutes the divine in you." The divine? It's so hard for us even to see the human. What have I to offer this young Native woman whose three decades of life bear the compressed torment of generations? An antidepressant capsule every morning, to be dispensed with her methadone, and half an hour of my time once or twice a month.

CHAPTER 5

Angela's Grandfather

With her straight bearing, oval face, dark eyes and long, black hair falling in waves to her shoulders, Angela McDowell is a Coast Salish princess, living the life of an exile in the Downtown Eastside. A long, horizontal scar mars her left cheek. "A girl cut me up when I moved into the Sunrise," she tells me in a matter-of-fact tone.

She's always late for appointments if she makes them at all. Often she endures withdrawal for a few days without methadone before she comes in for her prescription. Or she shoots up with street heroin.

A poet, Angela carries in her purse a pink notebook with a coiled wire spine. On each page, in finely articulated handwriting, are naïve rhymes of hope and loss, desolation and possibility. Some, I feel, are more authentic than others. *"One day with this addiction we fight / We all will win and see the light,"* she vows at the end of a poem about a life of abject drug seeking. I have my doubts: Are these her true feelings, or is she writing what she believes to be the appropriate sentiment?

Yet I can tell she's been somewhere real, and the truth she glimpsed there lends her authority. The joy she experienced long ago is present in her world-illuminating smile. When her lips part to laugh or smile, she reveals two rows of perfect, white teeth, remarkable in this corner of the world. Her eyes light up, the tension lines in her face soften and her scar grows faint. "Healing is in me," she tells me one day. "I've heard the voices of the ancient ones. I had a really powerful spirit as a child."

Angela was brought up, along with her brothers and sister, by her grandfather, a great shaman of her tribe. "He was the last surviving McDowell in his family. All his brothers and cousins and uncles and aunts were killed, so my grandfather was sent off to a boarding school to be raised from a very young boy. Grew up, married my grandmother and had all of his children—eleven girls, three boys. He carried the spirit from all of our ancestors. Every Native reserve has its own powers, spirits. We, the Coast Salish, we carry the gift of—I don't know how to say it—we almost can predict death. We see spirits. We see beyond. We see the other side." She shakes her head as if countering a misunderstanding on my part. "It's not like seeing a clear picture—more like when you see something from the corner of your eye. This is a gift I've been handed down."

A year before Angela's grandfather died, when Angela was seven, he set out to discover which of his descendants would continue to bear the gift. "He had to prepare us for his death and see which one of us was chosen. Every day for a year we went to the river, the same spot, and had a cedar bath—all the children."

The writer, cultural commentator, addict and bank robber Stephen Reid has explained to me that the Spirit Bath with cold water and cedar leaves is a sacred ceremony of the Coast Salish. Now serving out a long jail sentence at William Head Prison on Vancouver Island, he studies with a visiting Salish elder and feels highly honoured to be allowed to take part in the Spirit Bath. In both Stephen and Angela's telling, it sounds like a gruelling ritual, the purpose of which is spiritual cleansing.

At five o'clock in the morning, later in the winter, the old man and his wife led the children down to a stand of cedar trees by the riverside. Summer and winter, the children lay by the bank, stripped naked. The shaman chanted as their grandmother tore small branches from places where the rising sun was shining on the trees. Then, in absolute silence but for the rustling of the leaves and the murmuring of the stream, she dipped the boughs in the cold, rushing water. She bathed the children, brushing their bodies with the leaves. "They washed us off and cleansed us and strengthened us for our adult lives," says Angela, "to prepare us so we don't suffer broken bones and so when we're sick, we don't be sick for very long. And it's also a way for my grandfather to find out which one of us children is strong enough to carry on the spirituality. All of our ancestors are brought into the chosen one."

"How does he find out?"

"You're in ice-cold water and it feels like they're scraping your skin off you—it is not a fun thing for a little kid. We didn't believe what he was telling us it was for. But soon enough, I could hear drums—Native drums. After a while that's what soothed me, that's what I listened to. As my grandfather was praying and my grandmother was giving me the bath, I could hear drums. It was so cold and we had to lie still. I decided the only way I could get through it was not to pay attention to what my body was feeling. I would just lie there, listening to the drums, and let them do it. As time went on and it snowed, I began to hear singing—quiet, calm, beautiful singing in a language I'd never heard before. It was Native music. What was strange was that I didn't know how to speak Coast Salish at that time, but here I was singing along."

I listen to Angela with fascination alloyed with a vague longing—it's a sense of lost connection with past generations. I had no grandparents in my life. She is steeped in tradition and the spirit world. She's heard the voices of the ancients. I read the ancients but hear only my own thoughts.

"Where is the song coming from?" the shaman asked Angela one day when he observed his wife brushing the child with the cedar leaves and saw that she, the little girl, did not suffer. She was transported, he knew, and could now be his guide. The two of them walked slowly along the trail by the river, leaving Angela's brothers and sister and grandmother, until they were completely alone. And there in a clearing they sat, the shaman and his young granddaughter, and listened to the voices of the dead of their tribe. The dead of many generations keened and lamented and sang of their lives in an ancient tongue and told their stories and how they had worked, struggled and died since the coming of the white people, and even before. Angela received the stories and the teaching.

I see it in her. I've witnessed her speaking words of compassion and solace to other addicts in my office. I was also impressed by the quiet confidence with which she took the stage at a public event at the Central Branch of the Vancouver Library.

I was giving a talk on addiction. I'd invited Angela to read her poetry, and as usual, she arrived late. When I introduced her she strode purposefully to the podium from her place at the back. Unhurriedly she surveyed the audience of three hundred people and, as if it was a natural everyday practice for her, recited her works in a clear, resonant voice. It was a moving performance, rewarded with long and warm applause from her listeners.

That clearing by the river remains Angela's place of greatness, even though her connection with it was obscured by abuse later in her childhood. She has run far away from it and doesn't know if she'll ever return. No keeper of sacred tribal lore now, she lives in the Downtown Eastside as a cocaine-wired hustler and back-alley courtesan. "Blow for your dough / Play for your pay," she says in a poem.

But her joyous smile and patrician air of authority are born of her deep knowledge that such a place exists and that she has been there and heard the voices. They speak to her through all her misery. They still help her seek herself. "Mirror of my inner self, what do others see?" Angela asks in one of her verses. "Is it the truth in my heart, or human vanity? And what do I see?"

CHAPTER 6

—

Pregnancy Journal

This is the brief account of a pregnancy—and the birth of an opiate-dependent infant to an addicted mother. Despite her determination to face down her demons, the mother will not be able to keep the child. Her resources will not be adequate, and neither her pleas to the God-voice in her heart nor the support we at the Portland can provide will suffice to help her carry out her sacred intention to be a parent.

June 2004

I dash up to the fifth floor, where Celia is reported to be completely out of control and threatening to leap out the window. No idle threat, that—people have done it before. The reverberations of wall-piercing yells reach me in the stairwell two storeys below as I race toward the din.

I find Celia rampaging barefoot over broken glass, bleeding from several small cuts. The floor glitters with shards of shattered television screen, drinking glasses and crockery, lit up by a midday sun that throws its beams into the room at a sharp angle. The eviscerated TV console lies in the hall. Splattered food drips from the walls and from fragments of wooden chairs. Clothing is strewn all about. On the kitchen counter a small espresso machine gurgles and sizzles, filling the air with the pungent, acidic aroma of burnt coffee. A few blood-caked syringes rest on the table, the one piece of furniture still intact.

Celia stomps about, bellowing in a voice that's only semi-human: raspy, high and grating. Tears stream down her cheeks from her reddened eyes and quiver in droplets on her chin. She's wearing a dirty flannel nightgown. It is an unearthly scene to behold.

"I fucking hate him. Shitty, goddamn, fucking bastard." Seeing me, Celia slumps down on the ragged mattress in the corner. I kick aside a pile of towels and hunch against the balcony window. For now there is nothing to say. As I await some sign that she's ready for contact, I read the prayer she's written on the wall above her cot: "Oh, Great Spirit, whose voice I hear in the Winds and whose breath gives life to all the World around me, hear our cry, for we are small and weak." It ends with a plea: "Help me make peace with my greatest Enemy—myself."

June 2004: *next day*

Celia is quiet and even serene as she waits for her methadone script. She seems bemused by my astonishment.

"You say your room's back to normal?"

"Well, it's spotless."

"How can it be spotless?"

"Me and my old man put it together."

"The guy you hate?"

"I said I hate him, but I don't."

With her soft expression, clear eyes, straight brown hair and calm demeanour, Celia is an attractive thirty-year-old woman. It is impossible to recognize in her the raging harridan I saw less than twenty-four hours ago. "What do you suppose makes you fly off the handle like that?" I ask. "You were feeling upset, but there must have been some drug on board to make you that crazy. You were ripped on something."

"Well, yeah. Coke. It's very explosive. The less dope [heroin] I'm doing, the more stuff from the past surfaces. I don't know how to handle my feelings. With rock I get triggered, more sensitive—incredibly sensitive—to unresolved things in my life. Things I'm hurt about become overwhelming, to the point where I go from being completely devastated to desperate to almost volcanic—it's terrifying for me."

"So you've still been topping up your methadone with heroin. Why?"

"Because I want that coma state, where I don't feel anything." Reflective, cogent, articulate, Celia speaks slowly, even formally, in her low, husky voice. A gap in her teeth gives her a faint lisp.

"What is it you don't want to feel?"

"Every person I ever wanted to trust, I've been hurt by. I truly am in love with Rick, but for the life of me I can't bring myself to believe that he will not betray me. It stems right back to my sexual abuse."

Celia recalls being sexually exploited for the first time at the age of five, by her stepfather. "It went on for eight years. Recently I've been reliving the abuse in my dreams." In her nightmares, Celia is drenched in her stepfather's saliva. "That was a ritual," she explains with an almost flat matter-of-factness. "When I was a little girl, he would stand over my bed and spit all over me."

I shudder. After three decades as a doctor I sometimes believe I've heard every kind of depravity adults can inflict on the young and the unprotected. But in the Downtown Eastside new childhood horrors are always being revealed. Celia acknowledges my shock with a flicker of her eyelids and a nod and then continues. "Now my old man, Rick, was with the army in Sarajevo and he has post-traumatic stress. There's me, having sexual abuse dreams and waking up, and I've got him waking up screaming about guns and death. . . ."

"You do drugs to get away from the pain," I say after a moment, "but the drug use creates more pain. We can control your opiate addiction with the methadone, but if you want this cycle to stop, you'd have to be committed to giving up the cocaine."

"I am. I want this more than anything."

In the waiting area outside my office the patients are getting restless. Someone screams. Celia waves her hand dismissively.

I smile at her. "You didn't sound too different from that yesterday."

"I was a lot worse than that. I was completely insane."

The screaming resumes, this time louder. "Fuck off, you goddamn asshole," Celia shouts, her tone suddenly vicious. "I'm talking
with the doctor!"

August 2004

I like to have music playing on the small acoustic system behind my
desk. My patients, very few of whom are familiar with the classical
genre, often remark that they find it a welcome, soothing surprise.
Today it's *Kol Nidrei,* Bruch's setting of the Jewish soul's prayer for
atonement, forgiveness and unity with God. Celia closes her eyes.
"So beautiful," she sighs.

When the music is over, she stirs from her reverie and tells me
she and her boyfriend are making plans for the future.

"What about your ongoing addiction? Is it creating a problem for
you or him?"

"Well, yeah, because the whole me isn't there. . . . You don't get
the best of a person when there's an addiction, right?"

"Right," I concur. "I know something about that myself."

October 2004

Celia is expecting. Down here that's always a mixed blessing at best.
It may seem that a physician's first thought with a newly pregnant,
drug-dependent patient would be to counsel abortion. But the doctor's job—with this or any other population—is to ascertain the
woman's own preferences and, if appropriate, explain the options
without exerting any pressure to decide this way or that.

Many addicted women decide to have their babies, rather than
choose the route of an early abortion. Celia is determined to see
the pregnancy through and to keep the baby. "They've taken away
my first two kids; they'll never take this one," she vows.

A review of Celia's medical chart over the past four years reveals
nothing encouraging. Several suicide threats. Involuntary committal
to a psychiatric ward because, during a blaze at the Washington Hotel,

she would not come down from the fire escape. Numerous physical injuries—bone fractures, bruises, black eyes. Abscesses treated by surgical drainage, dental infections, episodes of pneumonia requiring hospitalization, a shingles outbreak, recurrent fungal infestations of the mouth, a rare blood infection—the manifestations of an immune system under siege by HIV and challenged to the limit by frequent drug injection. For a long time Celia did not comply with the pre-scribed antiviral treatments. Her liver is damaged by hepatitis C. The one hopeful note is that since being with Rick, her current "old man," she's been taking her HIV medications regularly, and her immune counts have climbed back up into the safe range. If she continues the treatment, her baby will not become infected.

Today she is here with Rick. The two snuggle close and give each other tender glances. It's the first prenatal visit, and Celia is recount-ing her previous childbearing history.

"I raised my first son for nine months. His father ended up leav-ing us . . . he was a good father . . . I was injecting. It was very irre-sponsible of me."

"So you understand why this baby might be taken away, too, if you continue using. "

Celia is emphatic. "Oh, yeah, definitely. I would never put a child in any position to suffer from my addiction . . . I mean it's easier to say than do . . . but . . ."

I look at Rick and Celia, sensing how fervently they want this child. Perhaps they see their baby as their saviour, as the force that will give them strength to hold their lives together. My concern is that they are engaged in magical thinking—like children, they believe that wishing something will make it happen. Celia is deeply entrenched in her addictions. Neither she nor Rick is close to resolving the traumas and psychological burdens that blight their relationship. I do not believe the stirring of this new life in Celia's womb will do for these parents what they have been unable to achieve for themselves. Freedom is not gained so easily.

Despite my doubts and misgivings, with all my heart I want them to succeed. Pregnancy has helped some addicts break away from their habits, and Celia would not be the first one to make it. Carol, the young woman with a crystal meth and opiate dependence quoted in Chapter 3, has given birth to a healthy infant, given up her addiction and moved to the B.C. interior to live with her grandparents. And there have been a few other success stories among my patients over the years.

"I'll give you whatever help I can," I say. "It's a chance for a new life, not just for the baby, but for you individually—and for the two of you together. But you know you have some obstacles to overcome."

The first item I bring up is Celia's addiction. Her opiate dependence can be taken care of by the methadone. Contrary to what Celia expects, we will not only maintain her on this drug but will likely increase the dose as the pregnancy proceeds. A fetus undergoing opiate withdrawal *in utero* may suffer neurological damage, so it's better for the baby to come into the world with an opiate dependence and to wean her from it gently *post partum*. Cocaine is another matter. Given how rabidly dysfunctional Celia is under the influence of this drug, it is inconceivable that she could comply with obstetrical care or, afterwards, maintain custody of her child unless she gives up the habit. I urge her to enter a recovery home, far from the Downtown Eastside.

"I can't be away from Rick," Celia replies.

"It's not about me," Rick says. "It's about you getting the recovery and stability you need."

"You said to me not long ago that you have trouble with trust," I remind Celia. "How clear are you that you trust Rick now?"

"Well, I'm seeing that he is very committed. But"—she takes a deep breath and looks directly at her partner—"I'm scared, because every time I have trusted in the past, I'm always . . . I'm always disappointed. So I'm scared, but I'm still willing to trust."

"If that's the case," I suggest, "then staying close to Rick physically . . ."

Celia completes the thought. "Then staying close to him physically is not going to change anything."

Outside the office the clamour of waiting patients is mounting. I promise to explore recovery options for Celia and hand her the standard blood test and ultrasound requisitions. When I rise to open the door, Celia does not budge from her chair. She hesitates and glances at Rick briefly before speaking. "You have to lighten up on me," she says to him. "I know it's very hard for you to see me doing dope when I'm pregnant . . ." She pauses and gazes at the floor. I urge her to continue.

"I need encouragement, not anger. Rick can be cutting with his words . . . very sharp." She faces him once more and addresses him deliberately and firmly. "You reinforce all the negative things people have said about me, accusing me . . . 'Yeah, they were right, they said this, they said that. Yeah, you are this, you are that,' and throwing in some more stuff that's nothing to do with me. I'm not promiscuous; I'm not a whore . . ."

Rick's fidgets and stares at his feet. "We still have a lot of work to do on our relationship," he says, "but we have a different motivation now."

"It's frustrating for you to watch Celia do drugs."

"Very frustrating. But that frustration is mine. It's my responsibility."

Rick, as an alcoholic, has done some Twelve-Step work. He is quick to understand and, like Celia, he is insightful and articulate. "There's a fine line," he offers, "between healthy boundaries and co-dependency, where you're just getting walked over. In the heat of the moment, it's so tough for me to discern that."

I momentarily permit myself some optimism. If anyone can make it, it's these two.

October 2004: later that month

Celia does not carry through with the recovery plan. In my office for her next methadone script, she confesses she is still smoking rock.

"It's almost for sure they will take the baby away," I remind her. "If you're using cocaine, they will not consider you a competent mother."

"That's one thing I'm going to be stopping. I'm trying my damn hardest. That's it. I'm stopping."

"It's your best chance of keeping the baby—your only chance."

"I know."

November 2004

Holding a wet compress to large welt above her right eye, Celia paces from door to window. "I got into a scrap with a girl. I'll be okay. But, hey, I did the ultrasound. I seen a little hand! It was so tiny."

I explain that the shadow on the ultrasound screen could not have been a hand: at seven weeks of gestation the limbs are not formed. But I'm moved by Celia's excitement and her evident bonding with the embryonic life she's carrying. She tells me she hasn't done cocaine for over a week.

November 2004: later that month

I don't know that I've ever seen such sadness as I see etched on Celia's features today. Her long, stringy hair is falling in front of her face as she bows her head and, from behind this veil, she speaks her words with painful slowness. Her voice is a keening, whimpering moan.

"He's told me to fuck off. . . . He made it more than clear he doesn't want anything to do with me anymore."

I feel dismayed, even irritated, as if Celia owed it to me personally to live out some happy, odds-defying fantasy of redemption. "Were those Rick's words or your interpretation?"

"No, he packed up all his stuff and didn't even have the heart to tell me what was going on, where he was, or anything. I ran into him this morning in the street and he screamed out a bunch of bullshit about how I cheated on him, which is complete crap. I have never cheated on him. But he's bounced. So that's my reality right now."

"You're hurt."

"I'm devastated. I've never felt so unwanted in my whole fucking life."

Yes, you have, I think to myself. You have always felt unwanted. And desperate as you are to offer your baby what you never experienced— a loving welcome into this world—in the end, you'll give her the same message of rejection.

It's as if Celia is reading my mind. "I'm still going to go through with the pregnancy," she says through pursed lips. "I could have an abortion, but no. This is my child; this is part of me. I don't care if I'm left standing alone or not. These things happen for a reason. God wouldn't give me anything more than I could handle. So I just have to have enough faith to believe that it's all going to come together in the right time. And the way it comes together is the way it's supposed to come together."

Celia has a strong spiritual bent. Will it see her through?

"I need to get into recovery. I need to get the hell out of here, tonight, even if it's just an emergency shelter for now; otherwise, I'm going to end up killing somebody. I just want to disappear . . ."

Once more, we make phone calls to various recovery homes. In the afternoon, two blocks away from the Portland, Celia jumps out of the cab driving her to the shelter the staff has arranged for her. Next morning she's back at the Portland, in a cocaine rage.

December 2004

Cocaine-free for a week, Celia is determined to stay clean. "I just can't incarcerate myself in some recovery place," she says, "but if I can keep away from the rock, I'll be all right." She is cheerful, clear-eyed and optimistic. The pregnancy is developing apace. As she gains weight, her somewhat sharp features fill out and she appears to be suffused by well-being. For obstetrical and HIV care, we've hooked her up with Oak Tree, a clinic associated with British Columbia Women's Hospital.

Seeing her like this, I'm reminded of Celia's strengths. In addition to her intelligence and her love-seeking nature, she has a sensitive, spiritually vibrant, artistic side. She writes poetry and paints and also has a beautiful mezzo singing voice. Staff members have been moved, hearing her sing her heart out to Bob Dylan and Eagles songs at the Portland music group and even in the hot tub–shower we have for our patients on the same floor as the clinic. If only her life-affirming tendencies could be kept active and in ascendance over her rigid, resigned, anxiety-ridden emotional mechanisms.

"You couldn't spare me a buck for a couple of cigarettes, could you, Doctor?"

"Tell you what," I say. "We'll go down to the corner and I'll get you a pack. Nicotine is harder to beat than cocaine."

Celia seems moved. "I can't believe you'd do that for me."

"Consider it a baby gift," I reply, "although it's not one I ever thought I'd give to a pregnant patient."

As I pay for the smokes and hand them to Celia, the salesclerk looks at me intently. "This is so great," Celia says. "I don't know how to thank you." Leaving the store, I hear the clerk echo her words in a low, mocking tone: " . . . so great. Don't know how to thank you." I turn around in the doorway and catch his expression. He is smirking. He knows exactly why, here on East Hastings, a reasonably well-dressed, middle-aged male would be buying a pack of cigarettes for a dishevelled young woman.

January 2005

Rick joins Celia for this office visit. They seem at ease, comfortable with each other.

"I can't keep up with this soap opera," I joke.

"I can't keep up with it either," says Rick, as Celia just hums to herself, a smile playing at the corners of her mouth.

She's been to the Oak Tree clinic. Her baby is growing, and the blood tests indicate that her immune system is in good shape. Although she's due in June, she'll soon be admitted for prenatal care, four months early, to Fir Square, the special unit at B.C. Women's Hospital for addicted mothers-to-be. Today she's here for a methadone script and, once more, requests some phone numbers of recovery homes. I provide both.

The two of them leave. Through the open door I see them stepping out the back entrance onto the sunlit porch, looking into each other's eyes, holding hands, walking calmly and peacefully.

It's the last time I'll see them together during the pregnancy.

January 2005: later in the month

One afternoon in late January Celia is voluntarily admitted to Detox, a first step toward entering a recovery program. By evening she's discharged herself. In the nightmare Celia lives out she is caught in a morass of pain, helpless, punished and utterly alone. She repeats her mantra: "I've never felt so abandoned in my whole fucking life." Her gaze, clouded and unfocused, is directed at the wall somewhere to the left of me. "How am I supposed to deal with it without a mountain of dope?"

Whatever answer I may have given to that question and whatever answers Celia struggled to give herself were not adequate. The remainder of her pregnancy can be summarized as brief episodes of hospitalization and escape; ongoing drug use; the frenzied pursuit of cocaine; and arrests. One arrest was for assault, when Celia spat on the nurses' desk in the admitting department. Of course, I recalled, she learned something about spitting in her childhood. But finally, she gave birth to a remarkably healthy infant girl who was easily weaned off her opiate dependence. In every other way the baby was fine. Unlike the opiates methadone and heroin, cocaine does not provoke dangerous physiological withdrawal reactions.

Rick, the father, was magnificent. Celia left hospital the day after delivery—her need to use overcame her determination to mother her newborn—but in a completely unprecedented break with policy, Rick was allowed to stay as an inpatient at the maternity ward. Greatly supported by hospital staff, he bottle-fed and nurtured the baby, bonding with her twenty-four hours a day for two weeks before taking her to his home. The nurses attending this father-infant pairing were astounded by his gentleness, love and devotion to his daughter.

Hostile and drug-addled, Celia was barred from visiting by court order. She was grief-stricken and infuriated. She believed she had been wilfully displaced in her newborn's affections. "It's my fucking baby," she screamed in my office, "my own little daughter. They've robbed me of the most precious thing in my life!"

December 2005

Rick drops in for a quick visit. I ask about his and Celia's child.

"She's in foster care right now," Rick says. "She came with me for a while, but then the home situation deteriorated because of the drug users in that house. They relapsed. And I relapsed with the alcohol, so they took the baby away. They got a child protection order." His shoulders tremble as he attempts to stifle his weeping. Then he looks up. "I saw her last month. I'm in the works of getting a new place for myself and I plan to take parenting groups and alcohol and drug counselling and everything. So far I'm doing pretty good."

January 2006

Celia is here for her monthly methadone script. The infant, now six months old, has been in a foster home. Celia is still dreaming about regaining custody of her daughter and of building a family life. But she's not capable of giving up cocaine.

"As much as you love your baby," I say to her yet again, "and as much as you want to love her, on crack you're not fit to be a mother. You yourself once said that you don't get the best of a person when there's an addiction. The child needs the best of you, needs you to be emotionally stable and present. Her sense of security depends on it. Her brain development thrives on it. You are no parent when you're controlled by your addiction. Don't you understand that?"

My voice is strained and cold; I can feel the tension in my throat. I'm angry with this woman. I'm trying force on her a truth that, as a workaholic doctor and in other ways, too, I tend to ignore in my own life.

Celia just stares her sullen, hard stare. I'm not telling her anything she hasn't told herself already.

—

As a human drama, this story does not have a happy finale—at least, not if we want our stories to have clear-cut beginnings and endings. Yet in the larger scheme, I choose to see a triumph in it: a demonstration of how life seeks life, how love yearns for love and how the divine spark that burns within us all continues to glow, even if it is unable to blaze into full, open flame.

What will happen to this infant, this being of infinite possibility? Given her dire beginnings, she may well lead a life of limitless sorrow—but she does not need to be defined by those beginnings. It depends on how well our world can nurture her. Perhaps our world will provide just enough loving refuge—enough "shelter from the storm" as Dylan has sung—so the baby, unlike her mother, can come to know herself as something other than her own worst enemy.

CHAPTER 7

—

Beethoven's Birth Room

L ittle do I know it, but Ralph and I are about to have an
engaging historical debate at this, our first meeting. A thin,
tall, middle-aged man with sagging cheeks, he limps into my
office, leaning on a cane. Much of his scalp is shaved, an inexpert
home salon job with uneven patches and razor nicks. A makeshift
mohawk of dyed jet-black hair adorns the crown of his head. The
Hitler moustache under his nose is no idle fashion statement as
our conversation will soon reveal.

The purpose of this visit is for me to gather his medical history,
prescribe medications and complete the welfare form that will enti-
tle Ralph to a monthly dietary supplement. His left ankle, injured in
an industrial accident, subsequently developed arthritis, and his
drug habit sabotaged proper medical treatment. His pain needs are
legitimate, and despite his substance dependence, I will not withhold morphine. In any case, stimulants are Ralph's drugs of choice,
cocaine being chief among them.

I'll soon come to know Ralph as one of the most intellectually
gifted people I have ever met. He is also profoundly sad—a lost
poetic soul with a hopeless, unrequited longing for human connection. Although his wide-ranging but undisciplined intellect is captive to whatever thought or emotion happens to possess it in the
moment, he also wields a sharp, self-mocking wit. He indulges in
highly aggressive and even violent behaviours when he's under the

influence of the uppers he uses. "I'm a schizo-affective, obsessive-compulsive, hyperactive paranoid delusional depressive with bipolar tendencies superimposed on antisocial personality disorder, and I also suffer from hallucinatory states triggered by drugs and especially by the hickey on my neck," he proclaims by way of introduction. "I've been given all those diagnoses by one psychiatrist or another," he goes on to explain. "I've seen many."

As for the dietary supplement, Ralph arrives with all the angles covered. "I need fresh meat, vegetables and fish, bottled water and vitamins. I have hepatitis C and diabetes."

The greater the number of medical conditions a person has, the greater the monetary support he receives. Addicts, who may spend a hundred dollars or more daily on their illicit drugs and who often miss health-related appointments, rarely fail to come in when it's time to have their papers filled out for the monthly twenty, forty or fifty bucks they receive for dietary support. I dutifully complete these forms, but with mixed feelings, because I know where the money will end up. There must be a better way, I think, to keep these malnourished people properly fed. To set up an alternative system we would need compassion, imagination and flexibility—qualities our social apparatus does not readily extend to the hardcore drug addict.

"Also, I need a low-sodium diet," says Ralph.

"Why?"

"I don't eat salt. I don't like salt. I always buy butter without salt . . . And what's dysphagia?" he asks, glancing at the list of supplement-approved conditions.

"From the Greek *phag,* to eat," I explain. "Dysphagia means difficulty swallowing."

"Oh, yeah, I have trouble swallowing. And I must have a gluten-free diet . . ."

"I can't do all this. I don't have any medical proof that you have diabetes, dysphagia or any salt- or gluten-related problem."

Ralph's rapid-fire, mumbled growl makes for a challenging listening experience. I can't make out the beginnings of his next phrase, which ends with "Rich American tourists laugh at us . . . American Jews . . ."

"American what?"

"American Jews."

I'm surprised at this turn in the conversation.

"What about them?"

"They laugh at us. They're so fuckin' malicious . . . eating the whole fuckin' world."

"American Jews are? . . . You're talking to a Canadian Jew."

"Hungarian Jew, I heard." Ralph's cloudy eyes emit a malevolent glimmer, and his glum frown turns into a smirk.

"Canadian and Hungarian Jew," I concede.

"Hungarian Jew," Ralph insists. "*Arbeit macht frei* . . . Heh, heh . . . do you remember what that means?"*

"Yes. You think that's funny?"

"Of course not."

"Do you know that my grandparents were killed in Auschwitz under that sign? My grandfather was a doctor. . . ."

"He starved the Germans to death," says Ralph as if stating an incontrovertible fact.

That ought to be my cue to end the exchange. I'm drawn in, however, by my determination to preserve my professional *sangfroid* and the therapeutic contact with the patient. Moreover, I'm curious to know just what this man is all about.

"My grandfather was a physician in Slovakia. How did he starve the Germans to death?"

Ralph's placid pseudo-rationality evaporates in a nanosecond. His sallow cheeks quiver with anger, his voice rises and the velocity of his speech accelerates with every word. "The Jews had all the gold, they took all the oil paintings . . . they took all the art . . . they were the police officers, judges, lawyers . . . and they starved the German people to fucking death. That Jew Stalin slaughtered 90 million Germans . . . the invasion of our fuckin' country . . . being fuckin' paralyzed, starved to death. You know that as well as I do. I got no remorse for you . . . I got no grief for you."

If as a Jew and infant survivor of genocide I can receive these ravings calmly, it's because I know they're not about me or my grand parents or even about World War II or Nazis and Jews. Ralph is

---

* *Arbeit macht frei* ("Work liberates") appeared on signs on the gates of Nazi concentration camps, including Auschwitz.

showcasing the terrible unrest of his soul. The suffering Germans and rapacious Jews in his narrative are projections of his own phantoms. The erratic mishmash he calls history reflects his inner chaos, confusion and fear. "I starved in Germany as a kid and I fuckin' starved in this country, too . . . Came here in 1961." (Ralph arrived as a teenager.) "Fuck Canadians. I hate Canadians."

It's time to leave ethnic relationships and history behind. "Okay," I say. "Let's see how the morphine works for you."

"How many do I have?"

"Four or five days' worth. Then I'll need to see you again."

"I hate going to the doctor's office all the time. I hate the doctor's office. It's a waste of time."

"I hate the gas station, too," I assure him, "but I go; otherwise, I run out of gasoline."

Ralph is conciliatory. "*Danke, mein Herr* . . . no hard feelings."

"No," I say.

We exchange cordial *auf Wiedersehens* to end this, our first encounter. There are many more to follow, several ending with Ralph hoisting the Nazi salute. Enraged when I refuse his demand for this or that drug, he screams, "*Heil Hitler!*" or "*Arbeit macht frei,*" or the ever-endearing "*Schmutzige Jude*—dirty Jew." Not that I have endless tolerance for Nazi slogans projected at me in idiomatic German. Generally I rise when the rant begins and open the door to signal the end of the visit. Ralph usually takes the hint, but on one occasion I threaten to call the cops if he doesn't expeditiously remove himself from my office.

—

The German Ralph speaks is not always full of hate-filled invective. He declaims staccato paragraphs of fluent German or lines from the *Iliad* in what sounds plausibly like ancient Greek. The second time we meet, he erupts in a storm of German recitation; the only word I recognize is "Zarathustra." "Nietzsche," he explains. "When Zarathustra was thirty years old he left his home and the lake of his home and went into the mountains. . . ."

These lines from Nietzsche roll rapidly off his tongue, as do quotations from other classics of his native country's literature. It's impossible to know how much truth there is in his idiosyncratic anecdotes, but his knowledge of culture is impressive—all the more so, since it seems largely self-acquired. His claims to have completed college here or there strike me as dubious. Diploma or none, he is well read.

"I love Dostoevsky," he informs me one day. I decide to test him.

"Perhaps my favourite author," I say. "What have you read by him?"

"Oh," says Ralph, nonchalantly rattling off several titles of the Russian author's novels and short stories: "*The Possessed, Crime and Punishment, The Gambler*—I liked that one especially, you know, being an addict—*Notes from the Underground* . . . Never got through *The Brothers Karamazov*. Too long."

Another time he tells me about an adventure he had as a youth, when he was back in Germany on a visit.

"I took this girl into Beethoven's *Geburtszimmer.*"

I recall my rudimentary childhood German—*geboren*, to be born, *Zimmer*, room. "Beethoven's birth room?"

"I took some wine and cheese and some salami and some marijuana. Yes, the room he was born in. We broke in, I jimmied the lock, took this girl up and I played his piano and had a great time."

"Ha," I say, raising a skeptical eyebrow. "What city was that in?" Another test.

"Bonn."

"Yes, Beethoven was born in Bonn," I murmur.

Ralph, a shade cocaine-manic, segues right into an entirely unexpected performance.

"Here's a poem I wrote you might like. It's called 'Prelude.'" His staccato recital is delivered in a low, grainy voice at a pace so fast that the listener is barely aware of his taking any breaths from beginning to end. The poem is composed of rhyming couplets in a steady pentameter. It speaks of loneliness, loss, fatalism.

"You wrote that?"

"Yes. I've written five hundred pages of poems. It was my life. Where they are now, I don't know. I was homeless for five years. I left my poems in a hostel where I stayed for a week. They wanted a hundred dollars to get my stuff back, but I couldn't afford it. Maybe it was auctioned off, maybe the security guard got it, maybe it went into the garbage. I don't know. I just remember a few pieces. It's all gone. I've lost everything."

Ralph is uncharacteristically pensive for a moment. Suddenly, his face lights up. "You'll recognize this," he says and declaims in rapidly spoken, rhyming German. Never fluent in the language, I'm unable to understand any of it, but I make a happy guess. "That sounds more like Goethe than Goebbels."

"It is," Ralph confirms triumphantly. "The final eight lines of *Faust*." Without missing a beat he recites in English:

> *All things transitory*
> *Are but a parable,*
> *Earth's insufficiency*
> *Here finds fulfillment.*
>
> *The ineffable*
> *Wins life through love.*
> *The eternal feminine*
> *Leads us above.*

He presents this poem without his customary hasty intensity; his voice is soft and gentle.

At home that evening I lift *Faust*, Part II, off the bookshelf and turn to the last page. There it is: Goethe's paean to spiritual enlightenment, the blessed union of the human spirit with the feminine principle, with divine love. Goethe, like Dante in *The Divine Comedy*, represents divine love as a feminine quality. I find Ralph's translation of Goethe, whether it's his own or memorized, more moving than the version I have in my hands.

As I read the great German's poet's verses in my comfortable home in an upscale, leafy Vancouver neighbourhood, I can't help thinking that at this very same moment Ralph, supported by his cane, is holding vigil somewhere in the dusky and dirty Hastings Street evening, hustling for his next hit of cocaine. And in his heart he wants beauty no less than I, and no less than I, needs love.

If I understand him well, above everything Ralph aches for unity with the eternal feminine *caritas*—blessed, soul-saving divine love. *Divine* here refers not to a supernatural deity above us but to the immortal essence of existence that lives in us, through us, beyond us. Religions may identify it with a god belief, but a search for the eternal extends far beyond formal religious concepts.

One consequence of spiritual deprivation is addiction, and not only to drugs. At conferences devoted to science-based addiction medicine, it is more and more common to hear presentations on the spiritual aspect of addictions and their treatment. The object, form and severity of addictions are shaped by many influences—social, political and economic status, personal and family history, physio-logical and genetic predispositions—but at the core of all addictions there lies a spiritual void. In the case of Serena, the Native woman from Kelowna, that void was generated by the unbearable abuse she suffered as a child—a theme I'll return to later. But for now, suffice it to say that if I hadn't already sensed Ralph's secret God-thirst from his Goethe recital, Ralph would, a few months hence, confirm it in so many words. In his soul of souls he longs to connect with the very same feminine quality within himself that his bellicosity and unbridled aggression trample so viciously underfoot.

Soon afterwards, perhaps at the very next visit, we are back to the *Arbeit macht frei*s, the *schmutzige Jude*s, the *Heil Hitler*s. "Stick your morphine up your ass," Ralph yells in his sandpaper voice. "Give me Ritalin. Give me cocaine. Give me Xylocaine!" He might as well be saying, "Give me liberty or give me death." Drugs are the only freedom he knows.

—

Blood-borne bacterial infections are frequent complications of drug use, especially given the poor hygienic state of many Downtown Eastside addicts. Last year Ralph was hospitalized, requiring two months of high-powered intravenous antibiotics to clear a life-threatening sepsis.

Toward the end of his treatment I visit him in his room on one of the medical wards of Vancouver Hospital. There I find a person very different from the enraged, hostile pseudo-Nazi who frequents my office. He's on his back, reclining on the half-elevated hospital bed, covered with a white sheet up to his midriff. His scrawny chest and upper limbs are bare. His salt-and-pepper hair is now evenly cut, forming a short tonsure above his shaven temples. He waves his left arm at me in greeting.

We begin with his medical status and post-discharge plans. My hope is to help him find housing away from the drug scene. Ralph expresses ambivalence at first but finally agrees that it would be a good idea to stay away from the Downtown Eastside.

"I'm glad you came out," he tells me. "Daniel came, too. We had a good conversation." At that time my son Daniel was employed as a mental health worker at the Portland Hotel. A musician and song-writer, he visited Ralph in hospital, and the two taped nearly an hour of Bob Dylan songs together. The recording consists mostly of Daniel strumming and picking along to Ralph's raw, coarse semi-baritone. As a singer, Ralph has a notably shaky grip on melody, but he has a feel for the emotional resonance of Dylan's lyrics and music.

"I apologized for what I said to Daniel and I apologize to you, for the *Arbeit macht frei* crap."

"I'm curious. What's that all about for you?

"It's just supremacy. I don't believe it anyway. No race is supreme. All people are supreme to God, or nobody is . . . It doesn't matter anyway. It's just stuff that goes through a person's mind. I grew up affected by National Socialism, as you did also, only you grew up on the other side of the table. It was an unfortunate situation. I apologize for everything I said against you and your son. I really wish to be out of here soon so Daniel and I can make more music."

"You know, what concerns me most is that it isolates you. I guess the way you learned to get along in the world is to be overly hostile."

"I guess that's the way it is." When Ralph becomes emotionally agitated, as he is now, the skin over his forearm muscles undulates like a bag of rolling marbles. "'Cause people treated me badly and . . . and you learn to treat them badly back. It's one of the ways. . . . It's not the only way. . . ."

"It's pretty common," I say. "And sometimes I can be pretty arrogant myself."

"Great. All I really want . . . It was all about drugs. I didn't want morphine . . . I wanted Xylocaine. That would have settled all my problems . . . There'd be nothing I'd be thirsting for, nothing I'd be in quest of. It would have solved everything."

Ralph embarks on a highly intricate explanation of how Xylocaine, a local anaesthetic, is prepared for inhalation by mixing it with baking soda and distilled water. The cooked product is breathed in through a piece of Brillo. He is very particular about the technique of inhalation, which, according to him, must end with the substance being slowly blown out through the nose. I listen in fascination to this extraordinary lecture in applied psychopharmacology.

"All these people on Hastings Street and Pender Street and all up and down the Downtown Eastside; they all blow it out their mouth. Ridiculous. It doesn't do anything. To metabolize properly it has to go through your smell glands to the brain. When it goes to the brain, it metabolizes and it freezes the little capillaries that go to the brain cells . . ."

"What do you feel when you do it?"

"It takes away my pain, my anxiety. It takes away my frustration. It gives me the pure essence of the Homunculus . . . you know, the Homunculus in *Faust*."

In Goethe's epic drama the Homunculus is a little being of fire conceived in a laboratory flask. He is a masculine figure, who voluntarily unites with the vast Ocean, the divine feminine aspect of the soul. According to mystical traditions of all faiths and philosophies, without such ego-annihilating submission it is impossible to attain spiritual enlightenment, "the peace of God, which passeth all understanding." Ralph yearns for nothing less.

"The Homunculus," he continues, "is the character that represents all I would have been, had it been possible for me to be that way. But it's not how I turned out. So now I use Xylocaine when I can get it or cocaine when I can't."

Ralph hopes to inhale peaceful consciousness through a glass pipe. I cannot be the Homunculus, he says, so I must be an addict.

"How long does that effect last?" I ask.

"Five minutes. It shouldn't have to cost forty bucks just to kill the pain for five minutes. And for five minutes of respite I slave my guts out up and down Hastings Street, up and down, talking to my buddies, extorting some money out of them. 'Look buddy, you've got to pay up some cash because if you don't, I'm going to lay a beating on you with my cane.'"

Under the sheet Ralph's belly, a little fuller after two months of rest and hospital fare, shakes with mirth as he recounts his outlandish bandy-legged banditry. "They laugh, and they lay some coin on me. I've got a lot of friends. And I beg, too. But I have to be out there hustling for hours and hours just to kill the pain for five minutes."

"So you work for hours to get five minutes' relief."

"Yes, and then I go out again, and go out again and again."

"What's the pain you're trying to kill?"

"Some of it physical, some of it emotional. Physical for sure. If I had some cocaine, I'd be out of this bed and outside smoking a cigarette right now."

I accept that Ralph finds some evanescent benefit from his substance use, and I tell him so. But does he not recognize the negative impact on his life? Here he is, two months in hospital, admitted within an inch of dying, to say nothing of his run-ins with the law and multiple other miseries.

"All that time and energy you have to spend chasing those five minutes—is it worth it? Let's face it, the way you're talking to me now is very different from the way you present yourself when you're downtown and using—miserable, unhappy and hostile. You provoke people's hostility toward you. Maybe it's not your intention, but that's what happens. It creates a huge negative impact. Is it worth it for those five minutes?

In his present drug-free state and benign mood Ralph puts up no argument. "I understand what you say and I agree one hundred per cent. I've approached things in an obtuse manner . . ."

"I wouldn't even call it obtuse," I reply. "I think you've approached things the way you've learned. My guess is that from a very early age, the world hasn't treated you very well. What happened to you? What made you so defensive?"

"I don't know . . . My father. My father is a mean, ugly person, and I hate his guts." Ralph spits out the words. Under the sheet his legs tremble violently. "If there is one man in this world I loathe, it's that man who had to be . . . *mein Vater*. Ah, it doesn't matter. He's an old man now and he can't pay for his crimes any more than he already has. He's paid for them a thousand times over."

"I think everybody does."

"I know that," Ralph growls. "I've paid for my crimes. Look at me. I can't even walk without this stupid stick. I want to fly and I'm stuck on the ground because . . . I'll tell you sometime . . ."

Another conversation then starts up between us. Ralph articulates a clever, intuitive and astute critique of workaday human existence and of our society's obsession with goals, the essence of which, he feels, varies little from his own pursuit of drugs. I see an uncomfortable truth in his analysis, no matter how incomplete a truth it is.

We part on good terms. "I'd love it if Daniel came back," Ralph tells me, "and I hope he brings a video recorder. Daniel could do an intro for a couple of songs and accompany me—I'm the better singer, you know. We could do more Dylan or 'Homeward Bound' by Simon and Garfunkel. They're all Jewish people. That's where my anti-Semitism disappeared into nothingness, because many of the greatest poetical minds were Jewish: Bob Dylan, Paul Simon, John Lennon—if it wasn't for these people, the world would be a far worse place."

I reluctantly inform him that John Lennon wasn't Jewish.

—

The plans for a new domicile didn't materialize. Shortly after our civilized Vancouver Hospital exchange, Ralph resumed his life in the Downtown Eastside. With the drugs back in his system, he has reverted to the volatile, embittered persona from which he emerges only fitfully. He visited my office not long ago to recite more poetry.

"Here's one you'll like," he says and starts in on his quick, mechanical drone.

I find myself loving the sordid honesty of Ralph's verses. The internal rhymes he takes care to include in every couplet reinforce the airtight and suffocating logic of the speaker's world: everything fits together: the futile search for companionship, sexual frustration, alienation, escape into drugs, grief, bathos, cynicism.

"Do you still write?" I ask.

"No." He waves a resigned hand across his face. "I haven't done it for a long time. Years, years. I've written everything I wanted to write. Every thought, every emotion I had, I wrote in poetry."

I glance at my watch, aware of the crowd of patients outside my office. "Wait," Ralph says quickly, "I have one more poem for you. It's called . . ." He searches his mind for the title, scratching his newly bald crown. His fingernails are lacquered with dark, purplish blue nail polish. Below the hem of his soiled T-shirt his forearm muscles are doing an agitated, serpentine dance.

"Oh, yes, it's called 'Winter Solstice.'" Again, Ralph recites in his inimitable, fast-drawl croak. He fixes his gaze directly at me, as if insisting on being heard. The poem ends with an eagle falling out of the sky, dead in mid-flight. I recall what Ralph said in hospital: "I want to fly and I'm stuck on the ground."

Two days later he returns, with unrealistic demands for medications and for assistance with food and housing I am in no position to provide. Out pours the rage, expressed with Ralph's uncensored Teutonic venom. "And there'll be some art for you later," he yells, stomping furiously out of the office into the waiting area, where his fellow addicts shake their heads in puzzlement and disapproval. "Can't be easy for you sometimes, working here," says my next patient, already walking in the door.

As I leave that afternoon, one of the Portland housekeeping staff, equipped with a bucket of soapy hot water and a scrub sponge, is washing a large, crudely drawn black swastika off the wall just beside the first-floor exit.

—

CHAPTER 8

There's Got to Be Some Light

In writing about a drug ghetto in a desolate corner of the realm of hungry ghosts, it's difficult to convey the grace that we witness—we who have the privilege of working down here: the courage, the human connection, the tenacious struggle for existence and even for dignity. The misery is extraordinary in the drug gulag, but so is the humanity.

Primo Levi, the insightful and infinitely compassionate chronicler of Auschwitz, called *moments of reprieve* those unexpected times when a person's "compressed identity" emerges and asserts its uniqueness even amid the torments of a man-made inferno. In the Downtown Eastside there are many moments of reprieve, moments when the truth of a person arises and insists on being recognized despite the sordid past or grim present.

—

Josh has been living at the Portland Hotel for about two years. He's a powerfully built young man with straight bearing, blue eyes, regular features, a blond beard and long hair to match. Because of his mental instability and drug use, his innate charm and sweetness are often lost on others. His intuition locks onto people's vulnerabilities with radar precision; his intelligence gives his language a knife edge that cuts deep. On a Friday morning, as I was preparing to incise and drain a large abscess on his leg, Josh spoke one disparaging word too many. It was not a good day—I was irritable and fatigued. My reaction was unrestrained and aggressive—to say that I lost it would be understatement.

That afternoon, ashamed, I trudged upstairs to Josh's room to make amends. As he listened to my apology, he looked at me in his customary intent and unblinking way, but with kindness in his eyes. Then, this man whose hostility causes others to cower in his presence and whose rampant, drug-fuelled paranoia can see ill will everywhere, said, "Thank you, but I meant to apologize to you. I see what it's like for you. You visited me in hospital last week and you were calm and attentive, an image of the good doctor. It must be hard for you in this place, all the negative energy down here and some of it comes from me—I see you absorb it, and I wonder how you hold it and still do your job. You're human, and something has to give sometime."

"People down here show a lot of insight," says Kim Markel, the vivacious, spike-haired Portland nurse, "but I still find it surprising when they express care about us. You think they're too into their head trips and drug trips and diseases to notice anything. Like, when I was having a couple of bad months in my personal life, I remember Larry coming up, and he's like 'Something's wrong with you. I can tell.' [Larry, a narcotic and cocaine addict, has lymphoma that could have been eradicated if his drug use hadn't sabotaged treatment. Now he's beyond cure.] 'You know what, Larry?' I said. "You're right. Something *is* wrong with me, and I'm working on that.' And he's like 'Okay . . . do you want to go out for a beer?' I said no, but I was touched. Despite their troubles, they pay enough attention that they actually know when we're having a hard time of it."

Kim combines professional efficiency with humour, down-to-earth presence and a refreshing openness to the novel and different. She is also kind. She witnessed my incident with Josh and gently massaged my shoulders after Josh left the examination room.

Josh had been homeless for three years before he moved into the Portland. His paranoia, violent outbreaks and drug addiction were so out of control that he couldn't be housed anywhere. Without the harm reduction facilities administered by the Portland Hotel Society and other organizations, many addicts and mentally ill people in the Downtown Eastside would be street nomads or, at best, migrants with five or six different addresses a year, being shunted from one dingy establishment to another. There are hundreds of homeless in the neighbourhood. As the 2010 Winter Olympics draw near, the city is predicting the numbers will rise—a prospect that some policymakers seem to regard more as a potential embarrassment than as a humanitarian crisis.

"When Josh first came, I couldn't even get into his room," Kim recalls. "Now, every time I go by, he wants me in to show me the mad space he lives in, and how he's cleaning it up. You know, he took me out last week for pizza. He had to buy me pizza. I was saying, 'No, no, I'll buy you lunch. I have more money.' He was adamant; this was his treat. It was the grossest pizza I've ever had," Kim laughs. "I had every bite and I was like 'Mmmm, thanks, man.' He still refuses his medications, and he's never going to be stable, but he's much more approachable."

—

The moments of reprieve at the Portland come not when we aim for dramatic achievements—helping someone kick addiction or curing a disease—but when clients allow us to reach them, when they permit even a slight opening in the hard, prickly shells they've built to protect themselves. For that to happen, they must first sense our commitment to accepting them for who they are. That is the essence of harm reduction, but it's also the essence of any healing or nurturing relationship. In his book *On Becoming a Person,* the great American psychologist Carl Rogers described a warm, caring attitude, which he called *unconditional positive regard* because, he said, "it has no conditions of worth attached to it." This is a caring, wrote Rogers, "[that] is not possessive, [that] demands no personal gratification. It is an atmosphere [that] simply demonstrates I care; not I care for you if you behave thus and so."[1]

Unconditional acceptance of each other is one of the greatest challenges we humans face. Few of us have experienced it consistently; the addict has never experienced it—least of all from himself. "What works for me," says Kim Markel, "is if I practise not looking for the big, shining success but appreciating the small: someone coming in for their appointment who doesn't usually come in . . . that's actually pretty amazing. At the Washington Hotel this client with a chronic ulcer on his shin finally let me look at his legs this week, after me harassing him for six months to have a peek. That's great, I think. I try not to measure things as good or bad, just to look at things from the client's point of view. 'Okay, you went to Detox for two days . . . was that a good thing for you?' Not, 'How come you didn't stay longer?' I try to take my own value system out of it and look at the value something has for them. Even when people are at their worst, feeling really down and out, you can still have those moments with them. So I try to look on every day as a little bit of success."

Kim had a very difficult time around Celia's pregnancy, as did many others among the female staff. "It was horrible to see," recalls Susan Craigie, Health Coordinator at the Portland. "Celia was beaten up in the street the day before she delivered her baby. There she was on the sidewalk, two black eyes and a bleeding nose, screaming 'The Portland won't give me taxi money to get to the hospital!' I offered to drive her. She insisted I give her ten bucks first so she could shoot up. I refused, of course, but my heart broke."

The three of us—Susan, Kim and I—are chatting in my office on a rainy November morning. It's "Welfare Wednesday," the second-to-last Wednesday of the month, when income assistance cheques are issued. In the drug ghetto it's Mardi Gras time. The office is quiet and will be until the money runs out on Thursday and Friday—and then a large group of hung-over, drug-withdrawn patients will descend upon the place, complaining, demanding and picking fights with each other. "Celia and her baby," says Kim, pursing her lips sadly. "One of the sweetest moments I've ever experienced was when I heard her singing one day. I was up on her floor doing my thing and she was having a shower. She began to sing. It was an awful country song, something I'd never listen to. But I had to stand still and listen. Celia's voice has a lot of purity in it. A pure, gentle voice. She was just belting it out. It seemed so clear to me all at once—the tone and the innocence behind it, that's the real Celia. She kept on singing and singing for fifteen or twenty minutes. It reminded me that there are all these different components to the people we work with. On a day-to-day basis we can really forget that.

"It also gave me this happy feeling that was tinged with a little bit of sadness. Her life could have been so different, I thought. I try not to have such thoughts in my day-to-day work . . . I try to take people as they are at any moment and support them that way. Not judge them or think of an alternative reality they could have, because we could all have alternative realities. I don't focus on my own 'What ifs' much, so I try not to focus on other people's. Only . . . there was this split second when I had two images in my brain: Celia at the worst moments I've seen her and then Celia singing to her kids, living on a farm somewhere with her family . . . And then I dropped both images and just listened to that lovely voice peacefully drifting towards me."

—

To Whom It May Concern:
You do not know me, although the name on the envelope might ring a Bell. I am the individual who took your son's life . . . on the 14ᵗʰ of May, 1994.

Remy's voice is tremulous with excitement or, perhaps, anxiety. He's a short, slender man with a pallid countenance peppered with grey stubbles to match his prematurely greying hair. He's standing in front of the open Hastings Street window. Over the hum of traffic that vibrates into the room, he reads the words from a crumpled and stained piece of foolscap. "Man," he says, "you don't know what this means to me, that I wrote this and that I can read it to you. Mind you, I don't know if I'll ever send it."

It took a Ritalin prescription to help Remy unburden his mind. He has severe Attention Deficit Hyperactivity Disorder (ADHD).

Never diagnosed before, he was dumbfounded when I told him about the lifelong patterns of physical restlessness, mental disorganization and impulse-regulation deficiencies that characterize the condition. "That's me all over," he kept repeating, hitting his forehead with his palm again and again. "How did you know that much about me? That's been me since I was ankle high to a flea!"

Remy's conversation is always an exercise in circumlocution. He launches into tirades on any topic, not recalling what he already said or where he was intending to go. He meanders, becoming snagged on the brambles of one thought, getting lost in the bushes of the next. He doesn't know how to stop the flow of words. Some authorities see ADHD as an inherited neurophysiological dysfunction, but in my view such psychological agitation has a deeper source. Remy's wandering speech patterns are attempts to escape an agonizing discomfort with his own self.

Now thirty-five, Remy has been an addict since his teenage years. His first drug of choice was cocaine. The heroin habit he acquired in prison is managed successfully with methadone, but he's rarely been off cocaine since his discharge. After I diagnosed his ADHD, he agreed to stay away from it—at least temporarily, so we could give him a trial of methylphenidate, better known by the trade name Ritalin.

He was astonished the first day he took this medication. "I'm calm," he reported. "My mind isn't going off like a machine gun. I'm thinking instead of just spinning. It's not fucking going sixty different miles an hour, in twenty different directions. I'm going, 'Hang on, I've gotta do one thing at a time here. Just let's slow down here.'"

A few days later, free from the agitating effects of cocaine and with his brain's hyperactivity soothed by methylphenidate, Remy returns to my office in a reflective frame of mind. "There's something I need to talk to you about."

I wait. Remy says nothing for a long time. Then: "I out and out fucking stabbed a guy once. I was up for four days, cocaine. I started drinking booze; I was a fucking mess. I was just the worst thing— I was a nightmare waiting to happen.

"I was in jail almost ten years. Ten years. All because of drugs. Every day I think about it. Every day, man. Every day . . . I won't tell it to other people. I'll just slough it off like it doesn't mean something. But it does mean something . . . I took some guy's life who did not deserve to die. 'Cause I was all fucked up on cocaine, and pills, and fucking booze . . . ."

Nothing in medical training prepares you to hear an admission like this. Remy was in my office seeking absolution as surely as if he were a penitent in a confession booth and I, a cassock-garbed priest.

"We all have moments in our lives that we wish we could relive . . . and do over again," I say. "But for you, this must be a big one."

"You know, I remember one thing my mom said to me. What it would take to straighten me out, she said, is if I ever began to listen to my heart. And I'm beginning to. That thing that I did, that terrible thing, is the only thing I have. That's reality, my reality. And I'm accepting it now."

"Can you forgive yourself?"

"Yeah, I can. I don't know how, but I can forgive myself. His family will never forgive me, though. They want to kill me. But myself, yeah, I will not let it bring me down. I've got to move on with my life. I mean, it'll always be there, but I've got to move on and stay positive and stay focused on living. I have to! I don't know if that's right or wrong, but I can't dwell in the past and let it bring me down. Otherwise, I'm fucked."

"Have you ever communicated with the family?"

"No. They're very, very prejudiced against white people. It was a Native guy I killed, and they're very, very prejudiced . . . ."

I suppress my urge to point out that a family's grief and anger or even vengeful feelings in such circumstances do not necessarily imply racial bigotry.

"Forgiveness is an important concept in the Native community."

"Yeah, not for this one. I know . . . That's why I left Saskatchewan. They're looking for me."

"Let me suggest something to you."

"You mean, write a letter to myself, to them? I know exactly what you're going to say!"

"That *is* what I was going to say. You see, you're listening to your heart."

"It makes sense, doesn't it," says Remy, enthused. "I could try that, just to see how it would make me feel. I'll bring it to you and you read it. We'll talk about it. . . . I'll take my medications. I like to write first thing in the morning. I've been thinking about it—as soon as you mentioned it, I knew what you were going to suggest. This might help clear my mind a little more. I think about it every day . . . I'm not into taking people's lives. You know, this happened eleven years ago." I've often seen Remy hyper but never so charged with purpose.

Later the same week, Remy is back in my office reading his composition, simultaneously nervous and triumphant. His rabbit eyes dart about, skipping from the paper he grasps in both hands to my face, constantly gauging my reaction. As he speaks, he sways, shifting his weight back and forth from one foot to the other.

To Whom It May Concern:
You do not know me, although the name on the envelope might ring a Bell. I am the individual who took your son's life . . . on the 14th of May, 1994.

The reason I'm writing this letter to you is just to let you know that there is not a day that has gone past since that tragic night took place, when I do not think of what I have done!!

I do not expect forgiveness on the Part of the family. But I feel I must write this to you to let you know how very sorry I am that it happened and that how wrong I was.

This has been eating away at me from 11 years now and I really don't think that the horrendous disregard and disrespect I have brought upon and done to your Son at such a young age by ending his life at 19 will ever leave my mind.

I'm hoping that the hatred you might have had for me is not as strong as it was in 1994! But if so I understand and can hold no ill feelings towards you or your Family for this.

I am truly and totally sorry for what I have done. I no longer drink alcohol, pop pills like there's no tomorrow. I don't do heroin anymore and I have finally given up cocaine, which is at the root of all evil.

Basically I'm writing to say I'm so very sorry for what I've done to you and your family and I hope one day you will find Peace.

Remy never did mail the letter. He gave it to me as a keepsake. I wish I could report that he successfully kept the cocaine monkey off his back. He has been unable to do that and, as a consequence, I had to discontinue his methylphenidate prescription. His intentions foundered when, shortly afterwards, he entered into a hopelessly overwrought relationship with a mentally unstable woman even more dependent on cocaine than he was.

There is in Remy an unquenchable optimism and a vital sense of humour. The light of possibility continues to glimmer in him, if only uncertainly. It's a spark, I'm convinced, that will never be extinguished. His confession and his letter, unsent though it remains, eased his burden. His contrition was deeply felt, his relief palpable. Although not free of cocaine, he says he's using much less than in the past. I believe him. Perhaps another conversation, another moment of contact with me or with someone else, will help him move forward again.*

—

"My mother calls me Canada's most famous junkie," says Dean Wilson sardonically. "I probably am." Dean is a well-known figure at political events and international conferences about drug addiction. One of the founders of VANDU, the Vancouver Area Network of Drug Users, he has been a tenacious and articulate advocate of decriminalization and harm reduction policies, a prime mover in the establishment of the pioneering Supervised Injection Site (also known colloquially as the Safe Injection Site). A Senate committee on addictions hailed his presentation as one of the most inspirational they had heard.

Dean is a thin, edgy figure with brimming-over energy that keeps him physically in motion even when he's sitting or standing. He speaks rapidly, leaping from one topic to another, interrupting himself only to chuckle at his own witticisms. He's fifty years old, but like many people with ADD, looks younger than his age. He

* As I do final revisions on the manuscript in October 2007, I'm happy to note that Remy has for the past two months stayed clear of cocaine and is doing well on methylphenidate.

knows I've also been diagnosed with Attention Deficit Disorder and laughs uproariously when I tell him my theory that we ADD folk look young because all the time we spend tuning out doesn't add to our years. Dean's fame spread after the international showing of filmmaker Nettie Wild's award-winning documentary *Fix: The Story of an Addicted City*. In the opening scene Dean, in business clothing, walks briskly down Hastings and tells how he once received a prize from IBM for selling more personal computers than any other salesperson in Canada. In the next scene, bare from the waist up, he displays his tattoo-covered torso and arms as he injects himself with pure heroin. "Sometime before this video's over, I will be straight," he promises the camera.

That hasn't happened. Dean has used: heroin intermittently and cocaine more consistently. He is on methadone. Occasionally he's tried to scam me—and at times he's likely succeeded in doing so—but now he's very direct in acknowledging his substance intake. "It's taken me a while to trust you," he says, "but I love it that when I'm fucking up I can tell you that I'm fucking up." (A statement which, for all I know, may be another scam.) More recently he's been clean of all injection drugs for a few months and is feeling optimistic and energized. "Tune in again next time for another exciting episode," he jokes about his ongoing battle.

Dean's one-room apartment at the Sunrise Hotel is a far cry from the expensive home he used to own in South Vancouver, when he was a single father bringing up his three children and earning hundreds of thousands of dollars a year. "I had a computer business," he says, "selling microcomputers back when they were $40,000 apiece. I would use my heroin in the morning and later at night. I did that for twelve years. Every second weekend, the kids would go see their mother. As soon as they were on that bus, I would shut the drapes, lock the doors and get totally wasted—until Sunday, when they came back. And then I would do the straight, blue-suit-and-tie thing and do the weekends with baseball and soccer for the next two weeks—just dying, just dying until I could close that door again and get high. It became harder and harder and harder to keep up the façade. I was lying to everybody, including myself. When I fell down, I really fell down. My wife [formerly a heavy drug user] finally straightened out, and the kids left to live with her. I immediately got back into cocaine. I hadn't used cocaine in thirteen years. . . . I blew $180,000 in six months, and before I knew it, I was living down here in the Cobalt Hotel."*

Despite silver-spoon early years in a wealthy adoptive family and a successful business life, Dean spent six years in prison for drug-related crimes. "What's the worst thing you've ever done?" I ask. Dean winces as he tells me about an incident in jail that still revolts him for its cruelty and physical sordidness—nothing would be served by repeating it here. "You're only the second person I've ever told this," he says. His long-time partner, Ann, was the first. "I saw and did some terrible things in jail. I could never talk about it. Ann finally told me to write it up. I wrote on for fifteen pages, couldn't stop. Three months later, she asked me to read it to her. I read it out: I finally voiced it. I turned and looked at her and said, 'You did it! You got it out of me.' It made it a lot easier. And then I burned those pages.

"As I purged that shit, I realized I had to bring light back into my life. Otherwise, all the horror I'd seen and done would have been for nothing. There's got to be some light. I believe there is a truth for lack of another word, I'll use 'spiritual' truth. It's not God or this or that, but the fact is, the world is good, it all equals up to good, and I want that goodness in me. . . .

"That's why I'm so into this activism part. The whole idea behind VANDU was to trust the untrustworthy, help the helpless. Then we became very political. We've taken on governments, changed politics in this city. I've led senators on a walkabout of this neighbourhood, showing them it's more than just drugs—it's a community. That so many political leaders now support harm reduction, that's our doing." Whether or not Dean's organization can take all the credit for this small but significant shift in the political wind, it's an initiative to be proud of.

"Former mayor Philip Owen at one point said all the addicts should be sent to the army base at Chilliwack. Two years later, he was advocating for the SIS [Supervised Injection Site]. We took

* The Cobalt is another Downtown Eastside residence, not under the Portland umbrella.

over City Hall and walked in with a coffin, to symbolize all the overdose deaths. Councillors said, 'Get them out of here.' I said, 'I just
need five minutes.' Mayor Owen gave us five minutes, and I have to
hand it to him—he listened to us. Now he's internationally known
for his leadership in harm reduction, and as a city, Vancouver is
known for that. And who were we? Just a bunch of junkies.

"The little bits of light in this community are not publicized
enough," Dean goes on. In his hotel there are three or four older
people. If Dean doesn't see them for twenty-four hours, he does a
room check. Others, he says, will look out for him. Many of the sex
trade workers are also part of a buddy system: if one doesn't show at
the end of the day, the buddy will set things in motion to find her.
"In the days when I used to live in the West End, I'd get into the
elevator and never look at anyone, just stare at the floor or the ceiling or the numbers as they lit up one after another. I didn't know
my neighbours. In my building I know everybody, and down here
it's like that everywhere."

In his hyperkinetic way, which makes him look as if he's jogging
even when he's sitting still, Dean continues. "Cynicism is rife down
here, but at the same time most of us want to see that we're looking
after each other. We have the feeling that no one else is going to
look after us—for most people down here, no one ever has—and so
we have to care for each other. It's done at the most basic level—
just, 'How are you, how are you getting along?' And then you leave
the person alone. We somehow balance all the ripping each other
off with the caring. There's a lot of warmth, a lot of support."

Dean knows that isolation is in the very nature of addiction.
Psychological isolation tips people into addiction in the first place,
and addiction keeps them isolated because it sets a higher value on
their motivations and behaviours around the drug than on anything
else—even human contact. "Rip-offs happen, but being part of the
community is important. Even if it's the poorest postal code in the
country, this is the last club. 'If you can't belong to this club,' I say,
'you can't belong to any club.'"

There are many volunteers, committed caregivers and support
groups in the Downtown Eastside. Innovative programs are often
initiated on shoestring budgets, with the participation of people

who were only recently wired to narcotics or other drugs. Judy, quoted in Chapter 3, has given up cocaine completely. She volunteers with other members of a night patrol, acting as guardian angels to sex trade workers. "We keep an eye on them. We speak with them, just to say hello or to kid around. We ask if they need any help. We give out condoms. We make them feel there's someone around they can turn to if they're in trouble." The transformation in Judy's self-perception, the rise in her self-esteem since she's begun to serve the needs of others in a genuine way is wondrous to behold. In a recent photograph she radiates a confidence and sense of purpose that were unimaginable just one year ago, when she was on IV antibiotics for a near-crippling spinal infection and had to wear a metal brace drilled into her skull.

"I've been through infections many times, but this was a really serious one," Judy told me shortly after her treatment was completed. "Having the steel halo on all that time and being limited and feeling screws bolted in my head—it was definitely an eye-opener. Yeah . . . every time I get any using thoughts I just remind myself what I went through for the last five months, and it's just not worth the chances.

"When I was using, I had tunnel vision," she now recalls. "I didn't really notice that life was still existing around me. I just knew my little world. What I wanted was what I revolved around—when was I going to have my next fix or next toke or whatever. Now I actually go for walks a couple of times a day, and I go out and I see all the people, and all the tourists. And I say, 'Hi . . . how you doing . . . ?' I don't know what's wrong with me . . . and it's so strange. . . . It's a good feeling, I'm liking it, but it's all so weird. Is this going to stop, is this going to change anytime soon? I'm not trying to be pessimistic. It's just that it's so unusual, so foreign to me."

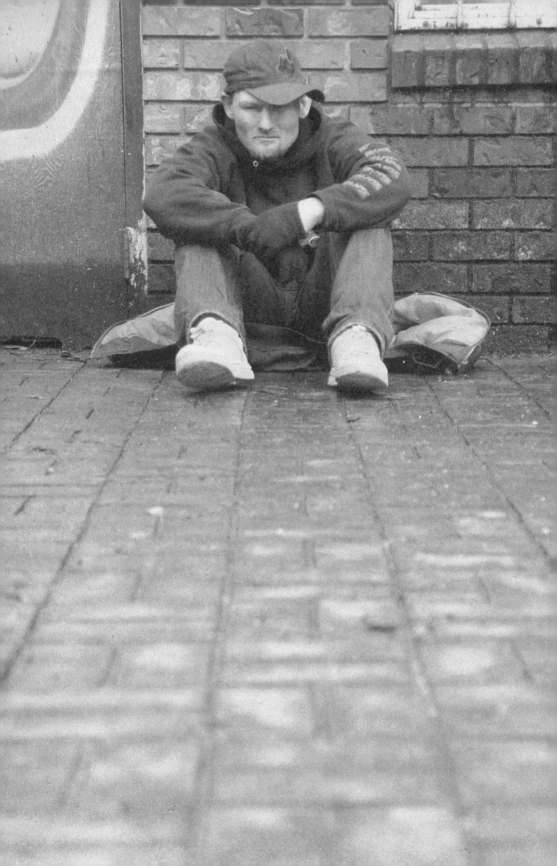

—

PART II

Physician, Heal Thyself

The meaning of all addictions could be defined as endeavours at controlling our life experiences with the help of external remedies. . . . Unfortunately, all external means of improving our life experiences are double-edged swords: they are always good and bad. No external remedy improves our condition without, at the same time, making it worse.

THOMAS HORA, M.D.

Beyond the Dream: Awakening to Reality

—

CHAPTER 9

Takes One to Know One

—

It's hard to get enough of something that almost works.
VINCENT FELITTI, M.D.

It's not one of my Portland days, but the work won't leave me alone. Susan, our health coordinator, rings me on my cell, sounding exasperated: "Mr. Grant is back here at the hotel. What should we do?" I stifle a profanity. I have no patience for treating addiction today; I'm supposed to be at home, writing a book about it.

"Mr. Grant" is Gary, a barrel-bellied, grey-bearded bear of a man, with HIV and diabetes—both risk factors for infection. Neither condition deters him from injecting any accessible vein in his foot with cocaine. His upper-arm vessels are too scarred and corroded by chemicals to serve. A large ulcer is eroding his right big toe, its black base oozing with the breakdown products of dead flesh. For two weeks we'd been urging Gary to accept hospitalization, since it was still possible that intravenous antibiotics could save his toe. "Yes, tomorrow," he'd say. But tomorrow never came.

Four days ago, late on Friday evening, I sought him out in his eighth-floor room. The homecare nurses treating the wound had called in desperation: "Would you commit him on mental health grounds?" Loath to use that ultimate weapon on someone in no way psychotic—just addicted—I promised to see what I could do. I was prepared to pull out the pink slip of involuntary committal, but only as a final resort.

Gary had just come in from scoring a deal. Like many in the Downtown Eastside, he supports his habit with what his long-time friend Stevie once mockingly called "a self-initiated, self-organized marketing endeavour." He makes just enough to keep himself in his substances of choice. Only two weeks before, Stevie had died of liver cancer. Gary had been very close to her—"a fellowship of free trade advocates" in Stevie's words. Intensely distressed by Stevie's demise, Gary had been on an extended cocaine binge since her death.

"Everybody's worried about you, Gary," I said. "That's why I'm here."

"Well, I'm worried about me, too."

Just then Kenyon appeared in the doorway, leaning on his cane. "Got any crystal, Gary?" he asked in his keening voice, slurring his words and seemingly oblivious of my presence. "Fuck off, you idiot. Can't you see the doctor's here?" "Okay," Kenyon replied, soothingly, as if humouring an obstreperous little child. "I'll be back." He hobbled off, the tap-tap of his wooden cane on cement echoing away down the hall.

"You could lose your foot," I resumed. "The gangrene is spreading."

"I can see that. If you tell me I have to go to hospital, I will. "

"I appreciate your confidence in my opinion. I only wish I could be equally confident in your capacity to fulfill your intentions, honourable as they are." The bite in my tone is deliberate. "You promised the same last week, and since then the ulcer has doubled in size. Will you go tonight?"

"Ah, not on a Friday night. I'll be in Emerg until the morning. Tomorrow."

"Gary, I hate to even say this, but if by tomorrow at eleven a.m. you haven't left for the E.R., I'm going to declare you mentally incompetent and commit you on the grounds that you're endangering your own health. You want the truth of it? I don't think for a minute you're crazy, but you're acting crazy. So I'll do it."

It's the same line I'd used on Devon a few months back when he'd refused treatment for a spinal abscess that could have left him quadriplegic. I rarely resort to such threats, as I find them ethically unjustifiable and, for the most part, valueless in practice. I did hospitalize Devon under duress, however, and he's thanked me for that since, many times over.

Next morning Gary did get himself to hospital, only to be discharged with an ineffective antibiotic. The hotel staff had not called me in time, and I'd had no opportunity to communicate with the E.R. physician. Arranging Gary's admission and linking him up with the appropriate specialists had been Sunday's work. And now, on Tuesday, he'd absconded from the HIV ward and fled back to the Portland. He'd passed the point of antibiotic salvage. Toe amputation was scheduled for Wednesday.

Although it's my mid-week writing morning, Susan believes Gary's situation is too delicate for the doctor who's filling in for me. I agree to drop in and, if compelled, to play the pink-slip card. I hear Susan's voice soften in relief. Heading downtown, I'm thrown a curveball by the addicted voice in my own head. "Sikora's? Just for a minute?" No, I tell myself, tempted as I am, that would be impossible to justify. I arrive at the Portland to find that Gary, mercifully, has returned to hospital in the nick of time, just before he would have lost his bed. Good, I think to myself. I'm tired of having to drag people to healing by the scruff of their neck. With that, I drive away from the Downtown Eastside, that woeful planet of drug users and dealers who hustle, grind, cheat and manipulate 24/7 to feed their habits.

I'm on my way to St. Paul's Hospital, where, in addition to my Portland work, I provide medical care to psychiatric inpatients. I take my usual route: exit the Portland parking garage, left out of the alley onto Abbott, right onto Pender. Two blocks past Abbott, my pulse quickens as I approach Sikora's—without doubt one of the world's great classical music stores.

Agitating my mind and body are thoughts of a CD of operatic favourites by the tenor Rolando Villazón. I listened to selections yesterday when I went to the store to pay off my latest debt, but resisted the urge to purchase. Today it's clamouring for me to return and pick it up. I must have it and I must have it now. The desire first arises as a thought and rapidly transforms itself into a concrete object in my mind, with a weight and a pull. It generates an irresistible gravitational field. The tension is relieved only when I succumb.

An hour later, I leave Sikora's with the Villazón disc and several others. Hello, my name is Gabor, and I am a compulsive classical music shopper.

A word before I continue: I do not equate my music obsession with the life-threatening habits of my Portland patients. Far from it. My addiction, though I call it that, wears dainty white gloves compared to theirs. I've also had far more opportunity to make free choices in my life, and I still do. But if the differences between my behaviours and the self-annihilating life patterns of my clients are obvious, the similarities are illuminating—and humbling. I have come to see addiction not as a discrete, solid entity—a case of "Either you got it or you don't got it"—but as a subtle and extensive continuum. Its central, defining qualities are active in all addicts, from the honoured workaholic at the apex of society to the impoverished and criminalized crack fiend who haunts Skid Row. Somewhere along that continuum I locate myself.

I've been to Sikora's several times a week in the past two months—not to mention brief forays to the Magic Flute on 4th Avenue and lightning visits to Sam the Record Man and HMV in Toronto during a recent speaking tour, to say nothing of the closing-out sale at Tower Records in New York. As of now, mid-February, I've blown two thousand dollars on classical CDs since the New Year. I've broken my word to stop bingeing, pledged with maximal contrition to my wife, Rae, after my thousand-dollar pre-Christmas and Boxing Day splurge. Day in, day out I've obsessed about what music to get and spent countless hours poring over write-ups on classical music websites—time that could have been devoted to family or to writing this book with its rapidly approaching deadline. But as soon as the reviewer says something like "no self-respecting lover of symphonic/choral/piano music should be without this set," I'm done for.

Suddenly I cannot imagine my life without this Dvořák symphony cycle or that version of Bach's Mass in B Minor, or this interpretation, on period instruments, of Haydn's Paris Symphonies. I cannot abide another moment without Rachmaninov's Preludes, or *Le Nozze di Figaro*, *Bachianas Brasileiras*, a collection of Shostakovich's chamber music; yet another fourteen-CD version—my fifth—of Wagner's Ring Cycle; new issues of Bach's solo violin or solo cello pieces. This very day I must have Locatelli's *L'Arte del Violino*, Rautavaara's *Garden of Spaces*, the Diabelli Variations, Pierre Hantaï's latest rendition of the Goldberg Variations on harpsichord, Schnittke's or Henze's or Mozart's complete violin concertos, my third version . . . I read and write, eat and even sleep with music in my ears. I cannot walk the dog without a sonata, a symphony, an aria sounding on the earphones. My thoughts and feelings and inner conversations about recorded classical music are what I wake up to in the morning, and they tuck me in at night.

Beethoven composed thirty-two piano sonatas. I own five complete recordings of them—having discarded twice as many, some repurchased and relinquished more than once. Stored away somewhere in our attic are two sets I will never listen to again. I have five complete versions of the sixteen Beethoven string quartets and six collections of the nine symphonies. At one time or another I've owned almost all the recorded Beethoven symphony cycles issued on CD, including the three out-of-favour sets also currently hiding in the attic. If at this very moment I were to begin to play all the collected Beethoven works on my shelves—and if I did nothing else—it would take me weeks to hear it all. And that's just Beethoven.

Many CDs on my shelves have made only cursory visits to my stereo's disc drive, if I've listened to them at all. Others have never had a hearing, languishing as orphans on my shelves.

Rae is suspicious. "Have you been obsessing and buying?" she's asked me a number of times in the past few weeks. I look directly at my life partner of thirty-nine years and I lie. I tell myself I don't want to hurt her. Nonsense. I fear losing her affection. I don't want to look bad in her eyes. I'm afraid of her anger. *That's* what I don't want.

I've given hints—almost as if I wanted to be caught. "You look stressed," Rae remarks one evening in early January. "Yes, it's all these CDs," I begin to reply. She eyes me: my embarrassment is instant and palpable. "I mean, all these CVs I have to email for my speaking engagements." A clumsy recovery. I'm guilty as sin and I must look it. How I manage to escape is beyond me. For a moment, I consider confessing as, eventually, I always do.

The following week, over morning coffee, I look up from the newspaper. "Ah," I remark to Rae, "the Vancouver Opera is doing *Don Giovanni* in March."

"*Don Giovanni,*" Rae muses. "I don't know that one. What's it about?"

"The Don Juan story. The obsessive womanizer. He's this creative, charming and energetic man. A daring adventurer, but a coward morally, who never finds peace within. His erotic passion is insatiable: no matter how often it's consummated, it leaves him restless and dissatisfied. And his poetic talent and his drive for mastery only serve his relentless need to possess. It's always about the next acquisition—he even keeps a notebook listing his amorous conquests. He has many, many opportunities for salvation, but he spurns them all. He torments others and sacrifices his own mortal soul. He scorns repentance, and in the end, he's dragged down to Hell."

Rae glances at me with something like surprise—or is it a knowing smirk? "You described that so eloquently," she says. "You brought the character alive. He's obviously close to your heart."

True, he is—I've purchased four versions of this Mozart masterpiece in the last month, adding to the two already in my collection. I've never listened to any of them from start to finish. And I've been lying, withholding all this from Rae. Actually, I'm a small-time, far less glamorous Don Giovanni—I cheat with operas, not women.

———

Some may find it difficult to understand how the desire to own six versions of *Don Giovanni* can be called an addiction. What's wrong with loving music, with having a passion for great art, with the search for the sublime in aesthetic experience? We humans need art and beauty in our lives. In fact, that's what makes us human. What distinguishes us from our defunct Neanderthal cousins is *Homo sapiens'* capacity for symbolic expression, our ability to represent our experience in abstract terms. That part of the prefrontal cortex didn't develop in the Neanderthal brain. Their species couldn't have produced a Mozart had they survived another million years. So, really, isn't it human to want beauty? To crave it, even?

And I do adore the music. It's both the most abstract form of art, capable of communicating without words or visual images, and the most immediate. For me at least, it's the purest form of artistic expression. With or without words, it speaks eloquently of loss and joy, doubt and truth, despair and inspiration, earthly lust and the transcendent divine. Music challenges me, thrills me, fills me, moves me, softens my heart. It releases streams of emotion in me that I dammed up long ago in the rest of my life. As Thomas De Quincey writes in *Confessions of an English Opium Eater,* music has the power to render life's passions "exalted, spiritualized, sublimed"— even if De Quincey thought he had to take opium to appreciate this.

So, yes, I am passionate about music—but I'm also addicted, which is an altogether different ontological boxed set.

Addictions, even as they resemble normal human yearnings, are more about desire than attainment. In the addicted mode, the emotional charge is in the pursuit and the *acquisition* of the desired object, not in the possession and enjoyment of it. The greatest pleasure is in the momentary satisfaction of yearning.

The fundamental addiction is to the fleeting experience of *not* being addicted. The addict craves the absence of the craving state. For a brief moment he's liberated from emptiness, from boredom, from lack of meaning, from yearning, from being driven or from pain. He is free. His enslavement to the external—the substance, the object or the activity—consists of the impossibility, in his mind, of finding within himself the freedom from longing or irritability. "I want nothing and fear nothing," said Zorba the Greek. "I'm free." There are not many Zorbas amongst us.

In my addicted mode the music still thrills, but it cannot release me from the need to pursue and acquire more and more. Its fruit is not joy but disaffection. With each CD I delude myself that now my collection will be complete. If only I could have *that* one—just one more, one more time, I could rest satisfied. So runs the illusion. "'Just one more' is the binding factor in the circle of suffering," writes the Buddhist monk and teacher Sakyong Mipham.[1]

My purest moment of freedom occurs after I park my car, hurry to Sikora's and, slowing down just before entering, draw a deep breath as I push the door open. For this nanosecond, life is limitless possibility. "We can perceive the infinite in music only by searching for this quality in ourselves," writes the pianist and conductor Daniel Barenboim.[2] Very true. But that's not the kind of infinite the addict seeks.

When you get right down to it, it's the adrenaline I'm after, along with the precious reward chemicals that will flood my brain when I hold the new CD in hand, providing an all too temporary reprieve from the stress of my driven state. But I've barely left the store before the adrenaline starts pumping through my circulation again, my mind fixated on the next purchase. Anyone who's addicted to any kind of pursuit—whether it's sex or gambling or shopping—is after that same fix of home-grown chemicals.

—

This behaviour has been recurring for decades, since my children were—

Wait. "The behaviour has been recurring?" What a neat way to put it outside of myself, as if it lived as an independent entity. *No, I have been doing this for decades, since my children were small.*

Many years I was spending thousands of dollars on compact discs. Dropping a few hundred dollars in an hour or two was no stretch. My all-time record came close to eight thousand dollars in one week. I was cushioned from economic disaster by the income I earned as one of the self-sacrificing—read workaholic—physicians much admired by the world at large. As I've written elsewhere, it was easy for me to justify all the spending as compensation for the hard work I was doing: one addiction providing an alibi for the other.*

The confusing part was this: both behaviour dependencies represented genuine aspects of me, each distorted out of proportion.

* This paragraph and several others in this chapter are adapted from *Scattered Minds*—the book I wrote about Attention Deficit Hyperactivity Disorder (ADHD) (Vintage Canada, 2000).

My addiction to music and books could masquerade as an aesthetic passion, and my addiction to work as a service to humanity—and I do have aesthetic passion, and I do wish to serve humanity.

I'm not the only person in the world intoxicated by classical music, and I'm far from alone in owning multiple sets of recorded masterpieces. So are all these other enthusiasts addicted, too? No, not all, but many of them are—I see them in the stores and read their comments on the World Wide Web. One addict knows another.

Any passion can become an addiction; but then how to distinguish between the two? *The central question is: who's in charge, the individual or their behaviour?* It's possible to rule a passion, but an obsessive passion that a person is unable to rule is an addiction. And the addiction is the repeated behaviour that a person keeps engaging in, even though he knows it harms himself or others. How it looks *externally* is irrelevant. The key issue is a person's internal relationship to the passion and its related behaviours.

If in doubt, ask yourself one simple question: given the harm you're doing to yourself and others, are you willing to stop? If not, you're addicted. And if you're unable to renounce the behaviour or to keep your pledge when you do, you're addicted.

There is, of course, a deeper, more ossified layer beneath any kind of addiction: the denial state in which, contrary to all reason and evidence, you refuse to acknowledge that you're hurting yourself or anyone else. In the denial state you're completely resistant to asking yourself any questions at all. But if you want to know, look around you. Are you closer to the people you love after your passion has been fulfilled or more isolated? Have you come more truly into who you really are or are you left feeling hollow?

The difference between passion and addiction is that between a divine spark and a flame that incinerates. The sacred fire through which Moshe (Moses) experienced the presence of God on Mount Horeb did not annihilate the bush from which it arose: *And YHWH's messenger was seen by him in the flame of a fire out of the midst of a bush. He saw: here, the bush is burning with fire, and the bush is not consumed!*[3] Passion is divine fire: it enlivens and makes holy; it gives light and yields inspiration. Passion is generous because it's not ego-driven; addiction is self-centred.

Passion gives and enriches; addiction is a thief. Passion is a source of truth and enlightenment; addictive behaviours lead you into darkness. You're more alive when you are passionate, and you triumph whether or not you attain your goal. But an addiction requires a specific outcome that feeds the ego; without that outcome, the ego feels empty and deprived. A consuming passion that you are helpless to resist, no matter what the consequences, is an addiction.

You may even devote your entire life to a passion, but if it's truly a passion and not an addiction, you'll do so with freedom, joy and a full assertion of your truest self and values. In addiction, there's no joy, freedom or assertion. The addict lurks shame-faced in the shadowy corners of her own existence. I glimpse shame in the eyes of my addicted patients in the Downtown Eastside and, in their shame, I see mirrored my own.

Addiction is passion's dark simulacrum and, to the naïve observer, its perfect mimic. It resembles passion in its urgency and in the promise of fulfillment, but its gifts are illusory. It's a black hole. The more you offer it, the more it demands. Unlike passion, its alchemy does not create new elements from old. It only degrades what it touches and turns it into something less, something cheaper.

Am I happier after one of my self-indulgent sprees? Like a miser, in my mind I recount and catalogue my recent purchases—a furtive Scrooge, hunched over and rubbing his hands together with acquisitive glee, his heart growing ever colder. In the wake of a buying binge, I am not a satisfied man.

Addiction is centrifugal. It sucks energy from you, creating a vacuum of inertia. A passion energizes you and enriches your relationships. It empowers you and gives strength to others. Passion creates; addiction consumes—first the self and then the others within its orbit.

The hit musical *Little Shop of Horrors* offers a brilliant metaphorical image of addiction. Seymour, a little nebbish of a flower shop clerk (played most famously in the 1986 film version by Rick Moranis) takes pity on a "strange and unusual" little plant that's dying of malnutrition. It brings the shop some much-needed business, but there's a problem. No one can figure out what the plant, named Audrey II after Seymour's sweetheart, needs for nourishment until one night Seymour accidentally pricks a finger and the plant hungrily swallows the drops of blood dripping from the wound. Only temporarily appeased, the plant wants more, and Seymour dutifully offers up another dose of his precious plasma. The plant then takes on a personality and voice of its own. Piteously the little plant pleads and cajoles, promising to be Seymour's slave. But then it issues an abrupt command: *"Feed me, Seymour!"* Terrified, Seymour does as he's told. The plant thrives and becomes huger and hungrier, and Seymour weakens and becomes anaemic—morally, as well as physically. When it looks as if he's going to be bled (literally) dry, Seymour stumbles on the idea of feeding the plant human corpses and is led into a new part-time vocation: murder. By the finale Seymour is forced to wage a heroic battle against the bloodthirsty Audrey II. Bent on conquest and power, the plant no longer even bothers to feign friendship.

So it is with addiction. Beginning with only the few drops of blood you're ready to donate at first, it soon consumes enough to dominate and rule you. Then it starts to prey on those around you, and you must struggle to extinguish it.

I lose myself when caught in one my addictive spirals. Gradually I feel an ebbing of moral strength and experience myself as hollow. Emptiness stares out from behind my eyes. I fear that even my friends at Sikora's, who sell me the goods, can see through my thin mask. There is nothing behind the façade but an organism palpitating for instant gratification. It's not a music lover standing at the counter but an abject weakling. I sense they pity me.

Everywhere I go, I find it an effort to impersonate myself. Nurses at St. Paul's Hospital ask me how I am. "Fine," I say. "I'm good." What I don't say is, "I'm obsessed. I just blew in from the record store and can hardly wait to get through my work here so I can rush down to the car to listen to this opera or that symphony. Then, unless I go to the store to pick up more stuff, I'll go home and lie to my wife. And I'm feeling guilty as hell. That's how I am." Self-deprecating, pessimistic or negative comments creep into my conversations. Someone on the ward compliments my work. I attempt a joke: "Oh, you can fool some of the people some of the time." No joke, that. They look at me strangely and protest that they meant it. Of course they did, but in my shame, I don't believe I deserve any praise. A secret addiction comes equipped with praise deflectors.

I become increasingly cynical about the world—politics, people, possibility, the future. Every morning I get into a hostile argument with the newspaper, resenting it for what it says or doesn't say. The *Globe and Mail,* in its news slant, editorials and choice of columnists, favours corporations, the mainstream parties and neo-con foreign policy makers. But the poor old *Globe* is just being true to its blue-blooded, capitalist self. It's still the best paper in Canada, and I'm the one who chooses to fund it with my subscription dollars. So why am I yelling at it over coffee? My negativity stems from my internal dissatisfaction, my harsh self-critique. The *Globe* doesn't speak the truth as I see it? Neither do I. The *Globe* justifies selfish acquisitiveness and exonerates dishonesty? Look who's talking.

Would that the spread of negativity were confined to my prickly relationship with print journalism. No, I become increasingly and reflexively critical, irritable and self-righteous with my teenaged daughter. The more I indulge myself, the more judgmental I am toward her. I can't be optimistic and believe in her growth and development when I know I'm sabotaging my own. How can I see the best in her when I'm blind to all but the worst in myself? Our interactions are tense. At age seventeen, she's at no loss for words or body language to communicate her displeasure.

My relationship with Rae loses vitality. Because my internal world is dominated by obsession, I have little to say and what I do say rings hollow in my own ears. Because my attention is pulled inward, the interest I offer her becomes dutiful, rather than genuine. When I'm in one of my addictive cycles, it's almost as if I were engaged in a sexual affair, with all the attendant obsession, lying and manipulation.

Above all, I'm absent. It's impossible to be fully present when you're putting up walls to keep from being seen. Intimacy and spontaneity are sacrificed. Something's got to give, and it does—sometimes for days, sometimes for weeks and months.

When they were much younger, I'd keep my children waiting or hurry them along to suit my purposes. If I could, I'd expunge from my personal history the time I left my eleven-year-old son at a comic-book shop after a soccer game, with one of his teammates. "I'll be back in fifteen minutes," I said. It was nearly an hour before I returned. I'd not only run to the store across the street; I'd also driven to another one, downtown, on my quest for whatever was at that moment my must-have-immediately recording. My son's face was clouded with anxiety and bewilderment when he finally saw me at the comic-book shop door.

I lied to my wife daily for weeks and months at a time. I'd rush into the house, stashing my latest purchases on the porch, pretending to be home and grounded. But inwardly I could think of nothing but the music. When the reckoning came, as it always did, I made guilty confessions and soon-to-be-broken promises.

I hated myself, and this self-loathing manifested itself in the harsh, controlling and critical ways I'd deal with my sons and my daughter. When we're preoccupied with serving our own false needs, we can't endure seeing the genuine needs of other people— least of all those of our children.

Perhaps the nadir, but certainly not the end, of my addictive years came when I left a woman in labour to run over the bridge, in midday traffic, to Sikora's. Even then, I would have had time to return to the hospital for the delivery had I not begun to cast about for other recordings to buy. I murmured apologies when I got back, but no explanations. Everyone was most understanding, even my disappointed patient. After all, Dr. Maté is a busy man. He can't be everywhere at once. I enjoyed a reputation in Vancouver as a physician who extended himself for his pregnant patients and would support them compassionately through their delivery. Not this time. This baby was born without me. (Her name is Carmela. She's a beautiful twenty-year-old dancer and university student. I told her mother, Joyce, the full story many years ago.)

This is not the first public "confession" I've made. I've written and spoken about my addictions before. And the truth is that as of this writing, neither my public acknowledgments of my behaviour nor my thorough understanding of its impact on myself and my family has stopped me from repeating the cycle. I've authored three books and receive letters and emails from readers the world over, thanking me for having helped them transform their lives. Yet I have continued to choose patterns that darken my spirit, alienate those closest to me and drain my vitality.*

—

In January 2006, when I'm in the midst of an extended CD obsession, Sean comes moaning into my office. "I'm messing up," he says. "I'm puking and shitting. I've been doing heroin . . . oh, man." Sean has been at a recovery home for months. I haven't seen him for a long time, but he did call regularly, proudly reporting on his progress and his determination to stay clean. Once, he left a voicemail: "I'm calling to say that I appreciate all your help. I just want to say thanks, man." Now he's back in the Downtown Eastside, pale, bedraggled, emaciated, unwashed. He's been living in the streets for weeks but plans to admit himself to a Christian rehabilitation camp.

"Don't you think you should be back on the methadone?" I suggest. Sean eagerly downs his first dose before recounting the details of this most recent relapse. "I don't know why, Doc. I thought I'd just use one time, just the one time. And that was it."

"So are you going through with the Christian rehab thing?"

"My family is pushing me, but I'm not up to it."

"Have you told them that?"

"No."

"What stops you from being straight with them?"

"Hurting them. They've helped me so much, and I turned around and failed so miserably."

I'm instantly filled with judgment. Annoyed by his neediness and weakness of will—that is, by my own—I want to teach him a lesson.

"I don't believe you," I counter. "Not that you don't mean it, but you're not being honest with yourself. You're not worried about hurting them—you're already hurting them."

* Since I wrote this chapter in February 2006, I have made significant changes in my relation to my addictive habits, as I will describe later.

"Yes, I am. But I don't want to go to this Christian place; I know what it's all about. It's really tough there—a complete schedule. It's harsh and rigid."

"That's not the point. I'm talking about telling your family the truth about how you feel and what you're up to. You just don't want to face the hassle of being clear with them. You're afraid of their judgment or of your own. You're too chicken to be honest."

Sean throws me a direct glance, an abashed smile on his face. "That's how it is, Doc."

"Well, then, get off it. Be open about what you want and what you don't want. That much you do owe your family."

"Doc," having pushed his addicted patient to tell the truth, will now go home and deceive his wife, his briefcase stuffed with the latest haul of Sikora's loot.

—

CHAPTER 10

Twelve-Step Journal: April 5, 2006

Tonight I will attend my first Twelve-Step group. I'm apprehensive. Do I belong there? What will I say? "Hi, I'm Gabor and I am a . . ." A what? An addict . . . or a voyeur?

I've never been hooked on substances. I've never tried cocaine or opiates, partly due to the fear that I'd like them too well. I've been drunk exactly twice in my life, during my college years. Both incidents ended with bouts of vomiting—the first time in the vehicle of Lieutenant Jeunesse, my company commander at the Canadian Officers Training Corps summer boot camp at Borden, Ontario. He was driving me and several comrades back to the barracks after an evening of carousing at the Officers' Club. "You made a mess of my car last night," the lieutenant shouted at me on the parade square early next morning. "Sorry, sir," I groaned by way of reply, drawing myself to full attention. "I wasn't thinking."

I expect to meet people at AA who, by and large, have had their lives devastated by alcohol or other drugs. For months or years at a time, their minds and bodies have been tortured by the craving for substances. They've been racked by withdrawal pangs, their throats parched, their brains beset by terrors and hallucinations. How can I compare myself with them? Will it feel like I'm slumming? How can I mention my petty dysfunctions alongside the tales of affliction I'm likely to hear tonight? What right do I have to claim even the dubious distinction of being a real addict? Calling myself an addict in such company may be nothing more than an attempt to excuse my selfishness and lack of discipline.

I fear being recognized. People may have seen me on TV or read something I've written. It's one thing to be on stage as an authority figure, addressing an audience on stress or ADHD or parenting and childhood development, and to acknowledge that I've had problems with impulse control over the years. In that context my public self-revelations are received as honest, authentic and even courageous. It's quite another matter to confess as a peer—to a group who have had a much closer confrontation with life's gritty realities than I have—that I'm "powerless," that my addictive behaviours often get the better of me. That I'm unhappy.

Of course, in my mind there also lurks a craving to be recognized. "If I'm not my public persona—doctor, writer—who am I?" it whispers. Without my achievements and the opportunity to display my status, intelligence and wit, I fear I do not cut a very impressive figure.

Wryly, I observe my ego do its frantic dance. It just can't get no satisfaction.

The meeting takes place in a church basement, which is surprisingly full. Behind a lectern at the front, a middle-aged woman whose amiable features reveal shyness mixed with authority calls to order a raucous, polyglot crowd of people seated on wooden chairs. I survey the audience through the gradually subsiding din: calloused hands; jeans; cowboy boots; ravaged faces; hardened looks; nicotine-stained teeth; whisky-gravel voices; earthy, back-slapping humour; easy camaraderie—a rough-edged, blue-collared, East Vancouver gathering. Young women sport green and pink neon stripes in spiky punk hairdos. Scruffy, middle-aged fellows exchange whispered jokes and toothless smiles. The scalp of the old man in front of me gleams between rows of thin, white hair like shiny furrows in a ploughed winter field.

I feel instantly at home and I realize why: the hyperkinetic, ADD-like energy of this bunch resonates with my own.

"Hi, I'm Maureen. I'm an alcoholic," the chairperson begins. "Hi, Maureen." The audience hails her from all sides of the room. A few more people are identified. "I'm Elaine, alcoholic . . . George, alcoholic. . . ." Loud cheers greet each name. Newcomers are invited to introduce themselves; I sit quietly.

"Welcome, all. The only requirement for membership is a desire to stop drinking." First I have to *start* drinking, I think. "We are here to surrender—to let go of the old ideas that keep us stuck." I don't do surrender. I'm not even sure what that means.

As if in response to my inner commentator, a tall, burly man strides to the lectern. He has a thick nose, and his oiled hair is slicked back into a ducktail. Looking at him, you feel you'd want to avoid him on a dark street. He speaks with the authority of someone who's looked himself in the eye without blinking. "I'm Peter, alcoholic." "Hi, Peter," the loud chorus responds.

"I'm here to tell you about surrender," he begins. "I'm here to tell you how hip, slick, cool I was when I first came to AA. You wouldn't believe how slick and cool." Snickers all round. "Anything I wanted, I could get with my mouth, and if I couldn't, I'd take it with my fists. I robbed my own mother once. That still hurts.

"When I first came here, all I wanted was to sober up enough so I could concentrate on my flourishing drug business. My last binge, six years ago, ended with three days in the bathroom where I kept puking, sweating and shitting myself. I didn't dare be more than a few feet away from the toilet or the shower." Boisterous laughter all around the room.

"After three days of bathroom living I reconnected the phone. Three messages. The first from my landlord: 'Peter, you're evicted.' The second from my mother: 'Peter, you can heal.' The third from my friend: 'Peter, I've surrendered and it works.' It's lining up perfect, I thought. If that jerk can surrender, so can I. I was still in my better-than phase." Nods of recognition, guffaws and applause.

"I looked around and asked myself what surrender would look like. In my case it looked like a large green Glad garbage bag into which I gathered all my drug paraphernalia, along with my little phone books of 'business contacts.' Wouldn't need them anymore. I chucked it all into the bin in the back alley."

I'm struck by that. Aha, surrender is not some abstract, airy-fairy, spiritual concept. It's individual, and it's practical. At the same time, I do feel like a voyeur here. My life and this man's cannot be measured on the same scale of suffering. I envy his serenity, humility and air of quiet command. (Thus speaks the automatic, mechanical voice of self-judgment in my mind.)

"Now my goal is only that each day I should become closer to the God that I understand. The greatest teaching I have received is that I can be happy without imposing my will on you or you or anyone else, even when I feel like doing so.

"You may not believe you can surrender, but as you do, there will be a shift. You'll know there's a shift because your heart changes. As you study the Big Book and you serve people and help the community, your heart softens. That's the greatest gift, a soft heart. I wouldn't have believed it."

Yes, a soft heart. How quickly my heart hardens. And how brittle a hard heart can be.

The last speaker is Elaine, alcoholic. "Hi, Elaine."

"In the eyes of the newcomers," she begins, "I see sadness, hunger, desperation. 'How will I ever have a life again? How will I get money, how will I build a relationship?'" Not my problems, I think. Still I wonder, What would she see in my eyes?

"Nothing's going to happen overnight for most of you. It took me a long time of coming to these meetings before I could hear anything, and that didn't sit well with me. Two things alcoholics hate is work and time. There has to be no effort involved, and you want the results right now." Chuckles and applause.

That's me. I resist emotional work and I do want immediate results. "A sense of urgency typifies attention deficit disorder," I wrote in *Scattered Minds*, "a desperation to have immediately whatever it is that one may desire at the moment, be it an object, an activity or a relationship." If it doesn't happen quickly for me, I feel like bailing, and unless I'm extraordinarily motivated, I often do.

"I used to be a militant party girl," Elaine continues in her Lauren Bacall voice, auburn-dyed bangs falling over her forehead above large, heavily painted eyes. "I wasn't going to take anything seriously except having a good time—and that meant being stone drunk.

"Three things that didn't help me were love, education and punishment. I didn't learn no matter how hard people tried to love me, no matter what facts I knew and no matter how many times life taught me harsh lessons. I didn't learn until I began to listen.

"The first time I listened was at an AA meeting in Toronto. A Native man in his sixties was speaking. 'I've been sober for two years now,' he said, 'and six months ago, I got my first job. If I had known how good it felt to work, I would have been done with drinking long ago. Five months ago I got my own place. Had I known how good that was, I would have gone sober long ago. Three months ago I got myself a girlfriend. Boy, if I'd known how great *that* was, I might never have drank in the first place.'" Merriment, chortles, the clapping of appreciative hands.

"'Now I'm sixty-four,' the man said, 'and I've just been told I have cancer. I have six months to live.'" Elaine pauses to look around the room as we take in this information. Silently, we wait for her conclusion. "I thought he's going to announce, 'I'm off on the biggest six-month drunk you can imagine. So the hell with you all and goodbye.' That's what I would have done with a death sentence hanging over me. But not this Native man. 'I'm just so grateful,' he said, 'so thankful that I'm sober, that I've had two years of sobriety and that I can look forward to the rest of my life in sobriety.'

"That's when I got that sobriety is more than just the absence of alcohol. It's a way of being. It's living life in its fullness."

Do I have to become an alcoholic, lose everything, puke my guts out and then get religion before I can experience the fullness of life, whatever the hell that means? I'm resentful. No, I'm anxious, fearful that it will never happen for me. That's what Elaine would have seen in my eyes. Or saw. Perhaps I was the newcomer she was talking about.

Elaine is about to leave the lectern amidst nods of approval, but she steps behind the microphone once more. "I don't mean," she says, "that my life is perfect. Sometimes it feels like things are completely falling apart, like this week. But I no longer confuse stuff that happens with my life. This moment is okay, even when things are coming apart at the seams. Right here, right now, at this moment, things are okay."

"Forget about your life situation for a while and pay attention to your life," writes the spiritual teacher Eckhart Tolle. "Your life situation exists in time—your life is now." I have read his book over and over, have underlined that phrase and understand it intellectually. This woman, Elaine, doesn't only understand it. She gets it. It's a truth she's discovered for herself.

"Surrender is the key," says Elaine. "Even now, whenever I try too hard, I mess it all up. Don't try. Just listen to God's directions."

Fuck. That God thing again. What God? Ever since I was a child, I've been shaking my fist at Heaven.

From the moment I had a mind of my own, I knew there was no all-knowing, all-powerful, all-loving God. In Eastern Europe under the Stalinist regimes there used to be a saying: "You can be honest or intelligent or be a member of the Communist Party. In fact, you can be any two of the three, but not all three at the same time." In the same way, I understood that God could be all knowing and all powerful, but not all-loving. How else to explain the murder of my grandparents in the gas chambers of Auschwitz or my own near-death as an infant in the Budapest ghetto? Or God can be all-loving and all-knowing, but not omnipotent. A milksop. A weakling. So what is this God whose directions I'm supposed to obey?

My moment of rebellion over, I know better and remember Peter's words: "My goal is only that each day I should become closer to the God that I understand." The God I understand? Not the wilful old man in the sky I've resented all my life. Truth. Essence. The inner voice I keep running away from. That's the God I've been resisting. If, Jonah-like, I'd rather hide in the stinking belly of a whale than face the truth I know so well, it's not because of intelligence but because of the refusal to surrender. To surrender, you have to give something up. I've been unwilling to do that. *And YHWH said to Moshe: "I see this people—and here, it is a stiff-necked people!"*

A few logistical details dealt with, chairs stacked, the meeting is over. I'm surprised by how quickly many people head for the exit. When I step outside, I see why—they're all in the parking lot, drawing puffs on their cigarettes and holding animated conversations in pairs or small groups. Smoke, bluish in the light thrown by the church windows, hangs in the air and dissipates slowly above them. I seek Peter, the burly former drinker and drug dealer. I feel drawn to him and believe he may have something to teach me.

He's conversing with two or three other men, their faces intermittently lit by cigarette glow. I'm too shy to approach.

As I stand there hesitating, I feel a hand on my shoulder. I turn my head. A woman is smiling at me. "Dr. Gabor Maté! I thought that was you! My name is Sophie. You delivered my baby nineteen years ago. You probably don't remember."

"I don't, but nice to see you." Sophie, she reminds me, was twenty-one years old when I attended the delivery of her child. As it turns out, far from feeling embarrassed at encountering a former patient at an AA event, I'm glad to be greeted by a friendly face. "Tell me something. Do I belong here?" I give the one-minute version of my history.

"You do belong." Sophie explains that the meeting is open to everyone. "If you have addictive behaviours, this is the right place for you. Unless it's marked with a C for 'Closed' in the AA schedule, anyone with a problem is welcome. The C meetings are for alcoholics only."

I will come back, I decide. What I've witnessed here are humility, gratitude, commitment, acceptance, support and authenticity. I so desperately want those qualities for myself.

"Nowhere do I see such power and grace as at my AA meetings," a writer friend has told me. A manic-depressive with a long history of alcoholism, she's been attending for fifteen years, and she's been urging me to do so. I finally get what she means.

As I walk to my car, I see Sophie approach a group of her friends. "You wouldn't believe who I just ran into," I hear her say.

I chuckle inwardly: my ego's yearning to be recognized, and the fear of it, realized at the last possible moment.

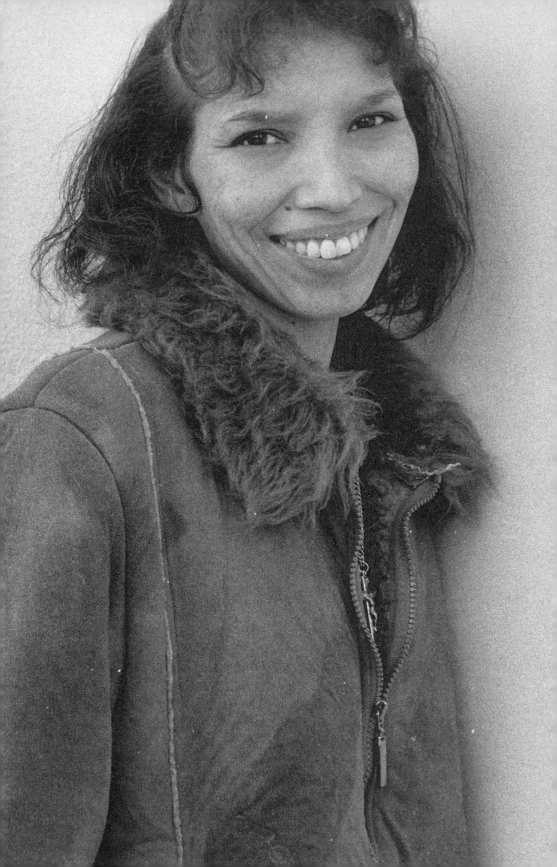

PART III

—

A Different State of the Brain

Recent brain imaging studies have revealed an underlying
disruption to brain regions that are important for the normal
processes of motivation, reward and inhibitory control in addicted
individuals. This provides the basis for a different view: that drug
addiction is a disease of the brain, and the associated abnormal
behavior is the result of dysfunction of brain tissue, just as cardiac
insufficiency is a disease of the heart.

DR. NORA VOLKOW

DIRECTOR, [U.S.] NATIONAL INSTITUTE ON DRUG ABUSE

—

CHAPTER 11

What Is Addiction?

Addicts and addictions are part of our cultural landscape and lexicon. We all know who and what they are—or think we do. In this section of the book we'll look at the subject from a scientific perspective, beginning with a working definition of addiction. We also need to dispel some common misconceptions.

In the English language addiction has two overlapping but distinct meanings. In our day, it most commonly refers to a dysfunctional dependence on drugs or on behaviours such as gambling or sex or eating. Surprisingly, that meaning is only about a hundred years old. For centuries before then, at least back to Shakespeare, addiction referred simply to an activity that one was passionate about or committed to, gave one's time to. "Sir, what sciences have you addicted yourself to," someone asks the knight Don Quixote in an eighteenth-century English translation of the Cervantes classic. In the nineteenth-century *Confessions of an English Opium Eater*, Thomas De Quincey never once refers to his narcotic habit as an addiction, even if by our current definition it certainly was. The pathological sense of the word arose in the early twentieth century.

The term's original root comes from the Latin *addicere*, "assign to."* That yields the word's traditional, innocuous meaning: a habitual activity or interest, often with a positive purpose. The

* From *dicere* ("to say") and the prefix *ad-* ("to").

Victorian-era British politician William Gladstone wrote about "addiction to agricultural pursuits," implying a perfectly admirable vocation. But the Romans had another, more ominous usage that speaks to our present-day interpretation: an *addictus* was a person who, having defaulted on a debt, was assigned to his creditor as a slave—hence, addiction's modern sense as enslavement to a habit. De Quincey anticipated that meaning when he acknowledged "the chain of abject slavery" forged by his narcotic dependence.

What, then, is addiction? In the words of a consensus statement by addiction experts in 2001, addiction is a "chronic *neurobiological disease* . . . characterized by behaviors that include one or more of the following: impaired control over drug use, compulsive use, continued use despite harm, and craving."[1] The key features of substance addiction are the use of drugs or alcohol despite negative consequences, and relapse. I've heard some people shrug off their addictive tendencies by saying, for example, "I can't be an alcoholic. I don't drink that much . . ." or "I only drink at certain times." The issue is not the quantity or even the frequency, but the impact. "An addict continues to use a drug when evidence strongly demonstrates the drug is doing significant harm. . . . If users show the pattern of preoccupation and compulsive use repeatedly over time with relapse, addiction can be identified."[2]

Helpful as such definitions are, we have to take a broader view to understand addiction fully. There is a fundamental addiction process that can express itself in many ways, through many different habits. The use of substances like heroin, cocaine, nicotine and alcohol are only the most obvious examples, the most laden with the risk of physiological and medical consequences. Many behavioural, nonsubstance addictions can also be highly destructive to physical health, psychological balance, and personal and social relationships.

Addiction is any repeated behaviour, substance-related or not, in which a person feels compelled to persist, regardless of its negative impact on his life and the lives of others. Addiction involves:

1. compulsive engagement with the behaviour, a preoccupation with it;

2. impaired control over the behaviour;
3. persistence or relapse, despite evidence of harm; and
4. dissatisfaction, irritability or intense craving when the object—be it a drug, activity or other goal—is not immediately available.

Compulsion, impaired control, persistence, irritability, relapse and craving—these are the hallmarks of addiction—any addiction. Not all harmful compulsions are addictions, though: an obsessive-compulsive, for example, also has impaired control and persists in a ritualized and psychologically debilitating behaviour such as, say, repeated hand washing. The difference is that he has no craving for it and, unlike the addict, he gets no kick out of his compulsion.

How does the addict know she has impaired control? Because she doesn't stop the behaviour in spite of its ill effects. She makes promises to herself or others to quit, but despite pain, peril and promises, she keeps relapsing. There are exceptions, of course. Some addicts never recognize the harm their behaviours cause and never form resolutions to end them. They stay in denial and rationalization. Others openly accept the risk, resolving to live and die "my way."

As we shall see shortly, all addictions—whether to drugs or to nondrug behaviours—share the same brain circuits and brain chemicals. On the biochemical level the purpose of all addictions is to create an altered physiological state in the brain. This can be achieved in many ways, drug taking being the most direct. So an addiction is never purely "psychological"; all addictions have a biological dimension.

And here a word about dimensions. As we delve into the scientific research, we need to avoid the trap of believing that addiction can be reduced to the actions of brain chemicals or nerve circuits or any other kind of neurobiological, psychological or sociological data. A multilevel exploration is necessary because it's impossible to understand addiction fully from any one perspective, no matter how accurate. Addiction is a complex condition, a complex interaction between human beings and their environment. We need to view it simultaneously from many different angles—or, at least, while examining it from one angle, we need to keep the others in mind. Addiction has biological, chemical, neurological, psychological, medical, emotional, social, political, economic and spiritual underpinnings—and perhaps others I haven't thought about. To get anywhere near a complete picture we must keep shaking the kaleidoscope to see what other patterns emerge.

—

Because the addiction process is too multifaceted to be understood within any limited framework, my definition of addiction made no mention of "disease." Viewing addiction as an illness, either acquired or inherited, narrows it down to a medical issue. It does have some of the features of illness, and these are most pronounced in hardcore drug addicts like the ones I work with in the Downtown Eastside. But not for a moment do I wish to promote the belief that the disease model by itself explains addiction or even that it's the key to understanding what addiction is all about. Addiction is "all about" many things.

Note, too, that neither the textbook definitions of drug addiction nor the broader view we're taking here includes the concepts of *physical dependence* or *tolerance* as criteria for addiction. Tolerance is an instance of "give an inch, take a mile." That is, the addict needs to use more and more of the same substance or engage in more and more of the same behaviour, to get the same rewarding effects. Although tolerance is a common effect of many addictions, a person does not need to have developed a tolerance to be addicted. And then there's physical dependence. As defined in medical terms, physical dependence is manifested when a person stops taking a substance and, due to changes in the brain and body, she experiences withdrawal symptoms. Those temporary, drug-induced changes form the basis of physical dependence. Although a feature of drug addiction, a person's physical dependence on a substance does not necessarily imply that he is addicted to it.

The withdrawal syndrome is different for each class of drug—in the case of opiates such as morphine or heroin it includes nausea, diarrhea, sweats, aches and pains and weakness, as well as severe anxiety, agitation and depressed mood. But you don't have to be addicted to experience withdrawal—you just have to have been taking a medication for an extended period of time.³ As many people have discovered to their chagrin, with abrupt cessation it's quite possible to suffer highly unpleasant withdrawal symptoms from drugs that are not addictive: the antidepressants paroxetine (Paxil) and venlafaxine (Effexor) are but two examples. Withdrawal does not mean you were addicted; for addiction, there also needs to be craving and relapse.

In fact, in the case of narcotics, it turns out that the addictive, "feel good" effect of these drugs seems to act in a different part of the brain than the effects that lead to physical dependence. When morphine is infused only into the "reward" circuits of a rat's brain, addiction-like behaviour results, but there's no physical dependence and no withdrawal.⁴

"Dependence" can also be understood as a powerful attachment to harmful substances or behaviours, and this definition gives us a clearer picture of addiction. The addict comes to depend on the substance or behaviour in order to make himself feel momentarily calmer or more excited or less dissatisfied with his life. That's the meaning I'll be referring to unless I am specifically describing *physical dependence,* the narrower medical phenomenon. Father Sam Portaro, author and former Episcopalian Chaplain to the University of Chicago, said it admirably well in a recent lecture: "The heart of addiction is dependency, excessive dependency, unhealthy dependency—unhealthy in the sense of unwhole, dependency that disintegrates and destroys."⁵

—

CHAPTER 12

From Vietnam to "Rat Park": Do Drugs Cause Addiction?

In the cloudy swirl of misleading ideas surrounding public discussion of addiction, there's one that stands out: the misconception that drug taking by itself will lead to addiction—in other words, that the cause of addiction resides in the power of the drug over the human brain. It is one of the bedrock fables sustaining the so-called "War on Drugs." It also obscures the existence of a basic addiction process of which drugs are only one possible object, among many. Compulsive gambling, for example, is widely considered to be a form of addiction without anyone arguing that it's caused by a deck of cards.

The notion that addiction is drug-induced is often reinforced. A celebrity, for instance, might announce when checking himself into a rehab centre, that he became hooked on narcotics after they were prescribed for, say, a back injury. "Making a career out of pratfalls eventually took a toll on Jerry Lewis," reported the Associated Press in April 2005:

> The entertainer said Sunday on ABC's This Week that he spent thirty-seven years in constant pain as a result of his trademark physical comedy, which led to an addiction to pills. "In 1965 they gave me one Percodan that took me through the day. And by '78, I was taking 13 a day, 15 a day. The addiction is devastating, because you're not even clear anymore why you're taking it. I had

already discussed a variety of options, one of which was to kill myself," he said.

I also took Percodan at one time, for a few days. After a wisdom-tooth extraction about thirty years ago I developed a condition called "dry socket syndrome," which I'd never heard about before and never wish to hear of again. The pain in my jaw was excruciating. I was swallowing Percodan in higher than recommended doses and more frequently than prescribed. Finally the third dental surgeon I consulted diagnosed the problem and cleaned and packed the infected socket. The pain then abated, and I've never taken Percodan or any other narcotic since.

Clearly, if drugs by themselves could cause addiction, we would not be safe offering narcotics to anyone. Medical evidence has repeatedly shown that opioids prescribed for cancer pain, even for long periods of time, do not lead to addiction except in a minority of susceptible people.[1]

During my years working on a palliative care ward I sometimes treated terminally ill cancer patients with extraordinarily high doses of narcotics—doses that my hardcore addict clients could only dream of. If the pain was alleviated by other means—for example, when a patient was successfully given a nerve block for bone pain due to malignant deposits in the spine—the morphine could be rapidly discontinued. Yet if anyone had reason to seek oblivion through narcotic addiction, it would have been these terminally ill human beings.

An article in the *Canadian Journal of Medicine* in 2006 reviewed international research covering over six thousand people who had received narcotics for chronic pain that was not cancerous in origin. There was no significant risk of addiction, a finding common to all studies that examine the relationship between addiction and the use of narcotics for pain relief.[2] "Doubts or concerns about opioid efficacy, toxicity, tolerance, and abuse or addiction should no longer be used to justify withholding opioids," concluded a large study of patients with chronic pain due to rheumatic disease.[3]

We can never understand addiction if we look for its sources exclusively in the actions of chemicals, no matter how powerful they are. "Addiction is a human problem that resides in people, not in the drug or in the drug's capacity to produce physical effects," writes Lance Dodes, a psychiatrist at the Harvard Medical School Division on Addictions.[4] It is true that some people will become hooked on substances after only a few times of using, with potentially tragic consequences, but to understand why, we have to know what about those individuals makes them vulnerable to addiction. Mere exposure to a stimulant or narcotic or to any other mood-altering chemical does not make a person susceptible. If she becomes an addict, it's because she's already at risk.

Heroin is considered to be a highly addictive drug—and it is, but only for a small minority of people, as the following example illustrates. It's well known that many American soldiers serving in the Vietnam War in the late 1960s and early 1970s were regular users. Along with heroin, most of these soldier addicts also used barbiturates or amphetamines or both. According to a study published in the *Archives of General Psychiatry* in 1975, 20 per cent of the returning enlisted men met the criteria for the diagnosis of addiction while they were in Southeast Asia, whereas before they were shipped overseas fewer than 1 per cent had been opiate addicts. The researchers were astonished to find that "after Vietnam, use of particular drugs and combinations of drugs decreased to near or even below preservice levels." The remission rate was 95 per cent, "unheard of among narcotics addicts treated in the U.S."*

"The high rates of narcotic use and addiction there were truly unlike anything prior in the American experience," the researchers concluded. "Equally dramatic was the surprisingly high remission rate after return to the United States."[5] These results suggested that the addiction did not arise from the heroin itself but from the needs of the men who used the drug. Otherwise, most of them would have remained addicts.

As with opiates so, too, with the other commonly abused drugs. Most people who try them, even repeatedly, will not become

* Remission: an abatement or reduction of symptoms in illness or addiction.

addicted.* According to a U.S. national survey, the highest rate of dependence after any use is for tobacco: 32 per cent of people who used nicotine even once went on to long-term habitual use. For alcohol, marijuana and cocaine the rate is about 15 per cent and for heroin the rate is 23 per cent.[6] Taken together, American and Canadian population surveys indicate that merely having used cocaine a number of times is associated with an addiction risk of less than 10 per cent.[7] This doesn't prove, of course, that nicotine is "more" addictive than, say, cocaine. We cannot know, since tobacco—unlike cocaine—is legally available, commercially promoted and remains, more or less, a socially tolerated object of addiction. What such statistics do show is that whatever a drug's physical effects and powers, they cannot be the *sole* cause of addiction.

—

For all that, there is a factual basis to the durable notion of certain drugs being inexorably addictive: *some people, a relatively small minority, are at grave risk for addiction if exposed to certain substances*. For this minority, exposure to drugs really will trigger addiction, and the trajectory of drug dependence, once begun, is extremely difficult to stop.

In the United States opiate relapse rates of 80 per cent to more than 90 per cent have been recorded among addicts who try to quit their habit. Even after hospital treatment the re-addiction rates are over 70 per cent.[8] Such dismal results have led to the impression that opiates themselves hold the power of addiction over human beings. Similarly, cocaine has been described in the media as "the most addictive drug on earth," causing "instant addiction." More recently, crystal methamphetamine (crystal meth) has gained a reputation as the most instantly powerful addiction-inducing drug—a well-deserved notoriety, so long as we keep in mind that the vast majority of people who use it do not become addicted.

* I'm not suggesting here that for those people who do not become addicted it's safe to use these drugs. I'm making a scientific case regarding the nature of addiction itself.

Statistics Canada reported in 2005, for example, that 4.6 per cent of Canadians have tried crystal meth, but only 0.5 per cent had used it in the past year.[9] If the drug by itself induced addiction, the two figures would have been nearly identical.

In one sense certain substances, like narcotics and stimulants, alcohol, nicotine and marijuana, can be said to be addictive, and it's in that sense that I use the term. *These are the drugs for which animals and humans will develop craving and which they will seek compulsively.* But this is far from saying that the addiction is caused directly by access to the drug. We will later explore why these substances have addictive potential; the reasons are deeply rooted in the neurobiology and psychology of emotions.

Because almost all laboratory animals can be induced into compulsive self-administration of alcohol, stimulants, narcotics and other substances, research has appeared to reinforce the view that mere exposure to drugs will lead indiscriminately to drug addiction. The problem with this apparently reasonable assumption is that animal laboratory studies can prove no such thing. The experience of caged animals does not accurately represent the lives of free creatures, including human beings. There is much to be learned from animal studies, but only if we take into account the real circumstances. And, I should add, only if we accept the tremendous suffering imposed on these involuntary "subjects."

Although there are anecdotes of animals in the wild becoming intoxicated, most of them are spurious, as is the case, for example, with stories of elephants getting "drunk" on fermenting marula fruit. There are no known examples of persistently addictive behaviours in the natural world. Of course, we cannot predict exactly what might happen if wild animals had free and easy access to addictive substances in the purified and potent forms administered in laboratories. What *has* been shown, however, is that conditions in the laboratory powerfully influence which animals will succumb to addiction. Among monkeys, for example, subordinate males who are stressed and relatively isolated are the ones more likely to self-administer cocaine. As I will later explain, being dominant leads to brain changes that give stronger monkeys some protection from an addictive response to cocaine.[10]

Bruce Alexander, a psychologist at Simon Fraser University in British Columbia, points out the obvious: laboratory animals in particular can be induced into addiction because they live under unnatural circumstances of captivity and stress. Along with other astute researchers, Dr. Alexander has argued that drug self-administration by these creatures may be how the animals "cope with the stress of social and sensory isolation." The animals may also be more prone to give themselves drugs because they are cooped up with the self-administration apparatus and cannot move freely.[11] As we will see, emotional isolation, powerlessness and stress are exactly the conditions that promote the neurobiology of addiction in human beings, as well. Dr. Alexander has conducted elegant experiments to show that even lab rats, given reasonably normal living situations, will resist the addictive appeal of drugs:

> My colleagues and I built the most natural environment for rats that we could contrive in the laboratory. "Rat Park," as it came to be called, was airy, spacious, with about 200 times the square footage of a standard laboratory cage. It was also scenic (with a peaceful British Columbia forest painted on the plywood walls), comfortable (with empty tins, wood scraps, and other desiderata strewn about on the floor), and sociable (with 16–20 rats of both sexes in residence at once).
>
> . . . We built a short tunnel opening into Rat Park that was just large enough to accommodate one rat at a time. At the far end of the tunnel, the rats could release a fluid from either of two drop dispensers. One dispenser contained a morphine solution and the other an inert solution.

It turned out that for the Rat Park animals, morphine held little attraction, even when it was dissolved in a sickeningly sweet liquid usually irresistible to rodents and even after these rats were forced to consume morphine for weeks, to the point that they would develop distressing physical withdrawal symptoms if they didn't use it. In other words, in this "natural" environment a rat will stay away from the drug if given a choice in the matter—even if it's already physically dependent on the narcotic. "Nothing that we tried," reported Bruce Alexander, "instilled a strong appetite for morphine or produced anything that looked like addiction in rats that were housed in a reasonably normal environment." By contrast, caged rats consumed up to twenty times more morphine than their relatively free living relatives.

Dr. Alexander first published these findings in 1981.[12] In 1980 it had already been reported that social isolation increased animals' intake of morphine.[13] Other scientists have since confirmed that some environmental conditions are likely to induce animals to use drugs; given different conditions, even captive creatures can resist the lure of addiction.

The Vietnam veterans study pointed to a similar conclusion: under certain conditions of stress many people can be made susceptible to addiction, but if circumstances change for the better, the addictive drive will abate. About half of all the American soldiers in Vietnam who began to use heroin developed addiction to the drug. Once the stress of military service in a brutal and dangerous war ended, so, in the vast majority of cases, did the addiction. The ones who persisted in heroin addiction back home were, for the most part, those with histories of unstable childhoods and previous drug use problems.[14]

In earlier military conflicts relatively few U.S. military personnel succumbed to addiction. What distinguished the Vietnam experience from these wars? The ready availability of pure heroin and of other drugs is only part of the answer. This war, unlike previous ones, quickly lost meaning for those ordered to fight and die in the faraway jungles and fields of Southeast Asia. There was too wide a gap between what they'd been told and the reality they witnessed and experienced. Lack of meaning, not simply the dangers and privations of war, was the major source of the stress that triggered their flight to oblivion.

—

Drugs, in short, do not make anyone into an addict, any more than food makes a person into a compulsive eater. There has to be a pre-existing vulnerability. There also has to be significant stress, as on these Vietnam soldiers—but, like drugs, external stressors by themselves, no matter how severe, are not enough. Although many Americans became addicted to heroin while in Vietnam, most did not.

Thus, we might say that three factors need to coincide for substance addiction to occur: *a susceptible organism; a drug with addictive potential; and stress.* Given the availability of drugs, individual susceptibility will determine who becomes an addict and who will not—for example, which two from among a random sample of ten U.S. GIs in Vietnam will fall prey to addiction.

In the rest of this section we'll investigate the roots of that susceptibility.

CHAPTER 13

A Different State of the Brain

"Addiction is mysterious and irrational," writes the psychiatrist Robert Dupont, who was the first director of the [U.S.] National Institute on Drug Abuse and White House drug czar under Presidents Nixon and Ford.[1]

Perhaps another view is possible. Addiction *is* irrational and at times the behaviour of addicts seems mystifying even to themselves. But what if we listen to addicts and hear their life histories as we began to do in the first part of this book? And what can we learn if we survey the brilliant and extensive scientific literature that has examined addiction from almost every conceivable angle? I believe that if we look with an open mind at this phenomenon called addiction, the sense of mystery will be replaced by an appreciation of complexity. We are left, above all, with awe for the amazing workings of the human brain and with compassion for those mesmerized by their addictive urges.

What does the research tell us?

—

As we have seen, laboratory animals can be led into drug and alcohol addiction. Hooked up to the appropriate apparatus and allowed unlimited access, many rats will self-administer intravenous cocaine to the point of hunger, exhaustion and death. Researchers even know how to make some laboratory creatures—rats, mice, monkeys and apes—more vulnerable to addiction by genetic manipulations or by interference with prenatal and post-natal development.

Animal experiments, some truly disturbing to read in detail, have allowed for finely tuned research into the relationships between brain circuitry, behaviour and addiction. Through new imaging methods we've been able to glimpse the human brain in action under the immediate influence of drugs and after long-term drug use. Radioactive techniques and magnetic frequencies enable researchers to measure blood flow to the brain and to gauge the level of energy used by brain centres during various activities or certain emotional states. Electroencephalograms (EEGs) have identified abnormal electrical brainwave patterns in some young people who are at greater-than-normal risk for alcoholism. Scientists have looked at the chemistry of the addicted brain, at its neurological connections and its anatomical structures. They've analyzed the workings of molecules, the membranes of cells and the replication of genetic material. They've investigated how stress activates the brain circuitry of addiction. Large-scale studies have examined what hereditary predispositions might contribute to addiction and how early life experiences may shape the brain pathways of addiction.

There are controversies, as we shall see, but everyone agrees that on the basic physiological level, addiction represents "a different state of the brain," in the words of physician and researcher Charles O'Brien.[2] The debate is over just exactly how that abnormal brain state arises. Are the changes in the addicted brain purely the consequence of drug use or is the brain of the habitual user somehow susceptible before drug use begins? Are there brain states that predispose a person to become addicted to drugs or to behaviours such as compulsive sexual adventuring or overeating? If so, are those predisposing brain states induced mostly by genetic inheritance or by life experience—or by some combination of both? The answers to these questions are crucially important for the treatment of addiction and for recovery.

The drug-addicted brain doesn't work in the same way as the nonaddicted brain and when imaged by means of PET scans and

MRIs,* it doesn't look the same. An MRI study in 2002 looked at the white matter in the brains of dozens of cocaine addicts from youth to middle age, in comparison with the white matter of nonusers. The brain's grey matter contains the cell bodies of nerve cells; their connecting fibres, covered by fatty white tissue, form the white matter. As we age, we develop more active connections and therefore more white matter. In the brains of cocaine addicts the age-related expansion of white matter is absent.[3] Functionally, this means a loss of learning capacity—a diminished ability to make new choices, acquire new information and adapt to new circumstances.

It gets worse. Other studies have shown that grey matter density, too, is reduced in the cerebral cortex of cocaine addicts—that is, they have smaller or fewer nerve cells than normal. A diminished volume of grey matter has also been shown in heroin addicts and alcoholics, and this reduction in brain size is correlated with the years of use: the longer the person has been addicted, the greater the loss of volume.[4] In the part of the cerebral cortex responsible for regulating emotional impulses and for making rational decisions, addicted brains have reduced activity. In special scanning studies these brain centres have also exhibited diminished energy utilization in chronic substance users, indicating that the nerve cells and circuits in those locations are doing less work. When tested psychologically, these same addicts showed impaired functioning of their prefrontal cortex, the "executive" part of the human brain. Thus, the impairments of physiological function revealed through imaging were paralleled by a diminished capacity for rational thought. In animal studies, reduced nerve cell counts, altered electrical activity and abnormal nerve cell branching in the brain were found after chronic cocaine use.[5] Similarly, altered structure and branching of nerve cells has been seen after long-term opiate administration and also with chronic nicotine use.[6] Such changes are sometimes reversible but can last for a long time and may even be lifelong, depending on the duration and intensity of drug use.

* PET: Positron Emission Tomography; MRI: Magnetic Resonance Imaging. Two recently developed, sophisticated imaging techniques that are now yielding new information about brain structure and functioning.

To write about the biology of addiction one must write about dopamine, a key brain chemical "messenger" that plays a central role in all forms of addiction. An imaging study of rhesus monkeys published in 2006 confirmed previous findings that the number of receptors for dopamine was reduced in chronic cocaine users.[7] Receptors are the molecules on the surfaces of cells where chemical messengers fit and influence the activity of the cell. Every cell membrane holds many thousands of receptors for many types of messenger molecules. Cells receive input and direction from other parts of the brain and the body and from the outside by means of messenger-receptor interactions. If it wasn't for their ability to exchange messages with their environment, cells could not function.

Cocaine and other stimulant-type drugs work because they greatly increase the amount of dopamine available to cells in essential brain centres. That sudden rise in the levels of dopamine, one of the brain's "feel-good" chemicals, accounts for the elation and sense of infinite potential experienced by the stimulant user, at least at the beginning of the drug habit.

As mentioned, it was already known that the brains of chronic cocaine users had fewer than normal dopamine receptors. The fewer such receptors, the more the brain would "welcome" external substances that could help increase its available dopamine supply. This recent primate study showed for the first time that the monkeys who developed a higher rate of cocaine self-administration—the ones who became more hardcore users—had a lower number of these receptors to begin with, *before* ever having been exposed to the chemical. This illuminating finding suggests that among rhesus monkeys, who are considered to be excellent models of human addiction, some are much more prone to extremes of drug dependence than others.

Stimulant drugs like cocaine and methamphetamine (crystal meth) exert their effect by making more dopamine available to cells that are activated by this brain chemical. Because dopamine is important for motivation, incentive and energy, a diminished number of receptors will reduce the addict's stamina and his incentive and drive for normal activities when not using the drug. It's a vicious cycle: more cocaine use leads to more loss of dopamine receptors. The fewer receptors, the more the addict needs to supply his brain with an artificial chemical to make up for the lack.

Why does chronic self-administration of cocaine reduce the density of dopamine receptors? It's a simple matter of brain economics. The brain is accustomed to a certain level of dopamine activity. If it is flooded with artificially high dopamine levels, it seeks to restore the equilibrium by reducing the number of receptors where the dopamine can act. This mechanism helps to explain the phenomenon of *tolerance,* by which the user has to inject, ingest or inhale higher and higher doses of a substance to get the same effect as before. If deprived of the drug, the user goes into withdrawal partly because the diminished number of receptors can no longer generate the required normal dopamine activity: hence the irritability, depressed mood, alienation and extreme fatigue of the stimulant addict without his drug: this is the *physical dependence* state discussed in Chapter 11. It can take months or longer for the receptor numbers in the brain to rise back to pre–drug use figures.

———

On the cellular level addiction is all about neurotransmitters and their receptors. In different ways, all commonly abused drugs temporarily enhance the brain's dopamine functioning. Alcohol, marijuana, the opiates heroin and morphine, and stimulants such as nicotine, caffeine, cocaine and crystal meth all have this effect. Cocaine, for example, blocks the reuptake, or re-entry, of dopamine into the nerve cells from which it is originally released.

Like all neurotransmitters, dopamine does its work in the space between cells, known as the synaptic space, or cleft. A synapse is where the branches of two nerve cells converge without touching, and it's in the space between them that messages are chemically transmitted from one cell to the next. That is why the brain needs chemical messengers, or neurotransmitters, to function. Released from a neuron, or nerve cell, a neurotransmitter such as dopamine "floats" across the synaptic space and attaches to receptors on a second neuron. Having carried its message to the target nerve cell, the molecule then falls back into the synaptic cleft, and from there it is taken back up into the originating neuron for later reuse; hence, the term reuptake. The *greater* the reuptake, the *less* neurotransmitter remains active between the neurons.

Cocaine's action may be likened to that of the antidepressant fluoxetine (Prozac). Prozac belongs to a family of drugs that increase the levels of the mood-regulating neurotransmitter serotonin between nerve cells by blocking its reuptake. They're called selective serotonin reuptake inhibitors, or SSRIs. Cocaine, one might say, is a dopamine reuptake inhibitor. It occupies the receptor on the cell surface normally used by the brain chemical that would transport dopamine back into its source neuron. In effect, cocaine is a temporary squatter in someone else's home. The more of these sites occupied by cocaine, the more dopamine remains in the synaptic space and the greater the euphoria reported by the user.[8]

Unlike Prozac, cocaine is not selective: it also inhibits the reuptake of other messenger molecules, including serotonin. By contrast, nicotine directly triggers dopamine release from cells into the synaptic space. Crystal meth both releases dopamine, like nicotine, and blocks its reuptake, like cocaine. The power of crystal meth to rapidly multiply dopamine levels is responsible for its intense euphoric appeal.

These stimulants directly increase dopamine levels, but the action of some chemicals on dopamine is indirect. Alcohol, for example, reduces the inhibition of dopamine-releasing cells. Narcotics like morphine act on natural opiate receptors on cell surfaces to trigger dopamine discharge.[9]

Activities such as eating or sexual contact also promote the presence of dopamine in the synaptic space. Dr. Richard Rawson, Associate Director of UCLA's Integrated Substance Abuse Program, reports that food seeking can increase brain dopamine levels in some key brain centres by 50 per cent. Sexual arousal will do so by a factor of 100 per cent, as will nicotine and alcohol. But none of these can compete with cocaine, which more than triples dopamine levels. Yet cocaine is a miser compared with crystal meth, or "speed," whose dopamine-enhancing effect is an astounding 1200 per cent.[10] It's easy to see why the crystal meth–addicted woman Carol spoke of the drug's effect as an "orgasm without sex." After repeated crystal meth use the number of dopamine receptors in crucial brain circuits will be reduced, just as with cocaine.

In short, drug use temporarily changes the brain's internal environment: the "high" is produced by means of a rapid chemical shift. There are also long-term consequences: chronic drug use remodels the brain's chemical structure, its anatomy and its physiological functioning. It even alters the way the genes act in the nuclei of brain cells. "Among the most insidious consequences to drugs of abuse is the vulnerability to craving and relapse after many weeks or years of abstinence," says a review of addiction neurobiology in a psychiatric journal. "The enduring nature of this behavioural vulnerability implies long-lasting changes in brain function."[11]

Since the brain determines the way we act, these biological changes lead to altered behaviours. It is in this sense that medical language refers to addiction as a chronic disease, and it is in this sense of a drug-affected brain state that I think the disease model is useful. It may not fully define addiction, but it does help us understand some of its most important features.

—

In any disease, say smoking-induced lung or heart disease, organs and tissues are damaged and function in pathological ways. When the brain is diseased, the functions that become pathological are the person's emotional life, thought processes and behaviour. And this creates addiction's central dilemma: if recovery is to occur, the brain, the impaired organ of decision making, needs to initiate its own healing process. An altered and dysfunctional brain must decide that it wants to overcome its own dysfunction: to revert to normal—or, perhaps, become normal for the very first time. The worse the addiction is, the greater the brain abnormality and the greater the biological obstacles to opting for health.

The scientific literature is nearly unanimous in viewing drug addiction as a chronic brain condition, and this alone ought to discourage anyone from blaming or punishing the sufferer. No one, after all, blames a person suffering from rheumatoid arthritis for having a relapse, since relapse is one of the characteristics of chronic illness. The very concept of choice appears less clear-cut if we understand that the addict's ability to choose, if not absent, is certainly impaired.

"The evidence for addiction as a different state of the brain has important treatment implications," writes Dr. Charles O'Brien. "Unfortunately," he adds, "most health care systems continue to treat addiction as an acute disorder, if at all."

—

CHAPTER 14

Through a Needle,
a Warm Soft Hug

All the substances that are the main drugs of abuse today originate in natural plant products and have been known to human beings for thousands of years.

Opium, the basis of heroin, is an extract of the Asian poppy *Papaver somniferum*. Four thousand years ago, the Sumerians and Egyptians were already familiar with its usefulness in treating pain and diarrhea and also with its powers to affect a person's psychological state. Cocaine is an extract of the leaves of *Erythroxyolon coca,* a small tree that thrives on the eastern slopes of the Andes in western South America. Amazon Indians chewed coca long before the Conquest, as an antidote to fatigue and to reduce the need to eat on long, arduous mountain journeys. Coca was also venerated in spiritual practices: Native people called it the Divine Plant of the Incas. In what was probably the first ideological "War on Drugs" in the New World, the Spanish invaders denounced coca's effects as a "delusion from the devil."

The hemp plant, from which marijuana is derived, first grew on the Indian subcontinent and was christened *Cannabis sativa* by the Swedish scientist Carl Linnaeus in 1753. It was also known to ancient Persians, Arabs and Chinese, and its earliest recorded pharmaceutical use appears in a Chinese compendium of medicine written nearly three thousand years ago. Stimulants derived from plants were also used by the ancient Chinese, for example in the treatment of nasal and bronchial congestion.

Alcohol, produced by fermentation that depends on microscopic fungi, is such an indelible part of human history and joy making that in many traditions it is honoured as a gift from the gods. Contrary to its present reputation, it has also been viewed as a giver of wisdom. The Greek historian Herodotus tells of a tribe in the Near East whose council of elders would never sustain a decision they made when sober unless they also confirmed it under the influence of strong wine. Or, if they came up with something while intoxicated, they would also have to agree with themselves after sobering up.

None of these substances could affect us unless they worked on natural processes in the human brain and made use of the brain's innate chemical apparatus. Drugs influence and alter how we act and feel because they resemble the brain's own natural chemicals. This likeness allows them to occupy receptor sites on our cells and interact with the brain's intrinsic messenger systems.

But why is the human brain so receptive to drugs of abuse? Nature couldn't have taken millions of years to develop the incredibly intricate system of brain circuits, neurotransmitters and receptors that become involved in addiction just so people could get "high" to escape their troubles or have a wild time on a Saturday night. These circuits and systems, writes a leading neuroscientist and addiction researcher, Professor Jaak Panksepp,* must "serve some critical purpose other than promoting the vigorous intake of highly purified chemical compounds recently developed by humans."[1] Addiction may not be a natural state, but the brain regions it subverts are part of our central machinery of survival.

I catch myself edging into a trap here. By writing that addiction "subverts" the brain, I realize I'm feeding the impression that addiction has a life of its own, like a virus invading the body, a predator ready to pounce or a foreign agent infiltrating an unsuspecting host country. In reality, the constellation of behaviours we call addiction is provoked by a complex set of neurological and emotional mechanisms that develop *inside* a person. These

* Head, Affective Neuroscience Research, Falk Center for Molecular Therapeutics, Northwestern University.

mechanisms have no separate existence and no conscious will of their own, even if the addict may often experience himself as governed by a powerful controlling force or as suffering from a disease he has no strength to resist.

So it would be more accurate to say: *addiction may not be a natural state, but the brain regions in which its powers arise are central to our survival.* The force of the addiction process stems from that very fact. Here's an analogy: let's say the section of someone's brain that controls body movements—the motor cortex—was damaged or did not develop properly. That person would inevitably have some kind of physical impairment. If the affected nerves managed nothing more than the motions of the little toe, any loss would hardly be noticeable. If, however, the damaged or undeveloped nerves governed the activity of a leg, the person would have a significant disability. In other words, the impairment would be proportional to the size and importance of the malfunctioning brain centre. So it is with addiction.

There is no addiction centre in the brain, no circuits designated strictly for addictive purposes. The brain systems involved in addiction are among the key organizers and motivators of human emotional life and behaviour; hence, addiction's powerful hold on human beings. Three major networks are involved. We'll look at the *opioid apparatus* in the rest of this chapter and, in Chapters 15 and 16, respectively, the *dopamine system* (which performs incentive-motivation functions) and the *self-regulation system* in the cortex, or grey matter. The defining molecules of the opioid apparatus are the brain's "natural narcotics"—the endorphins.

—

It was in the 1970s that an innate opioid system was first identified in the mammalian brain. The protein molecules that serve as the chemical messengers in this system were named endorphins by the U.S. researcher Eric Simon because they are endogenous—they originate within the organism—and because they bear resemblance to morphine. Morphine and its opiate cousins fit into the brain's endorphin receptors and thus, to quote a textbook on addiction research, the main endorphin receptor "represents the molecular gate for opioid addiction."[2] Humans are not the only creatures who have an innate opiate system. We share this pleasure with our near and distant relatives on the evolutionary ladder. Even one-celled organisms produce endorphins.

Not surprisingly, endorphins do for us exactly what plant-derived opioids can do: they're powerful soothers of pain, both physical and emotional. They grant, in the words of that opiate disciple Thomas De Quincey, "serenity, equipoise . . . the removal of any deep-seated irritation." For the distracted and soul-suffering person, a hit of endorphins, just like an infusion of opium products, "composes what has been agitated, concentrates what has been distracted."[3]

Beyond their soothing properties, endorphins serve other functions essential to life. They're important regulators of the autonomic nervous system—the part that's not under our conscious control. They affect many organs in the body, from the brain and the heart to the intestines. They influence mood changes, physical activity and sleep and regulate blood pressure, heart rate, breathing, bowel movements and body temperature. They even help modulate our immune system.

Endorphins are the chemical catalysts for our experience of key emotions that make human life, or any other mammalian life, possible. Most crucially, they enable the emotional bonding between mother and infant. When the natural opioid receptor systems of infant lab animals have been genetically "knocked out," they're unable to experience secure connection with their mothers. They're less distressed when separated from the mother, and this means they can't give her the signals she needs to act as their nurturer and protector. It's not that they can't feel discomfort or fear—they do when exposed to cold or to danger signals such as male mouse odours. But without opioid receptors they can't maintain the relationship with their mother, on whom their survival depends. They show no interest in their mother's cues.[4] Imagine the peril they would face if they acted indifferently to their mother in the wild. Conversely, young animals—dogs, chicks, rats and monkeys—who experience separation anxiety on being isolated from their mothers can be soothed by small, nonsedating doses of opiates.[5] Endorphins have been well described as "molecules of emotion."

The role of endorphins in human feelings was illustrated by an imaging study of fourteen healthy women volunteers. Their brains were scanned while they were in a neutral emotional state and then again when they were asked to think of an unhappy event in their lives. Ten of them recalled the death of a loved one, three remembered breakups with boyfriends and one focused on a recent argument with a close friend. Using a special tracer chemical, the scan highlighted the activity of opioid receptors in the emotional centres of each participant's brain. While the women were under the spell of sad memories, these receptors were much less active.[6]

On the other hand, positive expectations turn on the endorphin system. Scientists have observed, for example, that when people expect relief from pain, the activity of opioid receptors will increase. Even the administration of inert medications—substances that do not have direct physical activity—will light up opioid receptors, leading to decreased pain perception.[7] This is the so-called "placebo effect," which, far from being imaginary, is a genuine physiological event. The medication may be inert, but the brain is soothed by its own painkillers, the endorphins.

Opiate receptors can be found throughout the body and in each organ they play a specific role. In the nervous system they are tranquilizers and painkillers, but in, say, the gut, their role is to slow down muscle contractions. In the mouth, they diminish secretions. This is why narcotics taken for pain relief will cause unwanted side effects elsewhere in the body, such as constipation or a dry mouth. Why should there be so many different tasks for one class of natural chemicals? Because Nature, that thrifty homemaker, likes to preserve what is tried and true and to find as many uses as possible for each type of messenger protein. As evolution progressed, systems and substances that had a relatively narrow function in simpler organisms found new arenas of activity in the higher, more complex species that emerged.

Many other body chemicals serve multiple purposes—and the more evolved the organism, the more functions a particular substance will have. This is true even of genes: in one type of cell a certain gene will serve one function; elsewhere in the body, it will be assigned quite a different duty. In his book *Affective Neuroscience,* Dr. Jaak Panksepp gives a fascinating example of the role played in reptiles by vasotocin—a primitive version of the protein oxytocin, which triggers labour contractions and breastfeeding in female mammals.

> . . . Vasotocin is an ancient brain molecule that controls sexual urges in reptiles. This same molecule . . . also helps deliver reptilian young in the world. When a sea turtle, after thousands of miles of migration, lands on its ancestral beach and begins to dig its nest, an ancient bonding system comes into action . . . Vasotocin levels in the mother turtle's blood begin to rise as she digs a pit large enough to receive scores of eggs, and reach even higher levels as she deposits one egg after the other. With her labors finished, she covers the eggs, while circulating vasotocin diminishes to insignificant levels. Her maternal responsibilities fulfilled, she departs on another long sea journey.[8]

Mammalian mothers do not get off so easily—they stay with their helpless young. And oxytocin a more sophisticated version of vasotocin—plays a much more diverse role than its reptilian counterpart. It not only induces labour but also affects a mother's moods and promotes her physical and emotional nurturing of infants. In mammals of both sexes oxytocin also contributes to orgasmic pleasure and, more generally, may be considered one of the "love hormones." Just like opioids, oxytocin can reduce separation anxiety when infused into distressed young animals.

Significantly, oxytocin also interacts with opioids. It is not an endorphin, but it increases the sensitivity of the brain's opioid systems to endorphins—Nature's way of making sure that we don't develop a tolerance to our own opiates. (Remember that tolerance is the process by which an addict no longer feels the benefit of previously enjoyable doses of a drug and has to seek more and more.)

Why is it essential to prevent tolerance to our natural reward chemicals? Because opioids are necessary for parental love. The infant's well-being would be jeopardized if the mother became insensitive to the effects of her own opioids. Nurturing mothers experience major endorphin surges as they interact lovingly with their babies—endorphin "highs" can be one of the natural rewards of motherhood.

Given the many thankless tasks required in infant and child care, Nature took care to give us something to enjoy about parenting. Tolerance would more than rob of us those pleasures; it would threaten the infant's very existence. "It would be disastrous," writes Professor Panksepp, "if mothers lost their ability to feel intense social gratification from nurturance when children were still quite young."[9] By making our brain cells more sensitive to opioids, oxytocin allows us to remain "hooked" on our babies.

Opiates, in other words, are the chemical linchpins of the emotional apparatus in the brain that is responsible for protecting and nurturing infant life. *Thus addiction to opiates like morphine and heroin arises in a brain system that governs the most powerful emotional dynamic in human existence: the attachment instinct. Love.*

Attachment is the drive for physical and emotional closeness with other people. It ensures infant survival by bonding infant to mother and mother to infant. Throughout life the attachment drive impels us to seek relationships and companionship, maintains family connections and helps build community. When endorphins lock onto opiate receptors, they trigger the chemistry of love and connection, helping us to be the social creatures we are.

It may seem puzzling that Nature would have given one class of chemicals the apparently very different tasks of alleviating physical pain, easing emotional pain, creating parent–infant bonds, maintaining social relationships and triggering feelings of intense pleasure. In fact, the five roles are closely allied.

Opiates do not "take away" pain. Instead, they reduce our consciousness of it as an unpleasant stimulus. Pain begins as a physical phenomenon, registered in the brain, but we may or may not consciously notice it at any given moment. What we call "being in pain" is our subjective experience of that stimulus—i.e., "Ouch, that hurts"—and our emotional reaction to the experience.

Opiates help make some pain bearable. It has been suggested, for example, that high levels of endorphins help toddlers endure the many bumps and minor bruises they sustain on their rambunctious adventures. It's not that a toddler's injuries don't cause pain; they do. But partly because of endorphins, the pain isn't enough to discourage him. Without a high level of endorphins he might even want to stop his explorations of the world, so necessary for learning and development.[10] A child who complains bitterly of the slightest hurt and is often accused of being a "crybaby" is probably low on endorphins and is likely to be less adventurous than his peers.

Anatomically, physical pain is registered in one part of the brain, the thalamus, but its *subjective* impact is experienced in another part, the anterior cingulate cortex, or ACC. The brain gets the pain message in the thalamus, but "feels" it in the ACC. This latter area "lights up," or is activated, when we are reacting to the pain stimulus. And it's in the cortex—the ACC and elsewhere— that opiates help us endure pain by reducing not its physical but its emotional impact.

A recent imaging study showed that the ACC also "lights up" when people feel the pain of social rejection.[11] The brains of healthy adult volunteers were scanned as they were mentally participating in a game and then suddenly "excluded." Even this mild and obviously artificial "rejection" lit up the ACC and caused feelings of hurt. In other words, we "feel" physical and emotional pain in the same part of the brain—and that, in turn, is crucial to our bonding with others who are important to us. In normal circumstances, the emotional pain of separation keeps us close to each other when we most need that closeness.

Why did Nature make the mammalian opioid system responsible for our reactions to both physical and emotional pain? For a very good reason: the complete helplessness of the young mammal and its absolute dependence on nurturing adults. Physical pain is a danger alarm: if a child wakes up with a tummy ache, her ACC goes into overdrive and she'll give every possible signal to call her caregivers promptly to her side. For the infant mammal, emotional pain is an equally essential warning: it alerts us to the danger of separation from those we depend on for our very lives. Feeling this emotional pain triggers infant behaviours—ultrasonic vocalization in rat pups, pitiful crying in human babies—designed to bring the parent back.

The attentive presence of the nurturing adult will trigger endorphin release in the infant's brain, helping to soothe her.

A child can also feel emotional distress when their parent is physically present but emotionally unavailable. Even adults know that kind of pain when someone important to us is bodily present but psychologically absent. This is the state the seminal researcher and psychologist Allan Schore has called "proximal separation."[12] Given that the child's dependence is as much emotional as physical, in normal circumstances a child who senses emotional separation will seek to reconnect with the parent. Once more, the parent's loving response will flood the brain with endorphins and ease the child's discomfort. Should the parent not respond, or not respond adequately, endorphins won't be released, and the child will be left to his own inadequate coping mechanisms—for example, rocking or thumb-sucking as ways of self-soothing or tuning out to escape his distress. Children who have not received the attentive presence of the parent are, as we will see, at greater risk for seeking chemical satisfaction from external sources later in life.

In keeping with Nature's efficient, multipurpose "recycling" of chemical substances, endorphins are also responsible for experiences of pleasure and joyful excitement. Like infants and mothers, lovers, spiritual seekers and bungee jumpers—yes, bungee jumpers—all reach euphoric states in which endorphins play a key role. One study found that endorphin levels tripled in the blood of bungee jumpers for the half-hour following the leap and were correlated with the degree of reported euphoria: the higher the endorphin levels, the greater the euphoric feelings.[13]

While the brain's opiate receptors are the natural template for feelings of reward, soothing and connectedness, they are also triggered by narcotic drugs, and they play a role in other addictions, too. In a study of alcoholics, opioid receptor activity was diminished in several brain regions, and this was associated with increased alcohol craving.[14] The activation of opioid pathways and the resulting increased endorphin activity also enhances cocaine's effects.[15] As with alcohol, less endorphin activity means a greater desire for cocaine. Activation of opiate receptors contributes to the pleasures of marijuana use as well.[16]

In short, the life-foundational opioid love/pleasure/pain relief apparatus provides the entry point for narcotic substances into our brains. The less effective our own internal chemical happiness system is, the more driven we are to seek joy or relief through drug-taking or through other compulsions we perceive as rewarding.

The very essence of the opiate high was expressed by a twenty-seven-year-old sex trade worker. She had HIV and has since died. "The first time I did heroin," she said to me, "it felt like a warm soft hug." In that phrase she told her life story and summed up the psychological and chemical cravings of all substance-dependent addicts.

—

CHAPTER 15

Cocaine, Dopamine and Candy Bars: The Incentive System in Addiction

Lisa stands in the middle of my office and lifts her blouse to show the scattered red rash covering her abdomen, chest and back. Her body jerks around like a rigid puppet. In the crook of her right elbow she cradles a giant plastic bottle of orange drink as she would a baby or a doll. With her left hand she pulls at her hair. Although she's twenty-four years old, Lisa is so emotionally immature and physically childlike that often when I see her I think she belongs at home playing with dolls rather than here in the Downtown Eastside. Today her restless movements make her look even more childlike than usual. Her short stature, large eyes and puffy cheeks smeared with mascara and dried tears give her the look of an adolescent girl caught playing with her mother's makeup. She's high on cocaine.

"I've had this rash for three days. What is it, Doc?"

I ask her to sit so I can inspect her hands and feet. She pulls off her dirty white socks. The little red dots are visible on her palms and soles, as well.

"I'm afraid it's syphilis," I tell her. "You'll need a blood test."

In twenty years of family practice I never saw one case of syphilis; here in the Downtown East Side, it's diagnosed regularly.

As Lisa leaps to her feet, the plastic bottle clatters to the floor, spilling its contents. "How can it be syphilis?" she exclaims in a voice that mixes childish surprise with complaint. "I thought that was a sexual disease."

"It is."

"But can you get it when the guy just comes on your pussy?" For a moment her naïveté leaves me at a loss for words.

"Who was your partner?" I ask. "He ought to be tested as well."

"How should I know, Doc? It was in an alley. I was looking for coke money. It was the day before Welfare Wednesday and I couldn't wait anymore."

—

Many addicts have told me that cocaine is a tougher taskmaster than heroin, harder to escape. Although it doesn't cause physical withdrawal symptoms nearly as distressing, the psychological drive to use it seems more difficult to resist— even after it no longer gives much pleasure.

Cocaine increases brain levels of the neurotransmitter dopamine by blocking it from being transported back into the nerve cells that release it. (Recall that all drugs work by locking into receptor sites on cell surfaces.) Cocaine's effects wear off very quickly because it occupies its receptor sites for only a brief time. The urge to use, to get the next dopamine hit, then redoubles. Like other stimulant drugs—speed, nicotine and caffeine—cocaine taps directly into a brain system that, in its own way, is just as powerful as the opioid attachment/reward system described in the previous chapter. It plays a key role in all substance addictions and also in behavioural addictions.

There is an area in the midbrain which, when triggered, gives rise to intense feelings of elation or desire. It's called the ventral tegmental apparatus, or VTA. When researchers insert electrodes into the VTA of lab rats and the animals are given a lever that allows them to stimulate this brain centre, they'll do so to the point of exhaustion. They ignore food and pain just so they can reach the lever. Human beings may also endanger themselves in order to continue self-triggering this brain area. One human subject stimulated himself fifteen hundred times in a three-hour period, "to a point that he was experiencing an almost overwhelming euphoria and elation, and had to be disconnected despite his vigorous protests."[1]

Dopamine is the neurotransmitter chiefly responsible for the power of the VTA and its associated network of brain circuits. Nerve fibres from the VTA trigger dopamine release in a brain centre that plays a central role in all addictions: the nucleus accumbens, or NA, located on the underside of the front of the brain. Sudden increases in dopamine levels in the nucleus accumbens set off the initial excitement and elation experienced by drug users, and this is also what rats and people are after when they keep pushing those levers. All abusable substances raise dopamine in the NA, stimulants like cocaine most dramatically.

—

As in the case of the opioid apparatus, Nature did not design the VTA, the NA or other parts of the brain's dopamine system just so the addicts and drug users of the world could feel happier or more energized and focused. Indeed, the human brain's dopamine circuits are no less important to survival than its opioid system. If opioids help consummate our reward-seeking activities by giving us pleasure, dopamine initiates these activities in the first place. It also plays a major role in the learning of new behaviours and their incorporation into our lives.

Along with its connections in the forebrain and the cortex, the VTA thus forms the neurological basis of another major brain system involved in the addiction process: the incentive-motivation apparatus. This system responds to reinforcement, and reinforcers all have the effect of increasing dopamine levels in the nucleus accumbens.

Let's take a hypothetical situation involving a hypothetical "you." You see a chocolate bar in a Hallowe'en bag, and you're seized by a desire to munch on it: a classic example of a positively reinforced behaviour. That is, you've tasted a similar chocolate bar before and liked the experience. Now, when this new bar appears in your sight, dopamine is released in the NA, inciting you to take a bite. Your four-year-old daughter, to whom the bar belonged, accuses you of thieving. "The dopamine made me do it," you say in self-defence. Your daughter, nothing if not a reasonable preschooler, drops her resentment. "Of course, Daddy," she says sweetly, "because a cue associated with a previously pleasurable experience triggers a surge of dopamine in the NA and incites consummatory behaviour. Seeing my candy bar was your cue, and eating it was the consummatory behaviour. You have such a silly, predictable reinforcement system." "Wow," you say. "That's exactly right, honey. Will you share that last piece of chocolate with me?" "No way! Your dopamine circuits aren't my problem."

Environmental cues associated with drug use—paraphernalia, people, places and situations—are all powerful triggers for repeated use and for relapse, because they themselves trigger dopamine release. People trying to quit smoking, for example, are advised to avoid poker if they are used to having a cigarette while playing cards. Unless they move to a different area of town or to a recovery home, my Downtown Eastside patients find it virtually impossible to stop drug use, even when they form a strong intention to do so. Not only are drugs readily available, but everything and everyone in the environment reminds them of their habit.

Reinforcement is important in all addictions, drug-related or not. In my own case, it doesn't help matters that the Portland Hotel is located within a few blocks of those unscrupulous compact disc pushers at Sikora's, my favourite music haunt, and that I drive by there most days on my way to or from work. As I described earlier, I can feel excitement rising as I approach the store, even when I have no plan to go there, along with an urge to park the car and walk in. In my nucleus accumbens, the dopamine is flowing. The incentive is powerful.

Needless to say, life-essential reinforcers such as food and sex trigger VTA activation and dopamine release in the NA, since the performance of survival-related behaviours is the very purpose of the incentive-motivation system. Accordingly, this system is decisive in initiating activities such as foraging for food and other life-sustaining necessities, seeking sexual partners and exploring the environment. The VTA and NA and their connections with other brain circuits are also active when we explore novel objects and situations and evaluate them in light of previous reinforcing experiences. In other words, nerve fibres in the VTA are triggering dopamine release in the NA when a person needs to know, "Is this new whatever-it-is going to help me or hurt me? Will I like it or not?" The role of the dopamine system in novelty-seeking helps explain why some people are driven to risky behaviours such as street racing. It's one way to experience the excitement of dopamine release.

Dopamine activity also accounts for a curious fact reported by many drug addicts: that obtaining and preparing the substance gives them a rush, quite apart from the pharmaceutical effects that follow drug injection. "When I draw up the syringe, wrap the tie and clean my arm, it's like I'm already feeling a hit," Celia, the pregnant woman described in Chapter 6, once told me. Many addicts confess that they're as afraid of giving up the activities around drug use as they are of giving up the drugs themselves.

—

It is fascinating to look at some of the evidence linking the dopamine system to addictions. Animal experiments, distressing as they sometimes are to read about, can be stunning for their scientific ingenuity and technical expertise. Just how important dopamine receptors are to substance use was illustrated by a study of mice who had previously been trained to drink alcohol. They were given an "infusion" of dopamine receptors right into the nucleus accumbens. Before the infusion these rodents had fewer than normal dopamine receptors. The receptors were incorporated into a harmless virus that entered the animals' brain cells so that, temporarily, a normal range of receptor activity was achieved. As long as this artificial supply of dopamine receptors was available, the mice reduced their alcohol intake considerably—but they gradually became boozers again as the implanted receptors were lost to natural attrition.[2]

Why is this relevant? First, as I've already explained, chronic cocaine use reduces the number of dopamine receptors and thereby keeps driving the addict to use the drug simply to make up for the loss of dopamine activity. No wonder Lisa ended up with syphilis contracted in a back alley encounter. That was her way of obtaining the substance the incentive circuits in her brain were screaming for. (If she'd only had a nicotine addiction, she could have purchased a drug supplied by respectable manufacturers and dealers.) Dopamine receptor availability is also reduced in alcoholics, as well as in heroin and crystal meth addicts.[3]

More importantly, research now strongly suggests that the existence of relatively few dopamine receptors to begin with may be one of the biological bases of addictive behaviours.[4] When our natural incentive-motivation system is impaired, addiction is one of the likely consequences. But why would some creatures—human or non-human—have relatively few dopamine receptors? Why, in other words, would their natural incentive system be underfunctioning? I will soon present the evidence to show that such lacks are not random occurrences but have predictable—and preventable—causes.

—

As we have now seen, addiction inevitably involves both opioid and dopamine circuitry. The dopamine system is most active during the initiation and establishment of drug intake and other addictive behaviours. It is key to the reinforcing patterns of all drugs of abuse—alcohol, stimulants, opioids, nicotine and cannabis.[5] Desire, wanting and craving are all incentive feelings, so it is easy to see why dopamine is central to nondrug-related addictions, too. On the other hand, opioids—innate or external—are more responsible for the pleasure-reward aspects of addiction.[6]

Opioid circuits and dopamine pathways are important components of what has been called the limbic system, or the emotional brain. The circuits of the limbic system process emotions like love, joy, pleasure, pain, anger and fear. For all their complexities, emotions exist for a very basic purpose: to initiate and maintain activities necessary for survival. In a nutshell, they modulate two drives that are absolutely essential to animal life, including human life: attachment and aversion. We always want to move toward something that is positive, inviting and nurturing, and to repel or withdraw from something threatening, distasteful or toxic. These attachment and aversion emotions are evoked by both physical and psychological stimuli, and when properly developed, our emotional brain is an unerring, reliable guide to life. It facilitates self-protection and also makes possible love, compassion and healthy social interaction. When impaired or confused, as it often is in the complex and stressed circumstances prevailing in our "civilized" society, the emotional brain leads us to nothing but trouble. Addiction is one of its chief dysfunctions.

—

CHAPTER 16

Like a Child Not Released

Yesterday Claire sat in the hall area outside my office and howled bloody murder at the other patients awaiting their turns and, when I opened the door to let someone in, she aimed her invective at me. "You're not a doctor, you're the fucking Mafia!" was among the milder of the insults she hurled my way. There was no appeasing her. Kim, the Portland nurse, finally warned Claire that we'd call the police if she didn't leave off immediately. Sobbing, she made her way out the back door to the Portland's upper courtyard. At every step or two, she would turn around and scream hellishly at no one in particular, each epithet punctuated by a shower of spittle that sprayed from between her decayed teeth.

That's how Claire acts when she goes over to the dark side. She's one of the Portland's most challenging personalities. New staff are instructed never to let her into the reception office, no matter how positive she seems. One of her most recent borderline episodes counted a printer and the front desk phone system among its wounded.

Much of the time she ambles around like an overgrown child, craving love. "Dr. Maté, where's my hug?" she'll shout, running after me in the street. It's not personal to me; she begs for the same affection from Kim and many other Portland staff who have shown her kindness in the past. Her need for endorphins is as insatiable as is her need for the dopamine hits she gets from cocaine.

Today she's come to see me for a medical problem and we are calmly discussing the previous day's events.

"I can treat you in one of two ways," I say. "Like a totally mentally ill person, who's not responsible for what she does. Or I can treat you like you're not a mentally ill person, which is how I do try to relate to you. In that case you are responsible for what you do. Which do you prefer?"

"I don't know how to answer that," Claire smiles ruefully.

"Claire, it's not acceptable that you yell insults at me. It's not like anything even happened. Or whatever happened, happened in your mind, not in real life. You were screaming at me and at a whole bunch of other people who had as much right to see me as you did."

Claire bows her head. "I know, but I still don't know how to answer that."

"Was it cocaine?"

"Probably. I don't know." That means yes.

My voice loses some of its edge. "I really don't think you're in control when you're that way," I say. "I don't believe you're doing it deliberately."

Claire lifts her eyes to look straight at me. "Of course not," she says quietly.

"But what you do deliberately is that you use cocaine."

"Because I'm addicted to it."

"That's a choice you're making," I reply.

Even as the words leave my lips, I know I'm mouthing a platitude. From a certain point of view, everything we do is a choice. From a scientific perspective, though, Claire is closer to the mark. Her explanation that she is addicted—and that therefore her drug use is not the result of thoughtful deliberation—fits with the research evidence. It sounds like a cop-out, but in neurological terms, it's not.

—

"Recent studies have shown that repeated drug use leads to long-lasting changes in the brain that undermine voluntary control," says an article co-written by Dr. Nora Volkow, Director of the National Institute on Drug Abuse. "Although initial drug experimentation and recreational use may be volitional, once addiction develops this control is markedly disrupted."¹ In other words, drug addiction damages the parts of the brain responsible for decision making.

We've already seen that the brain circuits of motivation and of reward are recruited to serve addictive behaviours. In this chapter we'll consider scientific evidence suggesting that addiction also disrupts the *self-regulation circuits*—which the addict needs in order to choose *not* to be an addict.

We know which brain area controls actions like, say, the rotation of the thumb. If that area of the cortex is destroyed, the thumb doesn't move. The same principle applies to formulating decisions and regulating impulses. They, too, are governed by specific brain circuits and systems, but in a much more complex and interactive fashion than simple physical movements.

As with motor activities, we've discovered which parts of the brain are responsible for volition and choice by studying people whose brains have been injured. When certain brain areas are damaged, there are predictable patterns of impaired rational decision making and diminished impulse regulation. Brain-imaging studies and psychological testing indicate that *the same areas are also impaired in drug addiction*. And what is the result? If it wasn't enough that powerful incentive and reward mechanisms drive the craving for drugs, on top of that the circuits that could normally inhibit and control those mechanisms are not up to their task. In fact, they are complicit in the addiction process. A double whammy: the watchman is aiding the thieves.

—

To understand how this works, we need another glimpse at brain anatomy and physiology.

The human brain is the most complex biological entity in the universe. It has between 80 billion and 100 billion nerve cells, or neurons, each branched to form thousands of possible connections with other nerve cells. In addition, there are a trillion "support" cells, called glia, that help the neurons thrive and function. Laid end to end, the nerve cables of a single human brain would create a line several hundred thousand miles long. The total number of con-nections, or synapses, is in the incalculable trillions. The parallel and simultaneous activity of innumerable brain circuits and net-works of circuits produces millions of firing patterns every second of our lives. It's no wonder the brain has been described as a "super-system of systems."

In general, the higher in the brain we ascend physically, the more recent are the brain centres in evolutionary development and the more complex their functions. In the brain stem, automatic func-tions such as breathing and body temperature are regulated; the emotional circuits are higher up; and at the very top surface of the brain is the cortex, or grey matter. None of these areas works on its own; all are in constant communication with other circuits near and far, and all are influenced by chemical messengers from elsewhere in the body and brain. As a human being matures, higher brain sys-tems come to exert some control over the lower ones.

"Cortex" means bark and the multilayered cerebral cortex envelops the rest of the brain like the bark of a tree. About the size and thick-ness of a table napkin, it contains the cell bodies of neurons organ-ized into many essential centres, each with highly specialized functions. The visual cortex, for example, is in the occipital lobe at the back of the brain. If it sustains damage, as in the case of a stroke, vision is lost. The most recently evolved part of the cortex, distin-guishing us from other animals, is the prefrontal cortex, the grey mat-ter area in the front of the brain.

It's a simplification, but an accurate one, to say that the frontal cortex—and particularly its prefrontal portions—acts as the chief executive officer of the brain. It is here that alternatives are weighed and choices considered. It is also here that emotionally driven impulses to act are evaluated and either given permission to go ahead or—if necessary—inhibited. One of the most important duties of the cortex is "to inhibit inappropriate response rather than to produce the appropriate one," suggests neuropsychologist Joseph Ledoux.[2] The prefrontal cortex (PFC), writes psychiatrist Jeffrey Schwartz, "plays a central role in the seemingly free selection of behaviours" by inhibiting many of the alternative responses that arise in a situation, allowing only one to proceed. "It makes sense, then, that when this region is damaged patients become unable to stifle inappropriate responses to their environment."[3] In other words, people with impaired PFC function will have poor impulse control and will behave in ways that to others seem uncalled for, childish or bizarre.

It is also in the frontal cortex that social behaviours are learned. When the executive parts of the cortex have been destroyed in rats, they are still able to function—but only as immature youngsters who haven't acquired any social skills. They are impulsive, aggressive and sexually inappropriate. They behave very much like rats reared in isolation with no access to social play and other interactions.[4] Monkeys injured in the area of the right prefrontal cortex lose interactive skills such as the reading of emotional cues and the mutual grooming necessary for normal social contact. They soon come to be ostracized by their fellows. Human beings with prefrontal injuries also lose many of their social capacities. Here in the prefrontal cortex important nerve systems are implicated in addiction.

The executive functions of the prefrontal cortex are not restricted to any one area, and its proper workings depend on healthy connections and input from the emotional, or limbic, centres in lower parts of the brain. Conversely, dysfunction in the cortex helps to facilitate addictive behaviour. We'll now look at one particular prefrontal segment to understand how this happens.

—

Many studies link addiction to the orbitofrontal cortex (OFC), a cortical segment found near the eye socket, or orbit.[5] In drug addicts, whether they are intoxicated or not, it doesn't function normally. The OFC's relationship with addiction arises from its special role in human behaviour and from its abundant supply of opioid and dopamine receptors. It is powerfully affected by drugs and powerfully reinforces the drug habit. It also plays an essential supporting role in nondrug addictions. Of course, it doesn't function (or malfunction) on its own but forms part of an extensive and incredibly complex, multifaceted network—nor is it the only cortical area implicated in addiction.

Through its rich connections with the limbic (emotional) centres, the OFC is the apex of the emotional brain and serves as its mission control room. In normal circumstances in a mature human being, the OFC is among the highest arbiters of our emotional lives. It receives input from all the sensory areas, which allows it to process environmental data such as vision, touch, taste, smell and sound. Why is that important? Because it's the OFC's job to evaluate the nature and potential value of stimuli, based on present information—but also in light of previous experience. The neurological traces of early, formative events are embedded in the OFC, which, in turn, is connected with other memory-serving brain structures. So, for example, a smell that in early memory is associated with a pleasurable experience will likely be judged by the OFC in a positive way. Through its access to memory traces, conscious and unconscious, the OFC "decides" the emotional value of stimuli— for example, are we intensely drawn to or repelled by a person or object or activity, or are we neutral? It is constantly surveying the emotional significance of situations, their personal meaning to the individual. Through processes we are not consciously aware of, in microseconds the OFC decides our take on people or on a situation. Since our likes and dislikes, preferences and aversions strongly influence what we focus on, the OFC helps us decide to what or whom we should devote our attention at any given moment.[6]

The OFC—particularly on the right side of the brain—has a unique influence on social and emotional behaviours, including attachment (love) relationships. It is deeply concerned with the assessment of interactions between the self and others and plays a ceaseless (but fundamentally life-essential) game of "Who loves, who loves me not." It even gauges "How much does he/she love me or dislike me?"

While the explicit meaning of words spoken are decoded in specialized portions of the left hemisphere, the right OFC interprets the emotional content of communications—the other person's body language, eye movements and tone of voice. One cue the OFC watches for is the size of the other's pupils: in social interactions, especially in eyes set in a smiling face, dilated pupils mean enjoyment and delight. Babies are highly sensitive to such cues—as are aphasiac adults (people who, usually due to a stroke, have lost the ability to understand spoken language). Because they pay heed to physical/emotional rather than verbal messages, young children and aphasiacs have a much better sense of when they are being lied to than most of us.

These split-second analytic functions are unconscious. As in the old Mother Goose rhyme, we may be aware of the results but not of the process:

I do not like thee, Dr. Fell
The reason why I cannot tell.
But this I know, and know full well:
I do not like thee, Dr. Fell

In actual fact, the poor *doctor fell* victim to the anonymous poet's orbitofrontal cortex. Or, at the risk of completely alienating readers who aren't fond of word plays, Dr. Fell had a hard day at the OFC.

The OFC also contributes to decision making and to inhibiting impulses that, if allowed to be acted out, would be harmful—for example, inappropriate anger or violence. Finally, brain researchers have also linked the orbitofrontal cortex to our capacity to balance short-term objectives against longer-term consequences in the process of decision making.

Imaging studies consistently indicate that the OFC works abnormally in drug abusers, showing malfunctioning patterns in blood flow, energy use and activation.[7] No wonder, then, that psychological testing shows drug addicts to be prone to "maladaptive decisions when faced with short-term versus long-term outcomes, especially under conditions that involve risk and uncertainty."[8] Due to their poorly regulated brain systems, including the OFC, they seem programmed to accept short-term gain—for example, the drug high—at the risk of long-term pain: disease, personal loss, legal troubles and so on.

A regular finding of brain-imaging studies on drug addicts is *underactivity* of the OFC after detoxification.[9] In a similar vein, psychological testing of cocaine addicts has shown impaired decision making. In one study, some key aspects of their decision-making ability was a mere 50 per cent of normal. Only people with physical injury to the frontal cortex would score lower.[10]

It may seem paradoxical, but the OFC is also highly activated during craving—not to enhance decision making but to initiate craving itself. It turns out that different parts of the OFC have different functions: one part is involved in decision making; another in the automatic and emotional aspects of craving.[11] In imaging studies the OFC lights up when an addict so much as thinks about her drug.[12]

An abnormally functioning OFC has also been implicated in compulsive behaviours in both human and animal studies. A rat with a damaged orbitofrontal cortex will persevere in reward-seeking, addiction-type activities even after the rewards are removed. As the researchers comment, "these findings are reminiscent of the reports of drug addicts who claim that once they start taking a drug of abuse they cannot stop even when the drug is no longer pleasurable."[13]

—

If we consider the likelihood that Claire's apparatus for rational judgment and impulse control—including, prominently, the OFC—is impaired, we can begin to understand her aggressive behaviour the day before and also appreciate her argument that she does not "deliberately" use cocaine. With a malfunctioning OFC, she has little impulse inhibition. Instead, she carries immense, chaotic, ever-seething rage in her body and brain. Claire was raped repeatedly by her father over many years while her mother either didn't notice or looked away. Based on her history, it's certain that Claire also suffered psychological and physical abandonment almost from the moment of her birth. The emotional traces of those events are encoded in nerve patterns in her OFC, and that includes experiences she cannot consciously recall.*

* The brain structures for conscious recall develop during the first years of life, and aspects of the implicit memory system, which stores emotional memories, are present at birth. (And if they are present then, they likely existed before, as well.)

Cocaine disinhibits aggression. With little impulse control to begin with, under the influence of the drug Claire can become a rage machine—automatic, autonomic and, at such moments, virtually without conscious will.

But what about the "choice" I said she had when I was talking with her in my office— the choice to use cocaine the day before in the first place? Let's consider that question from the perspective of brain activity. It is not hyperbole to say that drugs have been the chief source of consolation that Claire, now in her thirties, has ever found. Ever since she began using in adolescence, they've offered her relief from searing emotional pain, loneliness, anxiety and a deep-seated fear of the world. As a result, her OFC has been trained to create a powerful emotional pull toward the drug from the second she even thinks about "fixing." Addiction research refers to this dynamic as *salience attribution:* the assignment of great value to a false need and the depreciation of true ones. It occurs unconsciously and automatically.

We can now reconstruct yesterday's events. When Claire sees the plastic bag with the white cocaine powder, the needle and the syringe—or when she so much as thinks about them—her brain will respond in a highly positive way. Owing to the OFC's influence on the incentive centres described in the last chapter, dopamine will start flowing in Claire's midbrain circuits. This causes the craving for the drug to intensify. Any thoughts of negative consequences are thrust aside: the part of the OFC that might speak up to warn her of these consequences is "gagged and bound." Thus Claire's OFC, impaired by years of drug use and perhaps even before then, encourages the self-harming activity, rather than inhibiting it. She injects.

Ten minutes later she takes her seat outside my office. Someone says the wrong thing—or she believes they do. Her OFC, unconsciously primed to recall the many times she has been attacked, insulted and injured, interprets this stimulus as a serious aggression. Claire is triggered. According to PET scans, the OFC distinguishes and reacts to angry, disgusted and fearful facial expressions in other people but not to neutral facial expressions.[14] Literally, all the "offending" person had to do was to look at Claire the wrong way.

After reading this description, you may think that I believe drug addicts bear no responsibility for their actions and have no choices. That is not my view, as I will explain later. I hope it's clear, however, that in the real world, choice, will and responsibility are not absolute and unambiguous concepts. People choose, decide and act in a context—and to a large degree, that context is determined by how their brains function. The brain itself also develops in the real world, influenced by conditions over which the individual, as a young child, had no choice whatsoever.

—

In this chapter we have seen that the orbitofrontal cortex, a central part of the brain system that regulates how we process our emotions and how we react to them, participates in substance dependence in a number of ways. First, it emotionally overvalues the drug, making it the chief concern of the addict—and often the only concern. It undervalues other objectives, such as food or health or relationships. By becoming triggered even at the thought of the drug (or activity) of choice, it contributes to craving. And finally, it fails at its task of impulse inhibition. It aids and abets the enemy.

All of this would explain an astonishing conversation with another patient, Don. It began with something he casually said as he sat down to wait for his methadone prescription.

"You what?"

Don sees my incredulity and gives me the sly smirk of a kid confessing a misdemeanour to an indulgent uncle. "You heard me. I pissed on the guy's leg, outside the pharmacy. The prick kept bothering me, so I said, 'George, you're talking a lot of bullshit. Is it wet enough for you?' And I took a leak on his pants."

I'm still shaking my head in disbelief. "You did that?"

"Yeah. I pissed on George's leg."

Don is in his thirties and, besides his methadone, he's on tranquilizing medications to control his behaviour. They do work well until he uses crystal meth. Then nothing works.

"All right, you did," I say. "Do you think that's appropriate?"

Today Don is clear of the drug, and he ponders my question for a moment before responding.

"No, it was pretty stupid . . . but . . . sometimes it's like . . . It's like, with my addiction . . . it's like I'm a child not released."

That's it—the neurobiology of addiction in a nutshell. Attacking energy, expressed as tantrums or aggression, rapidly erupts from a young child because the brain circuits that would allow him to resolve his frustrations in other ways are as yet unformed. The impulse control circuitry isn't connected yet either. Don, who has been a user since his adolescence, was never very mature to begin with. Decades of life as a drug addict have permitted very little continued maturation of either his behaviour or his brain. His experience tallies up with studies showing that the volume of drug users' grey and white matter is diminished and that this loss of cortical mass is correlated with length of drug use.[15]

Don has spent years living without any place to call home, surviving in the urban jungle by dint of street smarts, quick reflexes and intuition. Anywhere else he is out of his element. He's developed a cunning wisdom of sorts but never the capacity for self-control or normal social interaction or anything close to emotional balance. When his underdeveloped brain mechanisms are overwhelmed by drugs, he becomes—exactly as he says—a very young human being, not yet released from childhood.

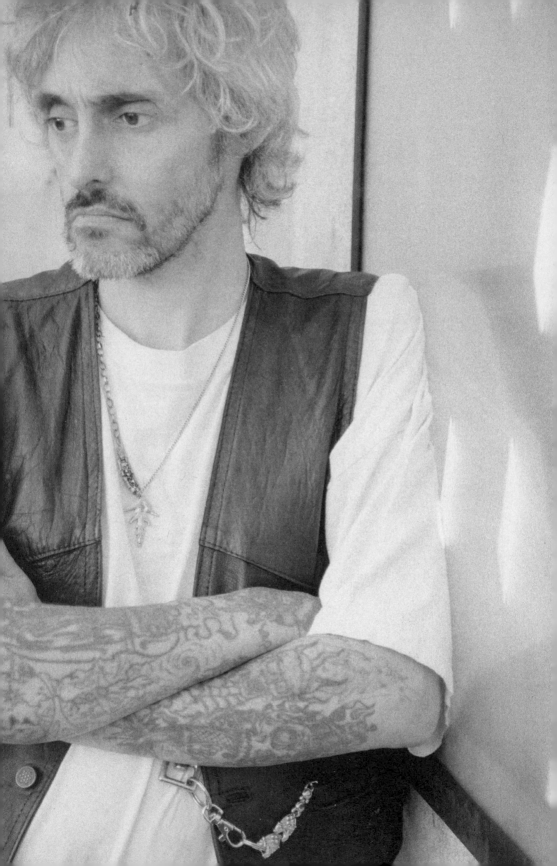

PART IV

—

How the Addicted
Brain Develops

If our society were truly to appreciate the significance of children's emotional ties throughout the first years of life, it would no longer tolerate children growing up, or parents having to struggle, in situations that cannot possibly nourish healthy growth.

STANLEY GREENSPAN, M.D.

CHILD PSYCHIATRIST AND FORMER DIRECTOR, CLINICAL

INFANT DEVELOPMENT PROGRAM, [U.S.] NATIONAL

INSTITUTE OF MENTAL HEALTH

—

CHAPTER 17

Their Brains Never Had a Chance

My first book, *Scattered Minds*, published in 2000, dealt with attention deficit disorder, a condition I myself have. It so happens that ADD is a major risk factor for addiction to a number of substances, including nicotine, cocaine, alcohol, cannabis and crystal meth, and also for gambling and other behavioural addictions—but that's not why I'm mentioning the book here. Rather, I want to tell an anecdote from just before its publication.

In *Scattered Minds*, I had laid out some well-established research evidence showing that the mammalian brain develops largely under the influence of the environment, rather than according to strict genetic predetermination—and that this is especially the case with the human brain. These findings were relatively recent but by then wholly uncontroversial, at least in brain science circles. They were not obscure academic secrets but had been the subjects of cover articles in both *Time* and *Newsweek*.

I was speaking on the phone with a young producer who had called me from Toronto to discuss a possible studio interview on a national television program. We were going over what material I might present on the air. I was just getting into some of the more fascinating of the research points when she interrupted me. "Wait. You mean to tell me that the size of a mother's pupils and how she looks at her baby will affect the chemistry of the kid's brain?" "Not only will it," I said, "it does so instantaneously!" I was on a roll, certain that this producer was just as enthralled as I with the insights of developmental neuroscience. "Over time, if there's a pattern of—"

"That's ridiculous," she said, interrupting a second time. "There's no way we can use that." And before I could ask her on what grounds she was rejecting the fruits of several decades of scientific investigation, she hung up.

That a TV producer, or any layperson for that matter, would have trouble accepting the new brain science is understandable, given the mind-body separation prevalent in our culture, and given, too, how long we've been taught that genes determine almost everything about a human being: personality traits, behaviour, eating patterns and all manner of disease. Much more perplexing is the fact that this new knowledge is virtually unfamiliar to the medical community. Despite the thousands of research papers published in leading scientific and medical journals, countless monographs and conference documents and several outstanding academic books on the subject, the role of the environment in brain development isn't taught in many medical schools.[1] It's not incorporated into our work with children or adults. Not only is brain development ignored in medical training, so is human psychological development. "It is astonishing to realize," remarks neurologist Antonio Damasio, "that [medical] students learn about psychopathology without ever being taught normal psychology."[2]

Such neglect is a loss for medical practice, and for millions of patients. Greater awareness of developmental influences on brain functioning and the personality would enrich and empower every field of medicine. And if more doctors knew what there is to know about this, I am convinced it would encourage a radical and overdue rethinking of social attitudes towards addiction.

Brain development in the uterus and during childhood is the single most important biological factor in determining whether or not a person will be predisposed to substance dependence and to addictive behaviours of any sort, whether drug-related or not. Startling as this view may appear to be at first sight, it is amply supported by recent research. Dr. Vincent Felitti was chief investigator in a landmark study of over seventeen thousand middle-class Americans for Kaiser Permanente and the [U.S.] Centres for Disease Control. "The basic cause of addiction is predominantly experience-dependent during childhood, and not substance-dependent," Dr. Felitti has written. "The current concept of addiction is ill-founded."[3]

To state that childhood brain development has the greatest impact on addiction is not to rule out genetic factors. However, the emphasis placed on genetic influences in addiction medicine—and in many other areas of medicine—is an impediment to our understanding.

—

"The human brain, a 3-pound mass of interwoven nerve cells that controls our activity, is one of the most magnificent—and mysterious—wonders of creation. The seat of human intelligence, interpreter of senses, and controller of movement, this incredible organ continues to intrigue scientists and laymen alike."

With these words President George H.W. Bush inaugurated the 1990s as "the decade of the brain." In the United States there followed an inspiring expansion of research into the workings and development of the brain. When the findings were collated, together with previously available information, a fresh and exciting view of brain development emerged. Old assumptions were discarded and a new paradigm established. Many of the details remain to be discovered, of course—the work of centuries, suggests Professor Jaak Panksepp in *Affective Neuroscience*—but the outlines are not in doubt. The view that genes play a decisive role in the way a person's brain develops has been replaced by a radically different notion: *the expression of genetic potentials is, for the most part, contingent on the environment.* Genes do dictate the basic organization, developmental schedule and anatomical structure of the human central nervous system, but it's left to the environment to sculpt and fine-tune the chemistry, connections, circuits, networks and systems that determine how well we function.

Of all the mammals, we humans have the least mature brain at birth. Early in their infancy other newborn animals perform tasks far beyond the capabilities of human babies. A horse, for example, can run on its first day of life. Not for a year and a half or more can most humans muster the muscle strength, visual acuity and neurological control skills—perception, balance, orientation in space, coordination—to perform that activity. In other words, the horse's brain development at birth is at least a year and a half ahead of our own—probably even more, in horse years.

Why are we saddled with such a disadvantage in comparison to a horse? We can think of it as a compromise imposed by Nature. Our evolutionary predecessors were permitted to walk upright, which freed forelimbs to evolve into arms and hands capable of many delicate and complicated activities. Those advances in manual versatility and dexterity required a tremendous enlargement of the brain, especially of its frontal areas. Our frontal lobes, which coordinate the movement of our hands, are much larger even than those of our closest evolutionary relative, the chimpanzee. These lobes, particularly their prefrontal areas, are also responsible for the problem solving, social and language skills that have allowed humankind to thrive. As we became a two-legged species, the human pelvis had to narrow to accommodate our upright stance. At the end of the nine months of human gestation the head forms the largest diameter of the body, the one most likely to get stuck in our journey through the birth canal. It's simple engineering: any further brain growth in the uterus and we couldn't be born.

To ensure that babies can make their way out of the birth canal, the bargain forced upon our ancestors was that the human brain would be relatively small and immature at birth. On the other hand, it would undergo tremendous growth outside the mother's body. In the period following birth, the human brain, unlike that of the chimpanzee, continues to grow at the same rate as in the womb. There are times in the first year of life when, every second, multiple millions of nerve connections, or synapses, are established. Three-quarters of our brain growth takes place outside the womb, most of it in the early years. By three years of age, the brain has reached 90 per cent of adult size, whereas the body is only 18 per cent of adult size.[4] This explosion in growth outside the womb gives us a far higher potential for learning and adaptability than is granted to other mammals. Were we born with our brain development rigidly predetermined by heredity, the frontal lobes would be limited in their capacity to help us learn and adapt to the many different environments and social situations we humans now inhabit.

Greater reward demands greater risk. Outside the relatively safe environment of the womb, our brains-in-progress are highly vulnerable to potentially adverse circumstances. Addiction is one of the possible negative outcomes—although, as we will see when we discuss genetic influences, the brain can already be negatively affected in the uterus in ways that increase vulnerability to addiction and to many other chronic conditions that threaten health.

The dynamic process by which 90 per cent of the human brain's circuitry is wired after birth has been called "neural Darwinism" because it involves the selection of those nerve cells (neurons), synapses and circuits that help the brain adapt to its particular environment, and the discarding of others. In the early stages of life, the infant's brain has many more neurons and connections than necessary—billions of neurons in excess of what will eventually be required. This overgrown, chaotic synaptic tangle needs to be trimmed to shape the brain into an organ that can govern action, thought, learning and relationships and carry out its multiple and varied other tasks—and to coordinate them all in our best interests. Which connections survive depends largely on input from the environment. Connections and circuits used frequently are strengthened, while unused ones are pruned out: indeed, scientists call this aspect of neural Darwinism *synaptic pruning*. "Both neurons and neural connections compete to survive and grow," write two researchers. "Experience causes some neurons and synapses (and not others) to survive and grow."[5]

Through this weeding out of unutilized cells and synapses, the selection of useful connections and the formation of new ones, the specialized circuits of the maturing human brain emerge. The process is highly specific to each individual person—so much so that not even the brains of identical twins have the same nerve branching, connections and circuitry. In large part, an infant's early years define how well her brain structures will develop and how the neurological networks that control human behaviour will mature. "Developmental experiences determine the organizational and functional status of the mature brain," writes child psychiatrist and researcher Bruce Perry.[6] Or in the words of Dr. Robert Post, chief of the Biological Psychiatry Branch of the [U.S.] National Institute of Mental Health: "At any point in this process you have all these potentials for either good or bad stimulation to get in there and set the microstructure of the brain."[7] And it is precisely here where the problem arises for young children who will, in adolescence and beyond, become chronically hooked on hard drugs: too much of what Dr. Post called bad stimulation. This is true of the hardcore intravenous drug users such as the ones I deal with in the Downtown Eastside. In many other cases it's not a question of "bad stimulation" but of a lack of sufficient "good stimulation."

Our genetic capacity for brain development can find its full expression only if circumstances are favourable. To illustrate this, just imagine a baby who was cared for in every way but kept in a dark room. After a year of such sensory deprivation the brain of this infant would not be comparable to those of others, no matter what his inherited potential. Despite perfectly good eyes at birth, without the stimulation of light waves, the thirty or so neurological units that together make up our visual sense would not develop. The neural components of vision already present at birth would atrophy and become useless if this child did not see light for about five years. Why? Neural Darwinism. Without the requisite stimulation during the critical period allotted by Nature for the visual system's development, the child's brain would never have received the information that being able to see is needed for survival. Irreversible blindness would be the result.

What is true for vision is also true for the dopamine circuits of incentive-motivation and the opioid circuitry of attachment-reward, as well as for the regulatory centres in the prefrontal cortex, such as the orbitofrontal cortex—in other words, for all the major brain systems implicated in addiction that we surveyed in the previous three chapters. In the case of these circuits, which process emotions and govern behaviour, it is the *emotional environment* that is decisive. By far the dominant aspect of this environment is the role of the nurturing adults in the child's life, especially in the early years.

The three environmental conditions absolutely essential to optimal human brain development are nutrition, physical security and consistent emotional nurturing. In the industrialized world, except in cases of severe neglect or dire poverty, the baseline nutritional and shelter needs of children are usually satisfied. The third prime necessity—emotional nurture—is the one most likely to be disrupted in Western societies. The importance of this point cannot be overstated: *emotional nurturance is an absolute requirement for healthy neurobiological brain development.* "Human connections create neuronal connections"—in the succinct phrase of child psychiatrist Daniel Siegel, a founding member of UCLA's Center for Culture, Brain and Development.[8] As we will soon see, this is particularly so for the brain systems involved in addiction. The child needs to be in an *attachment relationship* with at least one reliably available, protective, psychologically present and reasonably non-stressed adult.

Attachment, as we've already learned, is the drive to pursue and preserve closeness and contact with others; an attachment relationship exists when that state has been achieved. It's an instinctual drive programmed into the mammalian brain, owing to the absolute helplessness and dependency of infant mammals—particularly infant humans. Without attachment he cannot survive; without safe, secure and nonstressed attachment, his brain cannot develop optimally. Although that dependency wanes as we mature, attachment relationships remain important throughout our lifetime.

Daniel Siegel writes in *The Developing Mind*:

For the infant and young child, attachment relationships are the major environmental factors that shape the development of the brain during its period of maximal growth . . . Attachment establishes an interpersonal relationship that helps the immature brain use the mature functions of the parent's brain to organize its own processes.[9]

To begin to grasp the matter, all we need to do is picture a child who was never smiled at, never spoken to in a warm and loving way, never touched gently, never played with. Then we can ask our-selves: What sort of person do we envision such a child becoming?

Infants require more than the physical presence and attention of the parent. Just as the visual circuits need light waves for their development, the emotional centres of the infant brain, in particu-lar the all-important orbitofrontal cortex (OFC), require healthy emotional input from the parenting adults. Infants read, react to and are developmentally influenced by the psychological states of the parents. They are affected by body language: tension in the arms that hold them, tone of voice, joyful or despondent facial expressions and, yes, the size of the pupils. In a very real sense, the parent's brain programs the infant's, and this is why stressed par-ents will often rear children whose stress apparatus also runs in high gear, no matter how much they love their child and no matter that they strive to do their best.

The electrical activity of the infant's brain is exquisitely sensitive to that of the nurturing adult. A study at the University of Washington in Seattle compared the brainwave patterns of two groups of six-month-old infants: one group whose mothers were suffering postpartum depression and one group whose mothers were in normal good spirits. Electroencephalograms, or EEGs, showed consistent, marked differences between the two groups: the babies of the depressed mothers had EEG patterns characteris-tic of depression *even during interactions with their mothers that were meant to elicit a joyful response*. Significantly, these effects were noted only in the frontal areas of the brain, where the centres for the self-regulation of emotion are located.[10] How does this per-tain to brain development? Repeatedly-firing nerve patterns become wired into the brain and will form part of a person's habit-ual responses to the world. In the words of the great Canadian neu-roscientist Donald Hebb, "cells that fire together, wire together." The infants of stressed or depressed parents are likely to encode negative emotional patterns in their brains.

The long-term effect of parental mood on the biology of the child's brain is illustrated by several studies showing that concentra-tions of the stress hormone cortisol are elevated in the children of clinically depressed mothers. At age three, the highest cortisol levels were found in those children whose mothers had been depressed during the child's first year of life, rather than later.*[11] Thus we see that the brain is "experience-dependent." Good experiences lead to healthy brain development, while the absence of good experiences or the presence of bad ones distorts development in essential brain structures. Dr. Rhawn Joseph, a scientist at the Brain Research Laboratory in San Jose, California, explains it this way:

> [An] abnormal or impoverished rearing environment can decrease a thousand fold the number of synapses per axon [the long extension from the cell body that conducts electrical impulses toward another neuron], retard growth and eliminate billions if not trillions of synapses per brain, and result in the preservation of abnormal interconnections which are normally discarded over the course of development.[12]

Since the brain governs mood, emotional self-control and social behaviour, we can expect that the neurological consequences of adverse experiences will lead to deficits in the personal and social lives of people who suffer them in childhood, including, Dr. Joseph continues, "a reduced ability to anticipate consequences or to inhibit irrelevant or inappropriate, self-destructive behaviors."

Were these not exactly the dysfunctions we witnessed in Claire and Don in the previous chapter? It's what we see in all hardcore drug addicts.

We know that the majority of chronically hardcore substance-dependent adults lived, as infants and children, under conditions of severe adversity that left an indelible stamp on their development. Their predisposition to addiction was programmed in their early years. Their brains never had a chance.

---

* Such information ought to increase our respect for, and social and cultural support for, the parenting task. No one becomes depressed on purpose and, in my observation, depression in a new mother often reflects a lack of sufficient support in her environment.

—

CHAPTER 18

Trauma, Stress and the Biology of Addiction

The idea that the environment shapes brain development is a very straightforward one, even if the details are immeasurably complex. Think of a kernel of wheat. No matter how genetically sound a seed may be, factors such as sunlight, soil quality and irrigation must act on it properly if it is to germinate and grow into a healthy adult plant. Two identical seeds, cultivated under opposing conditions, would yield two different plants: one tall, robust and fertile; the other stunted, wilted and unproductive. The second plant is not diseased: it only lacked the conditions required to reach its full potential. Moreover, if it does develop some sort of plant ailment in the course of its life, it would be easy to see how a deprived environment contributed to its weakness and susceptibility. The same principles apply to the human brain.

The three dominant brain systems in addiction—the opioid attachment-reward system, the dopamine-based incentive-motivation apparatus and the self-regulation areas of the prefrontal cortex—are all exquisitely fine-tuned by the environment. To various degrees, in all addicted persons these systems are out of kilter. The same is true, we will see, of the fourth brain-body system implicated in addiction: the stress-response mechanism.

Happy, attuned emotional interactions with parents stimulate a release of natural opioids in an infant's brain. This endorphin surge promotes the attachment relationship and the further development of the child's opioid and dopamine circuitry.[1] On the other hand, stress reduces the numbers of both opiate and dopamine receptors. Healthy growth of these crucial systems—responsible for such essential drives as love, connection, pain relief, pleasure, incentive and motivation—depends, therefore, on the quality of the attachment relationship. When circumstances do not allow the infant and young child to experience consistently secure interactions or, worse, expose him to many painfully stressing ones, maldevelopment often results.

Dopamine levels in a baby's brain fluctuate, depending on the presence or absence of the parent. In four-month-old monkeys major alterations of dopamine and other neurotransmitter systems were found after only six days of separation from their mothers. "In these experiments," writes Dr. Steven Dubovsky, "loss of an important attachment appears to lead to less of an important neurotransmitter in the brain. Once these circuits stop functioning normally, it becomes more and more difficult to activate the mind."[2]

We know from animal studies that social-emotional stimulation is necessary for the growth of the nerve endings that release dopamine and for the growth of receptors to which dopamine needs to bind in order to do its work. Even adult rats and mice kept in long-term isolation will have a reduced number of dopamine receptors in the midbrain incentive circuits and, notably, in the frontal areas implicated in addiction.[3] Rats separated from their mothers at an early stage display permanent disruption of the dopamine incentive-motivation system in their midbrains. As we already know, abnormalities in this system play a key role in the onset of addiction and craving. Predictably, in adulthood these maternally deprived animals exhibit a greater propensity to self-administer cocaine.[4] And it doesn't take extreme deprivation: in another study, rat pups deprived of their mother's presence for only one hour a day during their first week of life grew up to be much more eager than their peers to take cocaine on their own.[5] So the presence of consistent parental contact in infancy is one factor in the normal development of the brain's neurotransmitter systems; the absence of it makes the child more vulnerable to "needing" drugs of abuse later on to supplement what her own brain is lacking. Another key factor is the *quality* of the contact the parent provides, and this, as we saw in the previous chapter, depends very much on the parent's mood and stress level.

All mammalian mothers—and many human fathers, as well—give their infants sensory stimulation that has long-term positive effects on their offspring's brain chemistry. Such sensory stimulation is so necessary for the human infant's healthy biological development that babies who are never picked up simply die. They stress themselves to death. Premature babies who have to live in incubators for weeks or months have faster brain growth if they are stroked for just ten minutes a day. When I learned such facts in the research literature, I recalled with appreciation a custom I had often observed among my Indo-Canadian patients during my years in family practice. As they were speaking with me during their early post-natal visits, these mothers would massage their babies all over their bodies, gently kneading them from feet to head. The infants were in bliss.

Humans hold and cuddle and stroke; rats lick. A 1998 study found that rats whose mothers had given them more licking and other kinds of nurturing contact during their infancy had, as adults, more efficient brain circuitry for reducing anxiety. They also had more receptors on their nerve cells for benzodiazepines, which are natural tranquilizing chemicals found in the brain.[6] I think here of my many patients who, on top of cocaine and heroin addictions, have been hooked since their adolescence on street-peddled "benzo" drugs like Valium to calm their jangled nervous systems. For a dollar a tablet, they get an artificial hit of the benzodiazepines their own brains can't supply. Their need for tranquilizers says much about their infancy and early childhood.

Parental nurturing determines the levels of other key brain chemicals, too—including serotonin, the mood messenger enhanced by antidepressants like Prozac. Peer-reared monkeys, separated from their mothers in laboratory experiments, have lower lifelong levels of serotonin than monkeys brought up by their mothers. In adolescence these same monkeys are more aggressive and are far more likely to consume alcohol in excess.[7] We see similar effects with other neurotransmitters that are

essential in regulating mood and behaviour, such as norepinephrine.[8] Even slight imbalances in the availability of these chemicals are manifested in aberrant behaviours like fearfulness and
hyperactivity, and increase the individual's sensitivity to stressors
for a lifetime. In turn, such acquired traits increase the risk of
addiction.

Another effect of early maternal deprivation appears to be a permanent decrease in the production of oxytocin,* which, as mentioned in Chapter 14, is one of our love chemicals.[9] It is critical to
our experience of loving attachments and even to maintaining committed relationships. People who have difficulty forming intimate
relationships are at risk for addiction; they may turn to drugs as
"social lubricants."

Not only can early childhood experience lead to a dearth of
"good" brain chemicals; it can also result in a dangerous overload
of others. Maternal deprivation and other types of adversity during
infancy and childhood result in chronically high levels of the stress
hormone cortisol. In addition to damaging the midbrain dopamine
system, excess cortisol shrinks important brain centres such as the
hippocampus—a structure important for memory and for the processing of emotions—and disturbs normal brain development in
many other ways, with lifelong repercussions.[10] Another major
stress chemical that's permanently overproduced after insufficient
early maternal contact is vasopressin, which is implicated in high
blood pressure.[11]

A child's capacity to handle psychological and physiological stress
is completely dependent on the relationship with his parent(s).
Infants have no ability to regulate their own stress apparatus, and
that's why they will stress themselves to death if they are never
picked up. We acquire that capacity gradually as we mature—or we
don't, depending on our childhood relationships with our caregivers.
A responsive, predictable nurturing adult plays a key role in the
development of our healthy stress-response neurobiology.[12]

---

* As noted earlier, oxytocin is not an opioid. Therefore, it has no relationship
  whatsoever with narcotic drugs like Oxycet or OxyContin; only the names are
  similar.

In the words of one researcher, "maternal contact alters the neu-robiology of the infant."* [13] Children who suffer disruptions in their attachment relationships will not have the same biochemical milieu in their brains as their well-attached and well-nurtured peers. As a result their experiences and interpretations of their environment, and their responses to it, will be less flexible, less adaptive and less conducive to health and maturity. Their vulnerability will increase, both to the mood-enhancing effect of drugs and to becoming drug dependent. We know from animal studies, for example, that early weaning can have an influence on later substance intake: rat pups weaned from their mothers at two weeks of age had, as adults, a greater propensity to drink alcohol than pups weaned just one week later. [14]

—

The statistics that reveal the typical childhood of the hardcore drug addict have been reported widely but, it seems, not widely enough to have had the impact they ought to on mainstream medical, social and legal understandings of drug addiction.

Studies of drug addicts repeatedly find extraordinarily high percentages of childhood trauma of various sorts, including physical, sexual and emotional abuse. One group of researchers was moved to remark that "our estimates . . . are of an order of magnitude rarely seen in epidemiology and public health." [15] Their research, the renowned Adverse Childhood Experiences (ACE) Study, looked at the incidence of ten separate categories of painful circumstances—including family violence, parental divorce, drug or alcohol abuse in the family, death of a parent and physical or sexual abuse—in thousands of people. The correlation between these figures and substance abuse later in the subjects' lives was then calculated. For each adverse childhood experience, or ACE, the risk for the early initiation of substance abuse increased two to four times. Subjects

* In the human context "maternal" does not necessarily refer to a female mothering figure or to a biological parent. It can also refer to primary caregivers of either gender.

with five or more ACEs had seven to ten times greater risk for substance abuse than those with none.

The ACE researchers concluded that nearly two-thirds of injection drug use can be attributed to abusive and traumatic childhood
events—and keep in mind that the population they surveyed was a
relatively healthy and stable one. A third or more were college grad-
uates, and most had at least some university education. With my
patients, the childhood trauma percentages would run close to one
hundred. Of course, not all addicts were subjected to childhood
trauma—although most hardcore injection users were—just as not
all severely abused children grow up to be addicts.

According to a review published by the [U.S.] National Institute
on Drug Abuse in 2002, "the rate of victimization among women
substance abusers ranges from 50% to nearly 100% . . . Populations
of substance abusers are found to meet the [diagnostic] criteria for
post-traumatic stress disorder . . . those experiencing both physical
and sexual abuse were at least *twice* as likely to be using drugs than
those who experienced either abuse alone."[16] Alcohol consumption
has a similar pattern: those who had suffered sexual abuse were
three times more likely to begin drinking in adolescence than those
who had not. For each emotionally traumatic childhood circumstance, there is a two- to threefold increase in the likelihood of early
alcohol abuse. "Overall, these studies provide evidence that stress
and trauma are common factors associated with consumption of
alcohol at an early age as a means to self-regulate negative or
painful emotions,"[17] write the ACE researchers.

It's just as many substance addicts say: they self-medicate to
soothe their emotional pain—but more than that, their brain
development was sabotaged by their traumatic experiences. The
systems subverted by addiction—the dopamine and opioid circuits, the limbic or emotional brain, the stress apparatus and the
impulse-control areas of the cortex—just cannot develop normally
in such circumstances.

We know something about how specific kinds of childhood
trauma affect brain development. For example: the vermis, a part of
the cerebellum at the back of the brain, is thought to play a key role
in addictions because it influences the dopamine system in the

midbrain. Imaging of this structure in adults who were sexually abused as children reveals abnormalities of blood flow, and these abnormalities are associated with symptoms that increase the risk for substance addiction.[18] In one study of the EEGs of adults who had suffered sexual abuse, the vast majority had abnormal brain-waves, and over a third showed seizure activity.[19]

These findings brought to mind a thirteen-year-old girl in my family practice who, apparently out of the blue, began to experience epileptic symptoms in the form of "absence spells." She would completely "zone out" for brief periods of time. Once, on a baseball diamond, she stared glassy-eyed and immobile, completely deaf to her teammates' shouts to swing the bat. She had similar spells in the classroom, lasting up to ten or twenty seconds. Her EEG was abnormal and the neurologist I consulted prescribed anticonvulsant medication. When I asked her in the privacy of my office if anything was stressing her, she simply said, "No."

Nine years later, no longer epileptic, she revealed to me that her seizures had begun during a period of repeated sexual abuse by a family member. Typically for sexually abused children, she felt there was no one to turn to for help, so she "absented" herself instead.

It gets worse. The brains of mistreated children have been shown to be smaller than normal by 7 or 8 per cent, with below-average volumes in multiple brain areas, including the impulse-regulating prefrontal cortex; in the corpus callosum (CC), the bundle of white matter that connects and integrates the functioning of the two sides of the brain; and in several structures of the limbic or emotional apparatus, whose dysfunctions greatly increase vulnerability to addiction.[20] In a study of depressed women who had been abused in childhood, the hippocampus (the memory and emotional hub) was found to be 15 per cent smaller than normal. The key factor was abuse, not depression, since the same brain area was unaffected in depressed women who had not been abused.[21]

I mentioned abnormalities in the corpus callosum, which facilitates the collaboration between the brain's two halves, or hemispheres. Not only have the CCs of trauma survivors been shown to be smaller, but there is evidence of a disruption of functioning there as well. The result can be a "split" in the processing of emotion: the two halves may not work in tandem, particularly when the individual is under stress. One characteristic of personality disorder, a condition with which substance abusers are very commonly diagnosed, is a kind of flip-flopping between idealization of another person and intense dislike, even hatred. There is no middle ground, where both the positive and the negative qualities of the other are acknowledged and accepted.

Dr. Martin Teicher, Director of the Developmental Biopsychiatry Research Program at McLean Hospital in Maryland, suggests the very intriguing possibility that our "negative" views of a person are stored in one hemisphere and our "positive" responses, in the other. The lack of integration between the two halves of the brain would mean that information from the two views, negative and positive, is not melded into one complete picture. As a result, in intimate relationships and in other areas of life, the afflicted individual fluctuates between idealized and degraded perceptions of himself, other people and the world.[22] This sensible theory, if proven, would explain a lot not only about drug-dependent persons, but also about many behavioural addicts.

Here I must admit to a shudder of recognition. I sometimes operate as if I were two different people: my view of things can be either very positive or highly cynical and pessimistic, and often dogmatically so. When I'm watching the happy channel, my negative perceptions seem like a crazy dream; when stuck in the dejected mode I can't recall ever having felt joy.

Of course, the moods and perceptions of my drug-addicted patients swing on pendulums far wilder and more erratic than mine. To some extent these extreme oscillations must be drug induced, but they also reflect the faulty brain dynamics that resulted from my patients' uniformly miserable childhood histories. Extreme circumstances breed extremist brains.

Such differences between a behavioural addict like me and the hardcore Skid Row addicts may place us worlds apart in social functioning and status, but the point remains that the chronic injection drug user is only at the far end of a continuum. Milder disruptions in early childhood experience and brain development can and do occur, and often result in "milder" forms of substance use or in non-drug, behavioural addictions.

—

Early trauma also has consequences for how human beings respond to stress all their lives, and stress has everything to do with addiction. It merits a brief look here.

Stress is a physiological response mounted by an organism when it is confronted with excessive demands on its coping mechanisms, whether biological or psychological. It is an attempt to maintain internal biological and chemical stability, or *homeostasis,* in the face of these excessive demands. The physiological stress response involves nervous discharges throughout the body and the release of a cascade of hormones, chiefly adrenaline and cortisol. Virtually every organ is affected, including the heart and lungs, the muscles and, of course, the emotional centres in the brain. Cortisol itself acts on the tissues of almost every part of the body—from the brain to the immune system, from the bones to the intestines. It is an important part of the infinitely intricate system of checks and balances that enables the body to respond to a threat.

At a conference in 1992 at the U.S. National Institutes of Health, researchers defined stress "as a *state of disharmony or threatened homeostasis.*"[23] According to such a definition, a stressor "is *a threat, real or perceived, that tends to disturb homeostasis.*"[24] What do all stressors have in common? Ultimately they all represent the absence of something that the organism perceives as necessary for survival— or its threatened loss. The threat itself can be real or perceived. The threatened loss of food supply is a major stressor. So is the threatened loss of love—for human beings. "It may be said without hesitation that for man the most important stressors are emotional," wrote the pioneering Canadian stress researcher and physician Hans Selye.[25]

Early stress establishes a lower "set point" for a child's internal stress system: such a person becomes stressed more easily than normal throughout her life. Dr. Bruce Perry is Senior Fellow at the Child Trauma Academy in Houston, Texas, and the former Director of Provincial Programs for Children's Mental Health in Alberta. As he points out, "A child who is stressed early in life will be more over-active and reactive. He is triggered more easily, is more anxious and distressed. Now, compare a person—child, adolescent or adult—

whose baseline arousal is normal with another whose baseline state of arousal is at a higher level. Give them both alcohol: both may experience the same intoxicating effect, but the one who has this higher physiological arousal will have the added effect of feeling pleasure from the relief of that stress. It's similar to when with a parched throat you drink some cool water: the pleasure effect is much heightened by the relief of thirst."[26]

The hormone pathways of sexually abused children are chronically altered.[27] Even a relatively "mild" stressor such as maternal depression—let alone neglect, abandonment or abuse—can disturb an infant's physical stress mechanisms.[28] Add neglect, abandonment or abuse, and the child will be more reactive to stress throughout her life. A study published in *The Journal of the American Medical Association* concluded that "a history of childhood abuse per se is related to increased neuroendocrine [nervous and hormonal] stress reactivity, which is further enhanced when additional trauma is experienced in adulthood."[29]

A brain pre-set to be easily triggered into a stress response is likely to assign a high value to substances, activities and situations that provide short term relief. It will have less interest in long-term consequences, just as people in extremes of thirst will greedily consume water knowing that it may contain toxins. On the other hand, situations or activities that for the average person are likely to bring satisfaction are undervalued because, in the addict's life, they have not been rewarding—for example, intimate connections with family. This shrinking from normal experience is also an outcome of early trauma and stress, as summarized in a recent psychiatric review of child development:

Neglect and abuse during early life may cause bonding systems to develop abnormally and compromise capacity for rewarding interpersonal relationships and commitment to societal and cultural values later in life. Other means of stimulating reward pathways in the brain, such as drugs, sex, aggression, and intimidating others, could become relatively more attractive and less constrained by concern about violating trusting relationships. The ability to modify behavior based on negative experiences may be impaired.[30]

Hardcore drug addicts, whose lives invariably began under conditions of severe stress, are all too readily triggered into a stress reaction. Not only does the stress response easily overwhelm the addict's already challenged capacity for rational thought when emotionally aroused, but also the hormones of stress "cross-sensitize" with addictive substances. The more one is present, the more the other is craved. Addiction is a deeply ingrained response to stress, an attempt to cope with it through self-soothing. Maladaptive in the long term, it is highly effective in the short term.

Predictably, stress is a major cause of continued drug dependence. It increases opiate craving and use, enhances the reward efficacy of drugs and provokes relapse to drug-seeking and drug-taking.[31] "Exposure to stress is the most powerful and reliable experimental manipulation used to induce reinstatement of alcohol or drug use," one team of researchers reports.[32] "Stressful experiences," another research group points out, "increase the vulnerability of the individual to either develop drug self-administration or relapse."[33]

Stress also diminishes the activity of dopamine receptors in the emotional circuits of the forebrain, particularly in the nucleus accumbens, where the craving for drugs increases as dopamine function decreases.[34] The research literature has identified three factors that universally lead to stress for human beings: *uncertainty, lack of information and loss of control*.[35] To these we may add *conflict that the organism is unable to handle* and *isolation from emotionally supportive relationships*. Animal studies have demonstrated that isolation leads to changes in brain receptors and increased propensity for drug use in infant animals, and in adults reduces the activity of dopamine-dependent nerve cells.[36,37] Unlike rats reared in isolation, rats housed together in stable social groupings resisted cocaine self-administration—in the same way that Bruce Alexander's tenants in Rat Park were impervious to the charms of heroin.[38]

Human children do not have to be reared in physical isolation to suffer deprivation: emotional isolation will have the same effect, as does stress on the parent. As we will later see, stress on pregnant mothers has a negative impact on dopamine activity in the brain of the unborn infant, an impact that can last well past birth.

—

Some people may think that addicts invent or exaggerate their sad stories to earn sympathy or to excuse their habits. In my experience, the opposite is the case. As a rule, they tell their life histories reluctantly, only when asked and only after trust has been established—a process that may take months, even years. Often they see no link between childhood experiences and their self-harming habits. If they speak of the connection, they do so in a distanced manner that still insulates them against the full emotional impact of what happened.

Research shows that the vast majority of physical and sexual assault victims do not spontaneously reveal their histories to their doctors or therapists.[39] If anything, there is a tendency to forget or to deny pain. One study followed up on young girls who had been treated in an emergency ward for proven sexual abuse. When contacted seventeen years later as adult women, 40 per cent of these abuse victims either did not recall or denied the event outright. Yet their memory was found to be intact for other incidents in their lives.[40]

Addicts who do remember often blame themselves. "I was hit a lot," says forty-year-old Wayne, "but I asked for it. Then I made some stupid decisions." (Wayne is the one who sometimes greets me with the bluesy chant "Doctor, doctor, gimme the news . . ." when I'm doing my rounds between the Hastings Street hotels.) And would he hit a child, I inquire, if that child "asked for it"? Would he blame that child for "stupid decisions"? Wayne looks away. "I don't want to talk about that crap," says this tough man, who has worked on oil rigs and construction sites and served fifteen years in jail for armed robbery. He looks away and wipes his eyes.

—

Grasping the powerful impact of the early environment on brain development may leave us feeling hopelessly gloomy about recovery from addiction. It so happens there are solid reasons not to despair. Our brains are resilient organs: some important circuits continue to develop throughout our entire lives, and they may do so even in the case of a hardcore drug addict whose brain "never had a chance" in childhood. That's the good news, on the physical level. Even more encouraging, we will find later that we have something in or about us that transcends the firing and wiring of neurons and the actions of chemicals. The mind may reside mostly in the brain, but it is much more than the sum total of the automatic neurological programs rooted in our pasts. And there is something else in us and about us: it is called by many names, "spirit" being the most democratic and least denominational or divisive in a religious sense. Later in this book, we will also examine its powerful transformational role.

As we conclude our tour of addiction's biological bases, however, we need to deal more directly with a topic I've already alluded to: the role of genes. Contrary to popular misconception, the truth about addiction is far from set in chromosomal stone; more good news, as we shall see presently.

CHAPTER 19

—

It's Not in the Genes

In 1990, newspapers and broadcast outlets across North America
reported that researchers at the University of Texas had identified the gene for alcoholism. This news was greeted with
tremendous interest, and the major media waxed enthusiastic with
pronouncements about the imminent end of alcoholism. *Time* magazine was among the foremost cheerleaders:

> The benefits from this line of research may be huge. In five years,
> scientists should have perfected a blood test for the gene, to help
> spot children at risk. And within a decade, doctors may have in hand
> a drug that either blocks the gene's action or controls some forms of
> alcoholism by altering the absorption of dopamine. Eventually, with
> genetic engineering, experts may find a way to eliminate altogether
> the suspect gene from affected individuals.[1]

The researchers in question had never made the claim that they
had discovered *the* "alcoholism gene," but they came close to making it. Some of their public statements fed that mistaken impression. Six years later the lead scientist, pharmacologist Kenneth
Blum, published a much more subdued assessment:

> Unfortunately it was erroneously reported that [we] had found the
> "alcoholism gene," implying that there was a one-to-one relation

between a gene and a specific behavior. Such misinterpretations are common—readers may recall accounts of an "obesity gene," or a "personality gene." Needless to say, *there is no such thing as a specific gene for alcoholism, obesity, or a particular type of personality* . . . Rather the issue at hand is to understand how certain genes and behavioral traits are connected.[2]

What the Texas group *had* located was a variation of the dopamine receptor gene (DRD2) that appears more commonly among alcoholics than nonalcoholics and "confers susceptibility to at least one form of alcoholism"—or so they thought after examining the brains of a few dozen corpses.[3] Even this more modest hypothesis, however, failed to stand up to future investigation. Subsequent studies were unable to confirm any association between the gene variant and alcoholism.[4] "The most important finding of research into a genetic role for alcoholism is that there is no such thing as a gene for alcoholism," writes the addiction specialist Lance Dodes. "Nor can you directly inherit alcoholism."[5]

Whatever problem we are hoping to resolve or prevent—be it war, terrorism, economic inequality, a marriage in trouble, climate change or addiction—the way we see its origins will largely determine our course of action. I present the case that the early environment plays a major role in a person's vulnerability to addiction not to exclude genetics but to counter what I see as an imbalance. Genes certainly appear to influence, among other features, such traits as temperament and sensitivity. These, in turn, have a huge impact on how we experience our environment. In the real world there is no nature vs. nurture argument, only an infinitely complex and moment-by-moment interaction between genetic and environmental effects. For this reason, as two psychiatrists at the University of Pittsburgh School of Medicine have pointed out, "the liability trait for alcoholism is not static." Owing to developmental and environmental factors, "the risk of alcoholism fluctuates over time."[6] Even if, against all available evidence, it was demonstrated conclusively that 70 per cent of addiction is programmed by our DNA, I would still be more interested in the remaining 30 per cent. After all, we cannot change our genetic makeup, and at this point, ideas of gene therapies to change human behaviours are fantasies at best. It makes sense to focus on what we *can* immediately do: how children are raised; what social support parenting receives; how we handle adolescent drug users; and how we treat addicted adults.

The current consensus—among those who accept a high degree of hereditary causation for alcoholism—is that predisposition to the disorder is about 50 per cent genetically determined.[7] Equally extravagant estimates are applied to other addictions. Heavy marijuana use is said to be 60–80 per cent heritable,[8] while the inherited liability to long-term heavy nicotine use has been calculated to be an astonishing 70 per cent.[9] Cocaine abuse and dependence are also reported to be "substantially influenced by genetic factors."[10] Some researchers have even suggested that alcoholism and divorce may share the same genetic propensity.

Such high figures are beyond possibility. The logic behind them rests on mistaken assumptions that owe less to science than to an exaggerated belief in the power of genes to determine our lives. In genetic theories of mental disorders, "unscientific beliefs play a major role," write the authors of a research review.[11]

—

It's not that genes do not matter— they certainly do; it's only that they do not and cannot determine even simple behaviours, let alone complex ones like addiction. Not only *is* there no addiction gene, there *couldn't* be one.

Until recently it was thought that there were one hundred thousand genes in the human genome. Even that number would have been inadequate to account for the unbelievable synaptic complexity and variability of the human brain.[12] However, it has now been discovered that there are only about thirty thousand gene sequences in our DNA—even less than in some lowly worms. "Our DNA is simply too paltry to spell out the wiring diagram for the human brain," writes UCLA research psychiatrist Jeffrey Schwartz.[13]

Far from being the autonomous dictators of our destinies, genes are controlled by their environment, and without environmental signals they could not function. In effect, they are turned on and off by the environment; human life could not exist if it wasn't so. Every cell in every organ in our bodies has exactly the same complement of genes, yet a brain cell does not look or act like a bone cell, and a liver cell does not resemble or function like a muscle cell. It is the environment within and outside the body that determines which genes are switched on, or activated, in which cell. "The cell's operations are primarily moulded by its interaction with the environment, not by its genetic code," the cell biologist Bruce Lipton has written.[14]

There is a new and rapidly growing science that focuses on how life experiences influence the function of genes. It's called *epigenetics*. As a result of life events, chemicals attach themselves to DNA and direct gene activities. The licking of a rat pup by the mother in the early hours of life turns on a gene in the brain that helps protect the animal from being overwhelmed by stress even as an adult. In rats deprived of such grooming, the same gene remains dormant. Epigenetic effects are most powerful during early development and have now been shown to be transmittable from one generation to the next, without any change in the genes themselves.[15] Environmentally induced epigenetic influences powerfully modulate genetic ones.

How a gene acts is called *gene expression*. It is now clear that "the early environment, consisting of both the prenatal and post-natal periods, has a profound effect on gene expression and adult patterns of behavior," to quote a recent article from *The Journal of Neuroscience*.[16] One example is related to alcohol consumption. A certain variation of a particular gene, found in some monkeys, reduces alcohol's sedative effects and also its disorganizing and unpleasant influence on balance and coordination. In other words, monkeys with this gene are less likely to feel semicomatose from drinking and less likely to lurch about like a drunken sailor. They have the capacity to imbibe greater amounts of alcohol without side effects and are more likely to drink until they're drunk. However, it was found that in mother-reared monkeys the gene was not expressed—that is, it had no impact on drinking behaviour. It did so only in monkeys who had been stressed in early life by being deprived of maternal contact and reared amongst peers.[17]

—

The overemphasis on genetic determination in addictions is based largely on studies of adopted children, especially of twins. I will not lay out here in detail the fatal scientific and logical flaws in such studies, but for those interested, I discuss them in Appendix I. The important point to explore here is how stresses during pregnancy can already begin to "program" a predisposition to addiction in the developing human being. Such information places the whole issue of prenatal care in a new light and helps explain the well-known fact that adopted children are at greater risk for all kinds of problems that predispose to addictions. The biological parents of an adopted child have a major epigenetic effect on the developing fetus.

The conclusions of many animal and human studies are best encapsulated by researchers from the Medical School at Hebrew University, Jerusalem:

> In the past few decades it has become increasingly clear that the development and later behaviour of an immature organism is not only determined by genetic factors and the postnatal environment, but also by the maternal environment during pregnancy.[18]

Numerous studies in both animals and human beings have found that maternal stress or anxiety during pregnancy can lead to a broad range of problems in the offspring, from infantile colic to later learning difficulties[19] and the establishment of behavioural and emotional patterns that increase a person's predilection for addiction. Stress on the mother would result in higher levels of cortisol reaching the baby and, as already mentioned, chronically elevated cortisol is harmful to important brain structures especially during periods of rapid brain development. A recent British study, for example, found that children whose mothers were stressed during pregnancy are vulnerable to mental and behavioural problems like ADHD or to being anxious or fearful. (ADHD and anxiety are powerful risk factors for addiction.) "Professor Yvette Glover of Imperial College London found stress caused by rows with or violence by a partner was particularly damaging," according to a BBC report. "Experts blame high levels of the stress hormone cortisol crossing the placenta. Professor Glover found high cortisol in the amniotic fluid bathing the baby in the womb tallied with the damage."[20] The study's results are consistent with previous evidence that stress on the mother during pregnancy affects the brain of the infant, with long-term and perhaps permanent effects.[21] This is where the father comes in, because the quality of the relationship with her partner is often a woman's best protection from stress or, on the other hand, the greatest source of it.

Women who were pregnant at the time of the 9/11 World Trade Center attacks and who suffered post-traumatic stress disorder (PTSD) as a result of witnessing the disaster passed on their stress effects to their newborns. At one year of age these infants had abnormal levels of the stress hormone cortisol. We might wonder if this was not a post-natal effect of the mother's PTSD. However, the greatest change was noted in infants whose mothers were in the last three months of pregnancy on September 11, 2001. So the fact that the *stage of pregnancy* a woman was at when the tragedy occurred was correlated with *the degree* of cortisol abnormality suggests that we are looking at an *in utero* effect.[22] It turns out that during gestation, just as after birth, brain systems undergo sensitive periods of development.

It has been demonstrated that both animals and humans who experienced the stress of their mothers during pregnancy are more likely to have disturbed stress-control mechanisms long after birth, creating a risk factor for addiction. Maternal stress during pregnancy can, for example, increase the offspring's sensitivity to alcohol.[23] As mentioned, a relative scarcity of dopamine receptors also elevates the addiction risk. "We've done work, and a lot of other people have done work showing that essentially the number and density of dopamine receptors in these receptive areas is determined *in utero,*" psychiatric researcher Dr. Bruce Perry told me in an interview.

For these reasons, adoption studies cannot decide questions of generic inheritance. Any woman who has to give up her baby for adoption is, by definition, a stressed woman. She is stressed not just because she knows she'll be separated from her baby, but primarily because if she wasn't stressed in the first place, she would never have had to consider giving up her child: the pregnancy was unwanted or the mother was poor, single or in a bad relationship or she was an

immature teenager who conceived involuntarily or was a drug user
or was raped or confronted by some other adversity. Any of these
situations would be enough to impose tremendous stress on any
person, and so for many months the developing fetus would be
exposed to high cortisol levels through the placenta. A proclivity for
addiction is one possible consequence.

It is commonly assumed, with no scientific basis, that if a condition "runs in a family," appearing in successive generations, it must
be genetic. Yet as we have seen, for example with my Downtown
Eastside patients, pre- and post-natal environments can be recreated
from one generation to the next in a way that would impair a child's
healthy development without any genetic contribution. Parenting
styles are often inherited epigenetically—that is, passed on biologically, but not through DNA transmission from parent to child.

—

Why, then, are narrow genetic assumptions so widely accepted and,
in particular, so enthusiastically embraced by the media? The neglect
of developmental science is one factor. Our preference for a simple
and quickly understood explanation is another, as is our tendency to
look for one-to-one causations for almost everything. Life in its wondrous complexity does not conform to such easy reductions.

There is a psychological fact that, I believe, provides a powerful
incentive for people to cling to genetic theories. We human beings
don't like feeling responsible: as individuals for our own actions; as
parents for our children's hurts; or as a society for our many fail-
ings. Genetics—that neutral, impassive, impersonal handmaiden
of Nature—would absolve us of responsibility and of its ominous
shadow, guilt. If genetics ruled our fate, we would not need to
blame ourselves or anyone else. Genetic explanations take us off
the hook. The possibility does not occur to us that we can accept
or assign responsibility without taking on the useless baggage of
guilt or blame.

More daunting for those who hope for scientific and social
progress, the genetic argument is easily used to justify all kinds of
inequalities and injustices that are otherwise hard to defend. It

serves a deeply conservative function: if a phenomenon like addiction is determined mostly by biological heredity, we are spared from having to look at how our social environment supports, or does not support, the parents of young children; at how social attitudes, prejudices and policies burden, stress and exclude certain segments of the population and thereby increase their propensity for addiction. The writer Louis Menand said it well in a *New Yorker* article:

> "It's all in the genes": an explanation for the way things are that does not threaten the way things are. Why should someone feel unhappy or engage in antisocial behavior when that person is living in the freest and most prosperous nation on earth? It can't be the system! There must be a flaw in the wiring somewhere.[24]

Succumbing to the common human urge to absolve ourselves of responsibility, our culture has too avidly embraced genetic fundamentalism. That leaves us far less empowered to deal either actively or pro-actively with the tragedy of addiction. We ignore the good news that nothing is irrevocably dictated by our genes and that, therefore, there is much we can do.

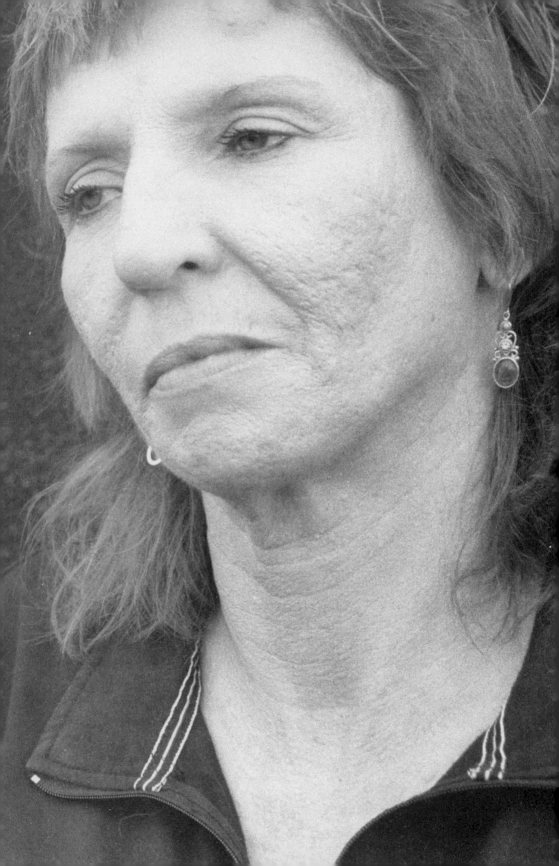

PART V

—

The Addiction Process and the Addictive Personality

Anyone who is not totally dead to himself will soon find that he is tempted and overcome by piddling and frivolous things. Whoever is weak in spirit, given to the flesh, and inclined to sensual things can, but only with great difficulty, drag himself away from his earthly desires. Therefore, he is often gloomy and sad when he is trying to pull himself away from them and easily gives in to anger should someone attempt to oppose him.

THOMAS À KEMPIS, FIFTEENTH-CENTURY CHRISTIAN MYSTIC
The Imitation of Christ

—

CHAPTER 20

"A Void I'll Do Anything to Avoid"

There are almost as many addictions as there are people. In the *Brahmajāla Sutta,* the spiritual master Gotama identifies many pleasures as potentially addictive.

. . . Some ascetics and Brahmins . . . remain addicted to attending such shows as dancing, singing, music, displays, recitations, hand-music, cymbals and drums, fairy shows; . . . combats of elephants, buffaloes, bulls, rams; . . . maneuvers, military parades; . . . disputation and debate, rubbing the body with shampoos and cosmetics, bracelets, headbands, fancy sticks . . . unedifying conversation about kings, robbers, ministers, armies, dangers, wars, food, drink, clothes . . . heroes, speculation about land and sea, talk of being and non-being . . . [1]

Gotama, known to us as the Buddha, lived and taught about twenty-five hundred years ago in what are now Nepal and northern India. Today he might also include in his sermon: sugar, caffeine, talk shows, gourmet cooking, music buying, right- or left-wing politics, Internet cafés, cell phones, the CFL or NFL or NHL, the *New York Times,* the *National Enquirer,* CNN, BBC, aerobic exercise, crossword puzzles, meditation, religion, gardening or golf. In the final analysis, it's not the activity or object itself that defines an addiction but our *relationship* to whatever is the external focus of

our attention or behaviour. Just as it's possible to drink alcohol without being addicted to it, so one can engage in any activity without
addiction. On the other hand, no matter how valuable or worthy an
activity may be, one can relate to it in an addicted way. Let's recall
here our definition of addiction: *any repeated behaviour, substance-
related or not, in which a person feels compelled to persist, regardless of its negative impact on his life and the lives of others.* The
distinguishing features of any addiction are: compulsion, preoccupation, impaired control, persistence, relapse and craving.

Although the form and focus of addictions may vary, the same set
of dynamics is at the root of them all. Dr. Aviel Goodman writes, "All
addictive disorders, whatever types of behaviors that characterize
them, share the underlying psychobiological process, which I call
the *addictive process.*"[2] It's just as Dr. Goodman suggests: addictions
are not a collection of distinct disorders but the manifestations of
an underlying process that can be expressed in many ways. The
addictive process—I will refer to it as the *addiction process*—
governs all addictions and involves the same neurological and psychological malfunctions. The differences are only a matter of degree.

There is plenty of evidence for such a unitary view. Substance
addictions are often linked to one another, and chronic substance
users are highly likely to have more than one drug habit: for example, the majority of cocaine addicts also have, or have had, active
alcohol addiction. In turn, about 70 per cent of alcoholics are
heavy smokers, compared with only 10 per cent of the general
population.[3] I don't believe I've ever seen an injection drug user at
the Portland Clinic who wasn't also addicted to nicotine. Often
nicotine was their "entry drug," the first mood-altering chemical
they'd become hooked on as adolescents. In research surveys more
than half of opiate addicts have been found to be alcoholics, as
have the vast majority of cocaine and amphetamine addicts, and
many cannabis addicts as well. Both animal and human researches
have demonstrated that common brain systems, brain chemicals,
and pharmacological mechanisms underlie alcohol and other substance addictions.[4]

All addictions, substance related or not, share states of mind
such as craving and shame, and behaviours such as deception,

manipulation and relapse. On the neurobiological level, all addictions engage the brain's attachment-reward and incentive-motivation systems, which, in turn, escape from regulation by the "thinking" and impulse control areas of the cortex. We explored this process in detail in the previous section on drug addiction. What does research show about the nonsubstance addictions?

Let's look at pathological gambling. Scientific work on this addiction is in its early stages, but as one researcher of pathological gambling writes, "preliminary results suggest the involvement of similar brain regions in drug- and non-drug-related urges."[5] Gamblers have abnormalities in the dopamine system, as well as in neurotransmitters other than dopamine. For example, like drug addicts, gamblers have diminished levels of serotonin—a brain chemical that helps to regulate moods and control impulses. One study compared physiological responses to a game of blackjack in two groups: pathological gamblers and casual players. Elevations of important neurotransmitters, especially dopamine, were much higher among the gamblers—that is, the brain's incentive-motivation system was much more activated, just as with drug addictions.[6] And the same areas "light up" on the brain imaging of gamblers as in drug addicts. Pathological gamblers behave like drug addicts—or, to a lesser extent, like me. "More than 40 people have been banned from B.C. casinos over the past three years for leaving their children alone in the car while they go inside," a Vancouver newspaper reported in July 2006. Some children were discovered in casino parking lots in this province as late as 3 a.m.[7]

It's safe to say that any pursuit, natural or artificial, that induces a feeling of increased motivation and reward—shopping, driving, sex, eating, TV watching, extreme sports and so on—will activate the same brain systems as drug addictions. In an MRI study, for example, playing with monetary incentives "lit up" the brain areas also aroused in the course of drug intake.[8] PET scanning revealed that the playing of video games raises dopamine levels in the incentive-motivation circuits.[9] Personal history and temperament will decide which activities produce this effect for any particular individual, but the process is always the same. For someone with a relative shortage of dopamine receptors, it's whichever activity best releases extra quantities of this euphoric and invigorating neurotransmitter that will become the object of addictive pursuit. In effect, people become addicted to their own brain chemicals. When caught in the urgent fever of my compact disc hunt, for instance, it's that hit of dopamine I'm after.

The evidence is compelling in the case of overeating, where we most clearly see that a natural and essential activity can become the target of faulty incentive-reward circuits, aided and abetted by deficient self-regulation. PET imaging studies in addictive eaters have, predictably, implicated the brain dopamine system. As with drug addicts, obese people have diminished dopamine receptors; in one study, the more obese the subjects were, the fewer dopamine receptors they had.[10] Recall that reduced numbers of dopamine receptors can be both a consequence of chronic drug use and a risk factor for addiction. Junk foods and sugar are also chemically addictive because of their effect on the brain's intrinsic "narcotics," the endorphins. Sugar, for example, provides a quick fix of endorphins and also temporarily raises levels of the mood chemical serotonin.[11] This effect can be prevented by an injection of the opiate-blocking drug Naloxone, the same substance used to resuscitate addicts who overdose on heroin.[12] Naloxone also blocks the comforting effects of fat.[13]

"It is becoming apparent that eating and drug disorders share a common neuroanatomic and neurochemical basis," conclude two experts on addiction and related disorders.[14]

Not only are the identical incentive-motivation and attachment-reward circuits impaired in the brains of overeaters and drug addicts, so are the impulse-regulating functions of the cortex. "Some evidence suggests a decision-making impairment in obese patients," a recent article in *The Journal of the American Medical Association* pointed out. "For example, very obese individuals score worse than substance abusers in the Iowa Gambling Test, a paradigm that also relies on the integrity of the right PFC [pre-frontal cortex] for execution."[15] The same authors noted that obese people are more prone to stress, since their hormonal stress-response apparatus is disturbed—another characteristic in common with other addicts.

Compulsive shoppers experience the same mental and emotional processes when engaged in their addiction. The thinking parts of the brain go on furlough. In a brain imaging study conducted at the University of Munster, Germany, scientists found "reduced activation in brain areas associated with working memory and reasoning and, on the other hand, increased activation in areas involved in processing of emotions," when even ordinary consumers were engaged in choosing between different brand names of a given product.[16] Under logo capitalism, it turns out, the vaunted "market forces" are largely unconscious—a feature of addiction that advertising agencies well understand. In previous work the electrical discharges of the brain circuits governing pleasure were also found to be in overdrive during shopping, in contrast to the rationality circuits. Neurologist Michael Deppe, the lead researcher, said that "the more expensive the product, the crazier the shoppers get. And when buying really expensive products, the part of the brain dealing with rational thought has reduced its activity to almost zero. . . . The stimulation of emotional centres shows that shopping is a stress relief."[17]

Addictions are often interchangeable—a fact that further buttresses the unitary theory that there's a common addiction process. Although my addictive tendencies are most obvious in my compact-disc-buying habit, I can shift seamlessly into other obsessive activities. The week we moved into our present home, twenty-four years ago, I attended the birthing of six babies, most of them at night. I'd accepted into my practice fifteen women whose due dates came that month, about ten too many for a busy family physician. I couldn't say no to being wanted. During the day, when not at the maternity hospital, I was working in my office. You can just imagine how much energy and presence I had left for my family. I have thrown myself equally blindly and avidly into political work and other pursuits. I've even had several of my addictions up and running at the same time. That is, the addiction process was active and looking for more and more external trophies to capture. For all that, the anxiety, ennui and fear of the void driving the whole operation rarely abated.

The less "respectable" and more harmful behavioural addictions play themselves out in the same way. Dr. Aviel Goodman has drawn this conclusion from research showing a significant overlap between his area of study (sex addiction) and other addictions, such as compulsive shopping, substance dependence and pathological gambling. In other words, many sex addicts will also have one or more of these superficially different addictions.[18] Pathological gamblers, too, are highly likely to fall under the sway of other destructive habits. About half of them are alcoholics and the vast majority are addicted to nicotine—and the more severe a person's gambling, the stronger the addiction to alcohol and smoking.[19]

Finally, the phenomena of tolerance and withdrawal are also connected with behavioural addictions, if not nearly to the same degree as with drug addictions. Tolerance means needing more and more of the same "hit" to get the same effect (that is, the same dopamine high). I usually begin my CD-buying binges with only one or two discs, but with each purchase the craving increases. In the end I'm hauling home hundreds of dollars' worth of recorded music every time I visit that den of iniquity, Sikora's music store. Withdrawal consists of irritability, a generally glum mood, restlessness and a sense of aimlessness. No doubt it has its chemical components: I'm experiencing the effect of diminished dopamine and endorphin levels. Other nonsubstance addicts experience similar symptoms after abruptly stopping whatever behaviour they were binging with. The journey from addictive self-indulgence to depression is rapid and inexorable.

"I'm working on sifting through my need for extremes in my life," the gifted writer Stephen Reid, now in jail for bank robbery, told me. Needing extremes, the addict leaps from one behaviour to another. There may be "a million stories in the Naked City," as an old New York cop program claimed, but there's only one addiction process.

—

While I was writing this book, my son Daniel served as my first editor. During the course of our mutual work we've had many discussions on addiction, and I asked him to write down his thoughts. His words illustrate how the addiction process can change its forms of expression without altering its basic nature. Whatever gets you through the night.

Dad,

I remember laughing derisively at age fourteen when you told me you were a CD addict: it sounded cushy, absurd. It also sounded like an excuse; suddenly you had a "problem," a pet alibi for being so erratic and absent-minded. The constant blare of classical music in our home was now further evidence of your pain; the Mahler shaking my bedroom ceiling was a reminder of your complexity. Was I supposed to feel sorry for you? I didn't know, nor did I care much to imagine, what void you were striving to fill. All I knew about it was what I inferred from the cycles of your behaviour: it was more important to you than the family was, than I was. I found this all a bit too pathetic, and I disdained this "addiction" business (because I thought it was bogus) and at the same time resented it (because I knew it was, on some level, valid).

So as you can imagine, I've never been eager to apply the term "addicted" to myself, even when the evidence points that way.

Part of the spin job is, "Hey, I can't be addicted. I don't have a central addiction, like my Dad." Maybe I've had a series of them, little ones, but they never last. They neither run nor ruin my life utterly. I imagine Woody Allen making comic hay out of that set-up: "Honest, sweetheart, I could never become an alcoholic; I'm horrible with commitment." I could even coin a new term. "ADD"iction: the inability to concentrate on one bad habit for any length of time.

I could name such seemingly innocuous things as a blog I kept in New York after I arrived there for grad school, and the series of personal development workshops I took several years ago. Those are just two recent examples. In each case my involvement started out as a very positive thing in my life, full of vigour and excitement, before it morphed into an all-consuming and counterproductive force.

The blog began as a way of channelling my excitement about being in a new environment.

During those nervous first months of grad school, I wrote in my blog sometimes for three or four hours a day—or night—instead of making time for social activities or exercise or sleep, or even schoolwork—in short, life. I felt compelled by some strange muse to push the blog envelope by including more and more private details about my life. It was like some wondrous Seussian contraption: I fed myself, like raw material, into the BlogMatic 3000 and out came a vivid, clever, sparkling artifact, so much more interesting and well-defined than my actual life as I knew it. I recall that even you and Mom, and many of my friends, lapped it up for a time, until it crossed that invisible line between self-expression and self-obsession—and then you let me know I'd crossed it. I'd surfed atop a wave of glowing attention, and so when it crashed I was genuinely perplexed.

Personal development took much the same course—no pun intended—except that it was even more positive off the top. It transformed my life in a number of wonderful ways, but then, it became my life in a way that didn't work. I got to the point where I was living only to have something to talk about in the workshops, which, for me, couldn't occur frequently enough to keep pace with my galloping conviction that I was a fraud. Meanwhile, I was trying to sell everyone on how transformed I was—and mightn't they, too, benefit from this? I knew the word among friends and family was that I was getting weird, but I saw no other way than to keep pushing.

When I'm addicted—there, I said it—there's a tremendous amount of drama, from the ecstatic rush of the honeymoon period all the way through to the crashing finale, when I realize this is "bad for me" and it's gotten "out of control" and I swear off it with a heroic mix of regret, shame, and sober-sounding resolve. This happened with the blog, my "transformational" crusade and plenty of other little episodes. That's certainly part of addiction's sick appeal: say what you want about it, it's pretty entertaining.

Oddly enough, the addiction really isn't over until I can see the emptiness (in a Buddhist sense) of the behaviour: not good, not evil, and certainly not exciting, just an outside "thing" I've been using unintelligently to dull the suffering edge of life. I say "unintelligently" because no addiction in the history of the world ever alleviated more suffering than it ended up causing.

So it turns out that I'm not so different from you, Dad. I, too, carry a void inside—nothing exotic, just an ordinary human despair-fear-anxiety factory—and mine will try to feed on anything that gives me an instant sense of self-definition, purpose or worth. (If I want to be quippy about it, it's a void I'll do anything to avoid.) I may not do it with drugs or gambling or, God forbid, Beethoven, but my way can be as noxious to me as yours is to you. If I've learned anything, it's that I have to be responsible for my own fear of emptiness. The fear is not personal—on the contrary it's pretty much universal—but I got the void I got and it's not going anywhere. When I can recognize that, I don't make the mistake of confusing it with who I am, or worse, expending a lot of energy trying to make it go away by any available means. Instead, I can be vigilant, patient and good-humoured with it.

Love, Daniel

—

CHAPTER 21

Too Much Time on External Things: The Addiction-Prone Personality

T here is something reassuring about bottoming out," says Stephen Reid wryly, "a sense that you can't fall any further." We are facing each other across a small, square wooden table. The metal frame chairs with plastic cushions are standard cheap cafeteria issue. Nothing distinguishes this room from other drab institutional cafeterias except the guard who monitors the prisoners and their guests from her elevated, windowed cubicle.

I am at William Head Institution on Vancouver Island to interview Reid, bank robber, self-described junkie and author. There are a few others in the cafeteria, some sipping coffee by themselves, some with visitors. At the table next to us a male prisoner is massaging his female visitor's shoulders, while the Native couple by the glass wall that faces the sea gaze in rapturous silence into each other's eyes. Outdoors on each side wild-growing shrubs of yellow Scotch broom populate the hill that slopes sharply down to the shore. Behind them gleams the metal mesh fence topped with coiled barbed wire.

In 1999 Stephen committed what he later described as "the worst bank robbery of my life," and was sent back to jail for eighteen years. With grey hair, round pink cheeks and walrus moustache he looks nothing like one would expect of a criminal who had perpetrated an act of violence he now speaks of with shame. He has gained a lot of weight in prison. He feels very much discouraged today, owing to a setback in his parole review process. "I binge eat when I try to deal with the impact of such disappointments," he says. To me he looks depressed.

We are conversing about our personal experiences of addiction and the hidden emptiness at the core, which our very different addictions always promise—but always fail—to fill. It may sound surprising to say this about a self-confessed junkie and coke-addled bank robber, but there is nothing Stephen reveals about his thoughts and emotions that I don't immediately recognize within myself.

His comment about bottoming out comes when I ask him about a passage in *Junkie,* an autobiographical essay he wrote for the anthology *Addicted: Notes from the Belly of the Beast:*

> Having fallen through the crust of this earth so many times, it seems that only on this small and familiar pad of concrete, where I can make seven steps in one direction, then take seven back, do my feet touch down with any certainty.[1]

Popular lore has it that the addict has to "hit bottom" before gaining the motivation to give up his habit. That may be true in some individual cases, but as a general rule it fails because what constitutes the lowest point is highly personal to each addict. For Stephen Reid, it's the bare, concrete floor of a prison. For me, it's the impact of my addictive behaviours on my family and the sense of alienation and shame that grows each time I indulge in a secretive purchasing binge. It's hard to imagine how anyone would define "hitting bottom" in the cases of my Portland Hotel patients who have lost all their earthly possessions, spouses, children, self-esteem, health and the possibility of living out anything close to a normal human life span. If freedom truly is another word for nothing left to lose, the hardcore hungry ghosts inhabiting Vancouver's Skid Row are very free indeed.

As I remarked earlier, the differences between my life and the lives of my Downtown Eastside patients are glaringly obvious. Less self-evident are the many similarities between my patterns and theirs: in the motivations that drive the addictions and in our actions around the addictive "object"—in their case and Stephen

Reid's, drugs; in mine, compact discs or public attention or the gratitude of patients or the self-oblivion of immersion in work or the constant need for consuming activity or mindless diversion. I've been as willing to sell my soul as they, only I charge a higher price. They settle for a bug-infested room on Hastings, my workaholism has bought me a lovely home; their object of addiction goes up their veins to be excreted by their kidneys or permeates their lungs and vanishes into the air, my shelves are lined with CDs, many of them unheard, and with books, many unread. Their addictions land them in jail; my obsessive striving for recognition and driven work habits have gained me admirers and a handsome income.

As to morality, duty and responsibility, if they have abandoned their children, I have also abandoned mine—by not being present for them and by placing a higher value on my perceived needs than on their real ones. If my patients have lied and manipulated, so have I. If they have obsessed about their next "hit," so have I. If they persist long after the negative consequences strike them, so have I. If they repeatedly make promises and resolutions only to relapse, it's nothing I haven't done. If Stephen Reid fell back into his drug addictions and ended up being physically separated from his children during their growing years, I repeatedly separated myself emotionally from my family. If drug addicts sacrifice love for immediate satisfaction, I have done so as well.

It may be argued that, at least so far as work is concerned, what I call my addictions have benefited other people. Even if that were true, it still wouldn't explain or justify addiction. The contributions I have made in a number of areas that I am passionate about could have been achieved without the addictive zeal that often drove me. There is no such thing as a good addiction. Everything a person can do is better done if there is no addictive attachment that pollutes it. For every addiction—no matter how benign or even laudable it seems from the outside—someone pays a price.

No human being is empty or deficient at the core, but many live as if they were and experience themselves primarily that way. Attempting to obliterate the *sense* of deficiency and emptiness that is a core state of any addict is like labouring to fill in a canyon with shovelfuls of dust. Energy devoted to such an endless and futile task is robbed from one's psychological and spiritual growth, from genuinely soul-satisfying pursuits and from the ones we love.

Stephen Reid has written about the "darkness . . . the secret self-loathing that pools in the heart of every junkie."[2] The shame arises because indulging the addiction process, even if with an ostensibly harmless object, only deepens the vacuum where connection with the world and a healthy sense of self ought to arise. The shame is that of self-betrayal. The utter insatiability of this sense of deficient emptiness hit home for me when I was invited to speak at IdeaCity, an annual conference about ideas, scientific advances and culture in Toronto. For years I looked at the list of presenters with bitterness. I was envious and longed to be invited—a longing that arose from my neediness around being wanted and recognized. Finally, I was asked to participate. My ego was satisfied—or so I thought. Once in Toronto, no sooner had I begun to enjoy the program and to relish meeting so many open-minded and fascinating people than the relentlessly possessive and ever-hungry ego voice in my mind began to agitate: "*Some of these speakers have been here two or even three times. Will you be asked again? You SHOULD be asked again. . . .*" I could only laugh. The ego can never get enough—it doesn't even know the concept.

When I tell my Portland patients about my addictive behaviour and how it feels on the inside—the craving, the unbearable urgency, the relapses, the shame—they all nod their heads and laugh in recognition. Stephen Reid also knows what I'm talking about. "I've spent too much time on external things," he says, "bouncing off other people . . . makes my teeth hurt, the work of pulling back from all those outside things and looking inside myself." His voice trails off as he says this, and then he adds: "It has seemed to me at times that you can be present in your life only as a kid or when you're on heroin." A credo of discouragement and defeat that many of us share: a child may be completely in the present moment, but an adult can get there only with artificial assistance.

—

Stephen's comment about his relentless focus on outside things touches upon the so-called addictive personality—or, to put it accurately, the addiction-prone personality. Is there such an entity? The answer is not a simple yes or no. No collection of personality traits will by themselves cause addiction, but some traits will make it much more likely that a person will succumb to the addiction process.

People are susceptible to the addiction process if they have a constant need to fill their minds or bodies with external sources of comfort, whether physical or emotional. That need expresses a failure of *self-regulation*—an inability to maintain a reasonably stable internal emotional atmosphere. No one is born with the capacity for self-regulation; as I've mentioned, the infant is completely dependent upon the parents to regulate his physical and psychological states. Self-regulation being a developmental achievement, we reach it only if the conditions for development are right. Some people never attain it; even in advanced adulthood they must rely on some external support to quell their discomfort and soothe their anxiety. They just cannot make themselves feel okay without such supports, whether they be chemicals or food or an excessive need for attention, approval or love. Or they seek to make their lives exciting by engaging in activities that trigger elation or a sense of risk. A person with inadequate self-regulation becomes dependent on "outside things" to lift his mood and even to calm himself if he experiences too much undirected internal energy. In my own case, I've binge-shopped CDs when I've felt down or restless or bored—but also when I've felt overly elated and didn't know what to do with myself.

Impulse control is one aspect of self-regulation. Impulses rise up from the lower brain centres and are meant to be permitted or inhibited by the cerebral cortex. A salient trait of the addiction-prone personality is a poor hold over sudden feelings, urges and desires. Also characterizing the addiction-prone personality is the absence of *differentiation*.[3] Differentiation is defined as "the ability to be in emotional contact with others yet still autonomous in one's emotional functioning." It's the capacity to hold on to ourselves while interacting with others. The poorly differentiated person is easily overwhelmed by his emotions, "absorbs anxiety from others and generates considerable anxiety within himself."[4]

Lack of differentiation and impaired self-regulation reflect a lack of emotional maturity.

Psychological maturation is the development of a sense of self as separate from inner experience—a capacity entirely absent in the young child. The child has to learn that she is not identical with whatever feeling happens to be dominant in her at any particular moment. She can feel something without her actions being automatically dictated by that feeling. She can be aware of other, conflicting feelings or of thoughts, values and commitments that might run counter to the feeling of the moment. She can choose. In the addict this experience of "mixed feelings" is often lacking. Emotional processes rule the addict's perspective: whatever she is feeling at the moment tends to define her view of the world and will control her actions.

The same applies in the realm of relationships: for maturation the child must become unique and separate from other individuals. She has to know her own mind and not be overwhelmed by the thoughts, perspectives or emotional states of others. The better differentiated she becomes, the more she is able to mix with others without losing her sense of self. The individuated, well-differentiated person can respond from an open acceptance of his own emotions, which are not tailored either to match someone else's expectations or to resist them. He neither suppresses his emotions nor acts them out impulsively.

Dr. Michael Kerr, a psychiatrist in Washington, DC, and director of the Georgetown University Family Center, distinguishes between two types of differentiation: *functional differentiation* and *basic differentiation,* which, from the perspective of health and stress are worlds apart. Functional differentiation refers to a person's ability to function *based on external factors.* The less basic differentiation a person has attained, the more prone he is to rely on relationships to maintain his emotional balance. When relationships fail to sustain such people, they may turn to addiction as the emotional crutch. Some of my Portland patients functioned reasonably well until, say, their marriages fell apart; then they spiralled rapidly into substance use. Even in the Downtown Eastside, their moods hit rock bottom or soar according to how they are doing with their current partners. They feel hurt easily and are quick to believe they are being rejected—and their level of drug use often hinges on what's happening in their relationships. When one relationship ends, they may immediately plunge into another. They are often unable to engage in a process of recovery because their partner is unwilling to join them; they see the relationship as being more important than their own healthy self. Poor differentiation also keeps people in destructive relationships, which themselves take on an addictive quality.

I, too, have had a tendency to look to outside sources of solace such as work and binge buying when there have been strains in my marriage—even when these strains originated in my own underdeveloped self-regulation and lack of basic differentiation.

These, then, are the traits that most often underlie the addiction process: poor self-regulation; lack of basic differentiation; lack of a healthy sense of self; a sense of deficient emptiness; and impaired impulse control. The development of these traits is not mysterious—or, more correctly, there is no mystery about the circumstances under which the positive qualities of self-regulation, self-worth, differentiation and impulse control fail to develop. Any gardener knows that if a plant hasn't grown, most likely the conditions were lacking. The same goes for children. The addictive personality is a personality that hasn't matured. When we come to address healing, a key question will be how to promote maturity in ourselves or in others whose early environment sabotaged healthy emotional growth.

—

CHAPTER 22

Poor Substitutes for Love:
Behavioural Addictions and Their Origins

D rug addicts have a limited stock of substances to choose from: they have fewer escape routes than those available to behavioural addicts. As a physician colleague in the Downtown Eastside put it: "They just have less in their kitbags than the rest of us." By comparison, the possibilities for behavioural addictions are almost infinite. How, then, is the "choice" made? Why self-improvement or blogging in my son's case and why sex or gambling for someone else? Why does buying compact discs set my dopamine circuits into action and why compulsive work? I put that question to Dr. Aviel Goodman, the authority on sexual addictions I've mentioned in earlier chapters. "It has a lot to do with which experience brings relief from whatever pains us," he said. "For a lot of people something like compact discs would not be high on the list, but my guess is that music means something deep for you, that for you it's a profound emotional experience."

And why might that be the case? "First, you may have a genetic sensitivity toward music," Dr. Goodman suggested, "and you may have been affected by the kind of music your parents listened to. But there could have been earlier influences—for example, whether in infancy you were often left in a room where you weren't cuddled but you were able to hear, so your auditory system became an important conduit of emotional connection with the world."

This Minnesota psychiatrist, who knew nothing about my background, came close to describing my early experience as I understand it.

I was born in Budapest in 1944, to Jewish parents, two months before the Nazis occupied Hungary. We endured the well-known set of calamities that war and genocide brought upon the Jews of Europe. For the first fifteen months of my life my father was away in a forced labour camp and for most of that time neither of my parents knew whether the other was alive or dead. I was five months old when my grandparents were killed at Auschwitz. Many years later, not long before her own death at age eighty-two in Vancouver, my mother told me that she was so depressed after her parents' murder that some days she got out of bed only to look after me. I was left alone in my crib quite often. I related some of this history in *Scattered Minds:*

Two days after the Germans marched into Budapest, my mother called the pediatrician. "Would you come to see Gabi," she requested, "he has been crying almost without stop since yesterday morning." "I'll come, of course," the doctor replied, "but I should tell you: all my Jewish babies are crying."

Now, what did Jewish infants know of Nazis, World War II, racism, genocide? What they knew—or rather, absorbed—was their parents' anxiety. . . . They inhaled fear, ingested sorrow. Yet were they not loved? No less than children anywhere.

When, owing to internal demons arising from their own childhoods or to external stressors in their lives, parents are unable to regulate—that is, keep within a tolerable range—the emotional milieu of the infant, the child's brain has to adapt: by tuning out, by emotional shutting down and by learning to find ways to self-soothe through rocking, thumb-sucking, eating, sleeping or constantly looking to external sources of comfort. This is the ever-agitated, ever-yawning emptiness that lies at the heart of addiction.

In the unbelievably overcrowded and unsanitary conditions of the Jewish ghetto of Budapest towards the end of the war, I became so ill that my mother feared I might die of disease or malnutrition.

In my twelfth month, she had me smuggled out to relatives who lived in hiding outside the ghetto. When she went out to the street to hand me to the kind but completely unknown Gentile visitor who was to take me away, she didn't know whether she would survive to the next day, let alone see me again. My relatives were caring people who looked after me as best they could, but I have to imagine that to a year-old infant, they were complete strangers. The small child's natural response to overwhelming emotional loss is a defensive shut-down. I've had a lifelong resistance to receiving love—not to *being* loved or even to knowing intellectually that I am loved, but to accepting love vulnerably and openly on a visceral, emotional level. People who cannot find or receive love need to find substitutes—and that's where addictions come in.

Music gives me a sense of self-sufficiency and nourishment. I don't need anyone or anything. I bathe in it as in amniotic fluid, it surrounds and protects me. It's also stable, ever-available and something I can control—that is, I can reach for it whenever I want. I can also choose music that reflects my mood, or if I want, helps to soothe it. As for forays to Sikora's, music-seeking offers excitement and tension that I can immediately resolve and a reward I can immediately attain—unlike other tensions in my life and other desired rewards. Music is a source of beauty and meaning outside myself that I can claim as my own without exploring how, in my life, I keep from directly experiencing those qualities. Addiction, in this sense, is the lazy man's path to transcendence.

The sources of my work addiction are clear to me. No matter how much she loves him in her heart—and my mother loved me with all of hers—a child with a depressed mother feels constant deprivation and deep distress. An eleven-month-old must sense a cataclysmic rupture in the order of things when he is given over to strangers and his mother abruptly disappears from his life. These sorts of experiences can also leave a deep impression in the psyche and create alterations in brain physiology that may—but do not necessarily, as we shall see—last a lifetime.

My sense of worth, unavailable to me for who I *am*, has come from work. And in the practice of medicine I found the perfect venue to prove my usefulness and indispensability. For a long time it was impossible for me to turn down work—the drug of being wanted was far too powerful to refuse and, in any case, I needed the flame of constant preoccupation to ward off the anxiety or depression or ennui that always lurked at the edges of my psyche. Like any addict, I used my addictions to help regulate my moods, my internal experience. On weekends when the beeper fell silent I felt empty and irritable—the addict in withdrawal.

—

The same dynamics come into play with eating disorders. How, we might ask, could an activity essential for survival become so distorted, undermining a person's health, sometimes to the point of shortening a person's life? Although it is commonplace to blame the current epidemic of obesity on junk food consumption and sedentary living, these are only the behavioural manifestations of a deeper psychological and social malaise.

In human development the ingestion of food has significance far beyond its obvious dietary role. Following birth the mother's nipple replaces the umbilical cord as the source of nutrients for the infant, and it is also a point of continued physical contact between mother and child. Proximity to a parent's body also meets emotional attachment needs that are as basic to the child as the need for physical sustenance.

When infants are anxious or upset, they are offered a human or a plastic nipple—in other words, a relationship with either a natural nurturing object or something that closely resembles it. That's how emotional nourishment and oral feeding or soothing become closely associated in the mind. On the other hand, emotional deprivation will trigger a desire for oral stimulation or eating just as surely as hunger. Children who continue to suck their thumbs past infancy are attempting to soothe themselves; it's always a sign of emotional distress. Except in rare cases of physical disease, the more obese a person is, the more emotionally starved they have been at some crucial period in their life.

As a novice family doctor I used to believe that all people needed was basic information. So all I had to do was to teach overweight individuals how excess body fat would overburden the heart, plug the arteries and raise the blood pressure, demonstrating my insights with naïve pencil drawings scratched on prescription pads, and they would leave the office grateful and transformed, ready for a new, healthier lifestyle. I soon found out that they left the office asking for their files to be transferred to some other physician less pedagogically zealous and more understanding about the ways of human beings. I learned that preaching at people about behaviours, even self-destructive ones, did little good when I didn't or couldn't help them with the emotional dynamics driving those behaviours.

Invariably, people who eat too much have not only suffered emotional loss in the past, but are also psychically deprived or highly stressed in the present. A woman might leave an unsatisfactory relationship, shed weight and gain confidence, only to become heavy again after going back to her partner. Emotional energy expended without perceived reward is compensated for by calories ingested. Similarly, many people who quit smoking begin to overeat because their craving for oral soothing is no longer eased by their cigarette and the loss of their stress reliever, nicotine, leaves them dopamine-deprived.

If children today are at greater risk for obesity than those of previous generations, it's not simply because they're less physically active as a result of being absorbed in TV or computers. It's primarily because under ordinary peacetime conditions there has never before been a generation so stressed and so starved of nurturing adult relationships. Of course, TV and computers have also become substitutes for the more constant real contact that parents used to provide when they worked near home or on the farm. These sources of entertainment are also used as substitutes for the sense of community formerly provided by large extended families or the clan, tribe or village. Children whose emotionally nourishing relationship with adults gives them a strong sense of themselves do not need to soothe themselves by passively taking in either food or entertainment.

The obesity epidemic demonstrates a psychological and spiritual emptiness at the core of consumer society. We feel powerless and isolated, so we become passive. We lead harried lives, so we long for escape. In Buddhist practice people are taught to chew slowly, being aware of every morsel, every taste. Eating becomes an exercise in awareness. In our culture it's just the opposite. Food is the universal soother, and many are driven to eat themselves into psychological oblivion.

The roots of sex addiction also reach back to childhood experience. Sex addiction authority Dr. Aviel Goodman points out that the vast majority of female sex addicts were sexually abused as children, as were up to 40 per cent of the men.[1] "Human beings are very adaptable," Dr. Goodman comments. Being held and cuddled is so important to us that we'll associate love with whatever gives us that warmth and contact. If a person feels wanted only sexually, as an adult she may look to sex to reaffirm that she is loveable and wanted. Sex addicts who were not abused as children may have had more subtle forms of sexualization projected on them by a parent or they may have felt so unloved or undesirable that they now look to sexual contact as a quick source of comfort.

The so-called nymphomaniac, the female sex addict, is not addicted to sex at all, but to the dopamine and endorphin rewards that flow from the feeling of being desired and desirable. Her promiscuity is not perversity but the outgrowth of a childhood adaptation to her circumstances. As with all addictions, sex addiction is a stand-in for nurturing the person was deprived of. The dopamine and endorphin rewards that love is meant to provide are obtained by having sex—but, as with all addictions, only temporarily. The craving for contact is, perversely, accompanied by a terror of real intimacy because of the painful instability of early relationships. That's why a relationship with a sex-addicted person won't last. "In a long term relationship you have to face yourself," says Monique Giard, a Vancouver psychologist with an interest in the treatment of sexual addiction. "It's very scary and potentially very painful to face one's deepest fears." By moving from one partner to another, a sex addict avoids the risk of intimacy, and just as with my constant quest for compact discs, the addict is always seeking the dopamine hit of the novel and the new.

Compulsive sexual roving, like all addictions, serves to help the addict avoid experiencing unpleasant emotions. "It takes a lot of discipline and courage to work through a negative thought and negative emotion," Ms. Giard points out. "Replacing a negative emotion with a positive one is the core of addictive behavior."[2]

Addictions can never truly replace the life needs they temporarily displace. The false needs they serve, no matter how often they are gratified, cannot leave us fulfilled. The brain can never, as it were, feel that it has had enough, that it can relax and get on with other essential business. It's as if after a full meal you were left starving and had to immediately turn your efforts to procuring food again. In a person with addictive behaviours, the orbitofrontal cortex and its associated neurological systems have been tricked from childhood onward into valuing false wants above real needs (this is the process we have identified as "salience attribution"). Hence, the desperation of the behavioural addict, the urgency to have that want answered immediately, as if it really were an essential requirement.

In addiction the Rolling Stones lyric is turned upside down: You can sometimes get what you want, but try as you might, you never get what you need.

—

As prisoner Stephen Reid listens to the story of my infancy during our exchange at the William Head Institution, he shakes his head and looks even more discouraged than before. "But you had these tragic beginnings," he says, "and yet you're free. You have a career. I had nothing like that happen to me, and here I am in jail again, where I've been most of my life due to my flaws and character weakness—my moral failure."

I see it differently, and not at all in terms of the harsh judgment Stephen has passed on himself. Apart from the severities we endured in my first year and a half or so, I was brought up in a stable, educated middle-class home by two parents who, for all their human flaws, gave loving, nurturing care to their children and to one another in the long term. Stephen, on the other hand, had a highly stressed and intimidated child for a mother, at least during his early years: he was born to a fifteen-year-old girl who was married to a raging alcoholic. His entire childhood was marked by poverty, shame, fear and emotional insecurity. "If anything disturbed my dad's world," he says, "he responded with blind fury."

Stephen was eleven years old when the town physician drove him out to the countryside, injected him with morphine and then initiated a relationship of drug-enabled sexual exploitation that persisted for many months. At the first hit of morphine the pre-adolescent Stephen was overawed by wonder as his brain flooded with opiates his own circuits could never produce. "What did that feel like?" I ask. "Like a warm, wet blanket," he replies, "a place of safety—the safety that came before pain and danger, before the enormity of being born, pushed and dragged, kicking and scream-ing into this world." The sex trade worker who told me that her first hit of heroin was like a warm, soft hug was fantasizing a state of infant joy. Stephen's "warm, wet blanket" harkens back even further, to the womb—perhaps the last time he'd had a sense of security.

I had a similar, if much milder, epiphany when in my mid-forties I was prescribed a serotonin-enhancing antidepressant. I was suf-fused by a sense of well-being I'd never imagined was possible. It's as if my brain cells were bathed in a normal chemical milieu for the first time. "So this is how human beings are meant to feel," I remarked to my sister-in-law. You don't know how depressed you've been until you know what it feels like *not* to be depressed. For both Stephen and me, given the early stresses that influenced our brain physiology, the newly experienced chemical state was a revelation.

How, then, to explain the addictions of people who, like my son Daniel, grew up in relatively comfortable circumstances, with par-ents who, contrary to being abusive or neglectful, did their best? To answer that question we need to revisit the issue of infancy and childhood, and the unique quality of *attunement* that optimal brain development requires.

Before we do, however, a few words on the touchy subject of "blaming the parent," a charge easily levelled at anyone who points to the crucial importance of the early rearing environment. The vigilance around parent blaming arises from people's natural defensiveness about anything that leaves them feeling accused of not loving their children or not doing their best. It's also part of a backlash against certain psychoanalytic theories and simplistic forms of pop psychology that flourished from the 1950s to at least the 1980s, which did encourage a blaming and even hostile attitude toward parents, especially mothers.

Yet the point is rarely that parents don't do their best no matter whom we consider: Stephen Reid's mother and father, or mine, or my wife and I as parents. As I've remarked before, even for my addicted patients, their greatest shame and regret is their failure to parent their own children, a sorrow that rarely fails to bring tears to their eyes. The point is that, as in the parenting my children received, our best is circumscribed by our own issues and limitations. In most cases, those issues and limitations originated in *our* childhoods—and so on down the generations. That parenting styles are passed on from one generation to the next is known both from human studies and animal experiments. In the latter, it has been shown that parental nurturing practices can be *biologically* inherited, not through genes but through molecular mechanisms. In other words, the parenting an infant receives can "program" her own brain circuitry in ways that will influence and may even determine how she will parent. The neurological basis of such transmission probably involves the oxytocin "love hormone" system, which is key in the mother-infant attachment relationship.[3] If we understand these facts, it's obvious that there is no one left to blame. I've remarked before that a blaming attitude is an entirely useless commodity. As the Sufi poet Hafiz writes, blame only perpetuates the "sad game."

I had an almost bizarre taste of the charge of parent bashing after the publication of *Scattered Minds,* my book on attention deficit disorder. In explaining my own ADD—a prime risk factor for addictions—I referred to the history of my infancy. "My mother and I had little opportunity for normal mother-infant experiences," I wrote. "These were hardly possible, given the terrible circumstances, her numbed mind state, and her having to concentrate her energies on basic survival. Attunement," I asserted, "can be severely interfered with despite the deepest feelings of love a mother may have."

The first review of *Scattered Minds* appeared in the *Toronto Star.* "Maté blames his mother," it said.

Blame, like beauty, is in the eye of the beholder.

—

Brain development can be affected adversely not only by "bad stimulation" coming in, to quote Dr. Robert Post but also by insufficient "good stimulation" occurring—by "nothing happening when something might profitably have happened," in the wonderful phrasing of the great British child psychiatrist D.W. Winnicott. Stressed parents have difficulty offering their children a specific quality required for the development of the brain's self-regulation circuits: the quality of *attunement*. Attunement is, literally, being "in tune" with someone else's emotional states. It's not a question of parental love but of the parent's ability to be present emotionally in such a way that the infant or child feels understood, accepted and mirrored. Attunement is the real language of love, the conduit by which a pre-verbal child can realize that she *is* loved.

Attunement is a subtle process. It is deeply instinctive and is easily subverted when the parent is stressed, depressed or distracted. A parent can be fully attached to the infant—fully "in love"—but not attuned. For example, the infants of depressed parents experience physiological stress not because they are not loved, but because their parents are not attuned with them—and attunement is especially likely to be lacking if parents missed out on it in their own childhoods. Children in poorly attuned relationships may feel loved, or be aware that love is there, but on a deeper and essential level they do not experience themselves as seen or appreciated for who they really are. Daniel, ever sensitive that something was lacking even if he couldn't exactly identify what, once wrote me a description of how he experienced his childhood:

> It seemed to me that I was growing up in a house where love was never in question; it was often affirmed. So I knew I was loved, but it came in shifting, confusing and unpredictable ways that left me on my guard about it, and always craving it in a simpler, more straightforward form. I felt I had to be crafty to catch it and get some for myself, to pin it down.

My son's recollection doesn't surprise me. My workaholism and other addictive behaviours left me only inconsistently present for my children, and the stresses in our marriage often meant that my wife and I were both preoccupied. It makes sense that Daniel would have felt he had to work for attention, that the love offered him was conditional and that his emotional terrain was often not appreciated, shared or mirrored by his parents.

Poorly attuned relationships provide an inadequate template for the development of a child's neurological and psychological self-regulation systems. In the words of child psychiatrist Daniel Siegel:

> From early infancy, it appears that our ability to regulate emotional states depends upon the experience of feeling that a significant person in our life is simultaneously experiencing a similar state of mind.[4]

Self-regulation does not refer to "good behaviour" but to the capacity of an individual to maintain a reasonably even internal emotional environment. A person with good self-regulation will not experience rapidly shifting extremes of emotional highs and lows in the face of life's challenges, difficulties, disappointments and satisfactions. She does not depend on other people's responses or external activities or substances in order to feel okay. The person with poor self-regulation is more likely to look outside herself for emotional soothing, which is why the lack of attunement in infancy increases addiction risk. It's what Stephen Reid meant when he said, "I've spent too much time on external things, bouncing off other people."

The importance of consistent, nonstressed parent–infant interactions was demonstrated in a primate experiment involving three groups of mother–infant pairs. The investigators set up three sets of conditions under which the mothers had to forage for food: a situation of high but predictable difficulty; one of consistently low difficulty; and the third of unpredictably varying difficulty: easy one time, difficult the next. They then observed the nature of mother–infant relationships during the test period, the "personality" traits that evolved as the three groups of infants matured and the biochemical status of the young monkeys' stress systems throughout their lifetimes.

It was not the high-difficulty foraging conditions that created stress for monkey moms and interfered with their parenting but the variable conditions, with their built-in unpredictability. These mothers exhibited "inconsistent and erratic, sometimes dismissive, rearing behavior." Their infants, unlike the ones in the other two groups, grew up to be anxious as adults, less social and highly reactive—traits known to increase addiction risk. Biologically, this group of monkeys had lifelong elevated levels of a major stress hormone in their spinal fluid, indicating an abnormality in their stress apparatus.[5] That also adds to the propensity for addiction, since both animals and humans use substances or other behaviours to modulate their experience of stress.[6] Obviously it's not a question of the mothers in the other two groups having been "better" parents but of the stresses afflicting the variable foraging mothers as they were nursing their infants—uncertainty being a trigger for physiological and emotional stress.

The lack of an emotionally attuned and consistently available parenting figure is a major source of stress for the child. Such a lack can occur when the parent is physically present but emotionally distracted—a situation that has been called *proximate separation*. Proximate separation happens when attuned contact between parent and child is interrupted due to stresses that draw the parent away from the interaction. The levels of physiological stress experienced by the child during proximate separation approach the levels experienced during physical separation.[7] The development of the brain's neurotransmitter and self-regulating systems and, in particular, the stress-control circuits, are then disrupted, and once entrenched, these physiological dysfunctions increase the risk for addictions. Addictive tendencies may already be seen in young children. In the absence of the biological mother, infant monkeys will become attached to an inanimate "surrogate mother" constructed of wire mesh, and human children lacking sufficient attuned parental contact may readily become addicted to television or to self-soothing behaviours such as eating.

The void is not in the parent's love or commitment, but in the child's perception of being seen, understood, empathized with and "gotten" on the emotional level. In our extraordinarily fragmented and stressed society, where parents often face the childrearing task without the support that the tribe, clan, village, extended family and community used to provide, misattuned parent–child interactions are increasingly the norm.

In contrast to the extensive research linking addiction to adverse childhood events—abuse, neglect and trauma—very little has been published on attunement outside specialized child developmental literature. I see two obvious reasons for this. First, the study of bad things that happened is fairly straightforward. It's much more difficult to research attunement, since few people can recall and few researchers can observe *what didn't happen but should have happened*. Second, a consciousness of even overt abuse is only slowly penetrating the addiction treatment community. So studies about the more subtle attunement issues are even further behind.

Poor attunement is also not something parents easily recall as they strive to understand the addictive behaviours of their adult children. As parents we make the natural mistake of believing that the intense love we feel for our kids necessarily means that they actually receive that love in a pure form. Further, parents who did not have attuned caring as small children may not notice their difficulty attuning to their own infants, just as people stressed from an early age may not realize just how stressed they often are. One couple I interviewed have two grown-up sons who both struggle with substance addiction. "Our boys' infancy and early childhood were the happiest years of our lives," the mother insisted. "There were no stresses for us then," the father added, "and we have always had a good marriage." It was after an hour of discussion that they disclosed that the man—a devoted parent and conscientious provider—had a cannabis habit all those years, well into his sons' adolescence. He did not perceive his habit as an addiction, nor that it created an emotional distance from his children. The mother, from a strict religious background, resented her husband's daily pot smoking and suppressed a rage that, until this very conversation, she had never expressed. Her belief, shared by many in our culture, was that if strong negative emotions like her anger remain under cover, the children will not suffer its effects.

While it's true that overt episodes of hostility between the parents may damage the child, so may repressed anger and unhappiness. As a rule, whatever we don't deal with in our lives, we pass on to our children. Our unfinished emotional business becomes theirs. As a therapist said to me, "Children swim in their parents' unconscious like fish swim in the sea." This mother and father were fully committed to their family and still are, but under such circumstances all the parental love in the world could not provide the children with a well-attuned, nonstressed, nurturing environment.

Thus it would be simplistic to claim that all hard-drug addictions originate in abuse or neglect and that all behavioural addictions are rooted in early stress and attunement problems. While generally true, in individual cases no clear divisions can be made. Many non-drug addicts were abused as children or suffered significant neglect. For example, there is a strong association between parental neglect and the later development of obesity.[8] Once more, neglect does not need to be intentional or overt: parental stress and depression during the child's early years will have the same effect, owing to the lack of attunement that follows. In the Adverse Childhood Experiences (ACE) Study it was found that childhood abuse was also a risk for adult obesity and that among the groups surveyed, the greater the weight, the greater was the percentage of adults who reported having been abused.[9] On the other hand, people can develop hardcore drug addictions without having been abused or neglected, as with the family we've just looked at. Also at risk are kids who fall under negative peer influence during the vulnerable teen years. In such cases, however, there is usually a disruption in the parent–child relationship before the peer effect can assert itself.[10]

—

Many phenomena in public life can be understood if viewed through the prism of addiction. As an illustration, we can look at the moral and legal demise of Conrad Black, Canadian-born business tycoon and international press baron, convicted in a Chicago court of fraud and obstruction of justice. If the media reports and biographical accounts are even remotely accurate, Black's behaviour closely resembles that of my drug-seeking patients, albeit on an infinitely grander scale. His actions have all the features of addictive drives. His childhood, emotionally impoverished and darkened by abuse, more than explains those drives."

Conrad Black is formally known by his British peerage title, Lord Black of Crossharbour—an honorific he craved and pursued. His high ambition was to hobnob with the elite of conservative political and business circles on both sides of the Atlantic, courting figures like Margaret Thatcher and Henry Kissinger as acquaintances. Following a spectacular rise to business and social prominence, he is now a convicted felon. In the words of an internal investigation at one of the companies he directed, his regime was one of "corporate kleptocracy." He has been described as unscrupulous, vain, arrogant and power hungry, with an insatiable appetite for cash. According to all of his biographers he has been relentlessly single-minded in his quest for power, status, financial gain and *haut monde* respectability. He is also blessed, or cursed, with a sharp intellect and an even sharper tongue, ever ready to cut down anyone who crosses him. The British magazine *New Statesman* praised one of the Black biographies as "a rounded portrait of a monster, albeit a self-conscious, even ironic monster."

All humans have the potential to behave monstrously or virtuously. The key question is how a child with great potential becomes an adult driven to engineer for himself such a dramatic rise and an even more dramatic descent. "Conrad has a lot going for him," *Globe and Mail* columnist Rex Murphy once wrote, referring to Black's ample blessings of natural abilities and social advantages. "What is perplexing is why a man so rich—in both senses of the term—would have chosen to go the way he has." Why would such a man define his ambitions "mainly in terms of that hollow word *more*. More money. More houses. More famous friends. Just more." I believe addiction best accounts for Conrad Black's otherwise perplexing life.

The addict is never satisfied. His spiritual and emotional condition is one of impoverishment, no matter how much he achieves, acquires or possesses. In the hungry-ghost mode, we can never be satiated. Scruples vanish in face of the addictive "need"—hence, the ruthlessness. Loyalty, integrity and honour lose meaning.

Black's wife, Barbara Amiel Black, has been his partner in insatiability. Formerly addicted to codeine, by the side of her wealthy husband Amiel became attached to luxury and limitless acquisition. Her closets reportedly house a collection of fashion shoes worth several hundred thousand dollars, rivalling Imelda Marcos's footwear storehouse, alongside "boxes of unopened panty hose, filed by color and make." "I have an extravagance that knows no bounds," Barbara Amiel told *Vogue* magazine in 2002—a self-parodying confession, perhaps, but accurate.

Black's childhood was the perfect crucible for an addict's mentality. According to his biographers the young Conrad was never close to his mother. In his autobiography, the warmest acknowledgment the hyper-eloquent Black could conjure up was that she was a "convivial and altogether virtuous person . . . as affable as he [Black's father] was prone to be aloof." It was the reclusive, often-absent, depressive and heavy-drinking father that Conrad idolized. The bookish, awkward, sensitive, intelligent child did not fit in with the easygoing jock camaraderie of the extended Black clan, and his parents acknowledged their inability to understand or relate to their precocious son. "We have this strange child—we don't know what to do with him," they told family friends.[12]

The young Black was abused, not at home, but at Toronto's Upper Canada College, the institution where the male scions of society's upper crust were educated in the ways of the world. Beatings by the instructors were indiscriminate and cruel. Black has described one thrashing at the hands of a teacher, using a heavy cane, as "a fierce and savage assault" that left him lacerated to a pulp. As a child and since then as well, Black has repeatedly likened UCC to a Nazi concentration camp. He referred to some of his teachers as *Gauleiters*—Nazi leaders in the Hitler mode, and to fellow students as *Sonderkommandos*—prisoners who collaborated with the SS guards. He had no one to turn to. So emotionally distant were his parents that, in his words, "they never really understood what I was so upset about in my school years."

In the recollection of a childhood friend the pre-adolescent Black exhibited behaviours that would lead most parents to request professional intervention: "he kicked holes in walls when he got upset as a child, threw knives around." At age twenty-five Conrad suffered bouts of severe anxiety, hyperventilation, insomnia and claustrophobia. All the ingredients for addiction were in the mix by the time he became an adult: parental non-attunement, psychological distress, impaired impulse control and emotional pain.

Under different social and economic circumstances, Conrad might well have sought solace in alcohol or hard drugs. Born into a world of privilege, however, and gifted with charisma, it was natural that power, wealth, status and "respect"—no matter how he acquired them—became the objects of his addictive pursuits.

Addicts respond with rage toward anyone who tries to deprive them of their drug, a rage that's fuelled by intense frustration. I have witnessed that rage in opiate seekers and have experienced it personally when, for example, my wife tried to stand in the way of my compulsive compact disc buying. Black's drugs of choice being power and *status*—social, economic, political and intellectual—we can understand the venom he directs at people who thwart him. Business associates who critiqued Black's operations as self-serving were, in his words, "corporate governance terrorists." The prosecutors conducting the legal case against him in Chicago were "Nazis." When historian Ramsay Cook gave Conrad's first book an unfavourable review, he called the distinguished academic "a slanted, supercilious little twit," possessing "the professional ethics of a cockroach." After the Catholic bishop of Calgary gave moral support to striking employees at the Black-owned *Calgary Herald,* the media mogul excoriated him as "a jumped-up little twerp of a bishop" and a "prime candidate for exorcism."

That sneering word "little" may articulate precisely how Conrad feels about himself at the core of his psyche—our sneers always tell us who we feel we are. A powerful person's self-esteem may appear to be high, but it's a hollow shell if it's based on externals, on the ability to impress or intimidate others. It's what psychologist Gordon Neufeld calls conditional or *contingent self-esteem:* it depends on circumstances. The greater the void within, the more urgent the drive to be noticed and to be "important," and the more compulsive the need for status. By contrast, *genuine self-esteem* needs nothing from the outside. It doesn't say, "I'm worthwhile because I've done this, that or the other." It says, "I'm worthwhile whether or not I've done this, that or the other. I don't need to be right or to wield power, to amass wealth or achievements."

Self-esteem is not what the individual consciously thinks about himself; it's the quality of self-respect manifested in his emotional life and behaviours. By no means are a superficially positive self-image and true self-esteem necessarily identical. In many cases they are not even compatible. People with a grandiose and inflated view of themselves are missing true self-esteem at the core. To compensate for a deep sense of worthlessness, they develop a craving for power and an exaggerated self-evaluation that may itself become a focus of addiction, as it appears to have done for the person who needed to become "Lord" Black. His bluster and pomposity, derided by some and resented by many, are compensations for what he lacks in self-acceptance, and, deeper, in spiritual fulfillment. The absurdist Austrian author Robert Musil wrote of one of his characters, "the whole ideology of the great man he lived by was only an emergency substitute for something that was missing."[13] It's a form of grandiosity I well know from within.

"Power is like a drug," wrote Primo Levi.

> The need for either is unknown to anyone who has not tried them, but after the initiation . . . the dependency and need for ever larger doses is born, as are the denial of reality and the return to childish dreams of omnipotence . . . The syndrome produced by protracted and undisputed power is clearly visible: a distorted view of the world, dogmatic arrogance, the need for adulation, convulsive clinging to the levers of command, and contempt for the law.[13]

Do not Levi's words apply to Lord Black and, perhaps, to many others in our culture?

I frequently hear one or another of my patients complain that his supposed friends are loyal, but only so long as he supplies them with drugs or money. A young Native man, who had been in jail for twelve years for armed robberies, disclosed that in the past year and a half he blew through $240,000 in personal inheritance and oil royalties from his reserve that accumulated during his incarceration.

"You must have supplied drugs to the whole world with that much money," I remarked. "Yeah," he said wryly, "I had many, many friends. And now I couldn't bum a loonie out there if I tried." The friendships of the super-rich may be just as materially based. Conrad Black has also bewailed being dropped by people whose good will he had long cultivated with lavish parties and dinner occasions, of being "spurned and shunned by persons who had personally accepted his hospitality in London, New York and Palm Beach."

It is surely no coincidence that Conrad has more than once likened himself to King Lear, the Shakespearean monarch who met his demise because he confused power and false adulation with love.

Addiction is always a poor substitute for love.

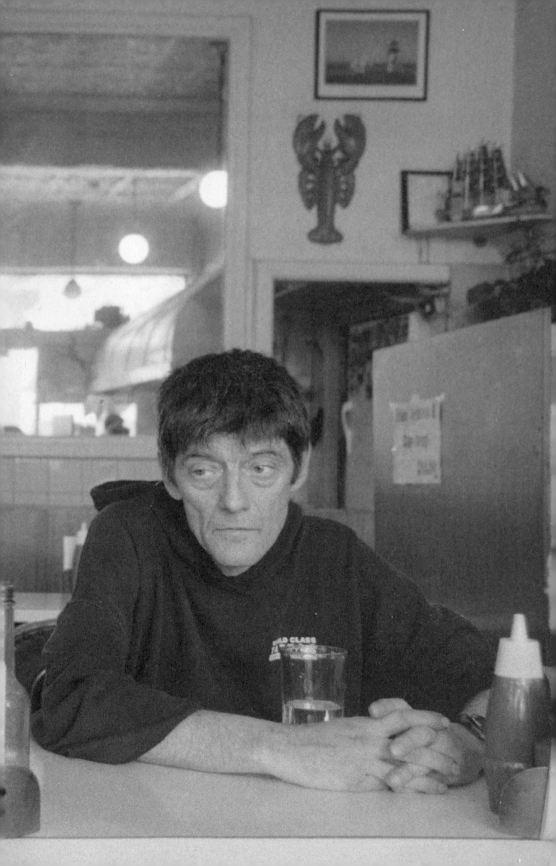

PART VI

Imagining a Humane Reality: Beyond the War on Drugs

What we are doing hasn't worked, it's never going to work and we
need to change our whole approach. Tinkering around the edges
isn't going to make a difference.

ALEX WODAK, M.D.

DIRECTOR, ALCOHOL AND DRUG SERVICE

ST. VINCENT'S HOSPITAL, SYDNEY, AUSTRALIA

—

CHAPTER 23

Dislocation and the
Social Roots of Addiction

—

I believe that to pursue the American Dream is not only futile
but self-destructive because ultimately it destroys everything
and everyone involved with it. By definition it must, because it
nurtures everything except those things that are important:
integrity, ethics, truth, our very heart and soul. Why? The reason
is simple: because Life/life is about giving, not getting.

HUBERT SELBY JR.
Requiem for a Dream (Preface, 2000)

Ralph, the God-starved, pseudo-Nazi poet, said something to
me in the hospital that ought to make many of us upstand-
ing, righteous citizens squirm. I was challenging his belief
in emancipation through drugs. "You talk about freedom. But how
much freedom can there be when you're chasing the drug the whole
day for just a few minutes of satisfaction? Where's the freedom in
that?"

Ralph shrugs his shoulders. "What else am I going to do? What
do *you* do? You get up in the morning, and somebody cooks you
bacon and eggs . . ."

"Yogurt and banana," I interject. "I prepare it myself."

Ralph shakes his head impatiently. "Okay . . . yogurt and banana.
Then you go to the office and you see a couple of dozen patients . . .

and all your money goes to the bank at the end of that, and then you count up your shekels or your doubloons. At the end of the day, what have you done? You've collected the summation of what you think freedom is. You're looking for security and you think that will give you freedom. You collected a hundred shekels of gold, and to you this gold has the capacity of keeping you in a fancy house or maybe you can salt away another six weeks' worth up and above what you already have in the bank.

"But what are you looking for? What have you spent your whole day searching for? That same bit of freedom or satisfaction that I want; we just get it differently. What's everybody chasing all the money for if not to get them something that will make them feel good for a while or make them feel they're free? How are they freer than I am?

"Everybody's searching for that feeling of well-being, that greater happiness. But I'd rather be a dog out in the street than do what many people go through to find their summation of freedom."

"There's a lot of truth there," I concede. "I can get caught up in all sorts of meaningless activities that leave me only temporarily satisfied, if that. Sometimes they leave me feeling worse. But I do believe there's a greater freedom than either your pursuit of the drug or my pursuit of security or success can provide."

Ralph looks at me as a benign but worldlywise uncle would gaze upon a naïve child. "And what would that freedom of pursuits be? What would be the ultimate freedom to be searching for?"

I hesitate. Can I authentically say this? "The freedom *from* pursuits," I say finally. "The freedom from being so needy that our whole life is spent trying to appease our desires or fill in the emptiness. I've never experienced total freedom, but I believe it's possible."

Ralph is adamant. "If it could be different, it would be. It is what it is. Let me put it to you this way: why is it that some people, through no merit whatsoever, get to have whatever they think will give them happiness? Others, through no fault of their own, are deprived."

I agree it's an unfair world in many ways.

"Then how can you or anyone else tell me that my way is wrong, theirs is right? It's just power, isn't it?"

I've often heard Ralph's worldview espoused by other drug addicts, if less eloquently. It's clear and obvious that his (and their) rationalization for addiction misses something essential. The defeatist belief that all pursuits arise from a selfish core in all humanity denies the deeper motives that also activate people: love, creativity, spiritual quest, the drive for mastery and autonomy, the impulse to make a contribution.

Although the cracks in his argument are easy to discern, perhaps it would be more worthwhile to consider what *realities* the drug-dependent Ralph might be articulating, and what we might see about ourselves in the dark mirror he holds up for us. Though we pretend otherwise, in our materialist culture many of us conduct ourselves as if Ralph's cynicism reflected the truth—that it's every man for himself, that the world offers nothing other than brief, illusory satisfactions. But from his pinched and narrow perch at the edge of society, the drug addict sees who we are—or more exactly, who we are *choosing to be*. He sees that we resemble him in our frantic material pursuits and our delusions and that we exceed him in our hypocrisies.

If Ralph's view is cynical, it's no more cynical than society's view of drug addicts as flawed and culpable, people to be isolated and shunned. We flatter ourselves.

And if I'm being honest, I might ask myself to what extent my insistence on that greater freedom is really not just the sentimentality of the privileged, pseudo-enlightened addict—a way for me to rationalize my own addictions: *I know I'm hooked, but I'm working on getting free, so I'm different from you.* If I really knew that kind of freedom, would I need to argue for it? Would I not just manifest it in my life and way of being?

—

At heart, I'm not that different from my patients, and sometimes I cannot stand seeing what little psychic space, what little heaven-granted grace, separates me from them—so I wrote in the first chapter. There are moments when I'm revolted by my patients' dishevelled appearance, their stained and decayed teeth, the look of insatiable hunger in their eyes, their demands, complaints and neediness. Those are times when I would do well to examine myself for irresponsibility in my own life, for self-neglect—in my case not so much physical but spiritual—and for placing false needs above real ones.

When I am sharply judgmental of any other person, it's because I sense or see reflected in them some aspect of myself that I don't want to acknowledge. I'm speaking here not of my *critique* of another person's behaviour in objective terms but of the self-righteous tone of personal *judgment* that colours my opinion. If, for example, I resent some person close to me as "controlling," it may be owing to my own inability to assert myself. Or I may react against another person because she has a trait that I myself have—and dislike, but don't wish to acknowledge: for example, a tendency to want to control others. As I mentioned in a previous chapter, some mornings I vituperate about right-wing political columnists. My opinion remains more or less constant: their views are based on a highly selective reading of the facts and rooted in a denial of reality. What does vary from day to day is the emotional charge that infuses my opinion. Some days I dismiss them with intense hostility; at other times I see their perspective as one possible way of looking at things.

On the surface, the differences are obvious: they support wars I oppose and justify policies I dislike. I can tell myself that we're different. Moral judgments, however, are never about the obvious; they always speak to the underlying similarities between the judge and the condemned. My judgments of others are an accurate gauge of how, beneath the surface, I feel about myself. It's only the wilful blindness in me that condemns another for deluding himself; my own selfishness that excoriates another for being self-serving; my lack of authenticity that judges falsehood in another. It is the same, I believe, for all moral judgments people cast on each other and for all vehemently held communal judgments a society visits upon its members. So it is with the harsh social attitudes toward addicts, especially hardcore drug addicts.

—

"What characterizes an addiction?" asks the spiritual teacher Eckhart Tolle. "Quite simply this: you no longer feel that you have the power to stop. It seems stronger than you. It also gives you a false sense of pleasure, pleasure that invariably turns into pain."[1]

Addiction cuts large swaths across our culture. Many of us are burdened with compulsive behaviours that harm us and others, behaviours whose toxicity we fail to acknowledge or feel powerless to stop. Many people are addicted to accumulating wealth; for others the compulsive pull is power. Men and women become addicted to consumerism, status, shopping or fetishized relationships, not to mention the obvious and widespread addictions such as gambling, sex, junk food and the cult of the "young" body image. The following report from the *Guardian Weekly* speaks for itself:

> Americans now [2006] spend an alarming $15 billion a year on cosmetic surgery in a beautification frenzy that would be frowned upon if there was anyone left in the U.S. who could actually frown with their Botox-frozen faces. The sum is double Malawi's gross domestic product and more than twice what America has contributed to AIDS programs in the past decade. Demand has exploded to produce a new generation of obsessives, or "beauty junkies."[2]

Beauty Junkies is the title of a recent book by *New York Times* writer Alex Kuczynski, "a self-confessed recovering addict of cosmetic surgery." And, with our technological prowess, we succeed in creating fresh addictions. Some psychologists now describe a new clinical pathology—Internet sex addiction disorder.

Physicians and psychologists may not be all that effective in treating addictions, but we're expert at coming up with fresh names and categories. A recent study at Stanford University School of Medicine found that about 5.5 per cent of men and 6 per cent of women appear to be addicted shoppers. The lead researcher, Dr. Lorrin Koran, suggested that compulsive buying be recognized as a unique illness listed under its own heading in the *Diagnostic and Statistical Manual of Mental Disorders,* the official psychiatric catalogue. Sufferers of this "new" disorder are afflicted by "an irresistible, intrusive and senseless impulse" to purchase objects they

do not need. I don't scoff at the harm done by shopping addiction—
I'm in no position to do that—and I agree that Dr. Koran accurately describes the potential consequences of compulsive buying:
"serious psychological, financial and family problems, including
depression, overwhelming debt and the breakup of relationships."[3]
But it's clearly not a distinct entity—only another manifestation
of addiction tendencies that run through our culture, and of the
fundamental addiction process that varies only in its targets, not
its basic characteristics.

In his 2006 State of the Union address, President George W.
Bush identified another item of addiction. "Here we have a serious
problem," he said. "America is addicted to oil." Coming from a man
who throughout his financial and political career has had the closest possible ties to the oil industry, this stark admission might have
been transformational. Unfortunately, Mr. Bush framed the problem purely in geopolitical terms: the U.S. finds itself dependent on
a resource from abroad, a resource that "the enemies of freedom"
would deny its citizens. Hence, the country needs to develop other
sources of energy. So the problem is not the addiction itself, only
that the supply of the substance in question may be jeopardized:
typical addict's logic, of course.

Whether we tally health expenditures, loss of human life, economic strain or any other measure, the "respectable" addictions,
around which entire cultures, industries and professions have been
built, leave drug addiction in the dust.

We've already defined addiction as any relapsing behaviour that
satisfies a short-term craving and persists despite its long-term negative consequences. The long-term ill effects of our society's addiction, if not to oil then to the amenities and luxuries that oil makes
possible, are obvious. They range from environmental destruction,
climate change and the toxic effects of pollution on human health to
the many wars that the need for oil, or the attachment to oil wealth,
has triggered. Consider how much greater a price has been exacted
by this socially sanctioned addiction than by the drug addiction for
which Ralph and his peers have been declared outcasts.

And oil is only one example among many: consider soul-, body-
or Nature-destroying addictions to consumer goods, fast food,

sugar cereals, television programs and glossy publications devoted to celebrity gossip—only a few examples of what American writer Kevin Baker calls "the growth industries that have grown out of gambling and hedonism." The metropolis of gambling and hedonism, Las Vegas, received nearly 40 million visitors in 2006, and its local population base has increased by 18 per cent since 2000. The highest-grossing independent restaurant in the U.S. is the Tao Las Vegas. It features seminaked women, gaming consoles, poolside plasma TV screens, preprogrammed iPods, all amid a "proliferation of Buddhas, pulsating music and sensuous décor."[4] I doubt either owners or customers are alive to the absurdity of co-opting the Tao, the ancient Chinese wisdom path of nonattachment and surrender, to support addiction, or of using images of Buddha, the teacher of serene mindfulness, to shill food, liquor and games of chance.

We need hardly mention legally permissible substance dependencies on nicotine and alcohol: in terms of scale, their negative consequences far surpass the damage inflicted by illicit drugs. And what do the mass marketing and advertising of these often-lethal substances reflect if not addiction? Exactly like drug pushers who are themselves addicted, tobacco companies behave as if they, too, were driven by addiction: in their case, to profit.

In August 2006 U.S. District Judge Gladys Kessler ruled that the big tobacco companies had deceived the public concerning the health effects of their product:

[The] defendants have marketed and sold their lethal product with zeal, with deception, with a single-minded focus on their financial success, and without regard for the human tragedy or social costs that success exacted.[5]

Treating smoking-related illnesses has incurred costs in the multiple hundreds of billions of dollars. According to the *New York Times*, there are currently 44 million adult smokers in the U.S., and four out of five are addicted to tobacco. "Tobacco kills 440,000 smokers every year in the United States, and secondhand smoke inhaled by bystanders claims another 50,000."[6]

How can we compare the misdemeanours of my patients—petty dealers thrown against the wall and frisked by police in the back alleys of the Downtown Eastside—with those of their respectable counterparts in corporate boardrooms? In May 2007, Purdue Pharma, a giant drug manufacturer, pleaded guilty to criminal charges that the firm had "misled doctors and patients" in claiming that their product, OxyContin, was less addictive than other opiate medications. "That claim," said the *New York Times,* "became the linchpin of an aggressive marketing campaign that helped the company sell over $1 billion of OxyContin a year . . . But both experienced drug abusers and novices, including teenagers, soon discovered that chewing an OxyContin tablet—or crushing one and then snorting the powder, or injecting it with a needle—produced a high as powerful as heroin."[7]

We see that substance addictions are only one specific form of blind attachment to harmful ways of being. Yet we condemn the addict's stubborn refusal to give up something deleterious to his life or to the lives of others. Why do we despise, ostracize and punish the drug addict when as a social collective we share the same blindness and engage in the same rationalizations?

To pose that question is to answer it. We despise, ostracize and punish the addict because we don't wish to see how much we resemble him. In his dark mirror our own features are unmistakable. We shudder at the recognition. This mirror is not for us, we say to the addict. You are different, and you don't belong with us. Ralph's critique, for all its flaws, is too close for comfort. Like the hardcore addict's pursuit of drugs, much of our economic and cultural life caters to people's craving to escape mental and emotional distress. In an apt phrase, Lewis Lapham, long-time publisher of *Harper's Magazine,* derides "consumer markets selling promises of instant relief from the pain of thought, loneliness, doubt, experience, envy, and old age."[8]

According to a Statistics Canada study, 31 per cent of working adults aged nineteen to sixty-four consider themselves workaholics, who attach excessive importance to their work and are "overdedicated and perhaps overwhelmed by their jobs." "They have trouble sleeping, are more likely to be stressed out and unhealthy, and feel they don't spend enough time with their families," reports the *Globe and Mail.* Work doesn't necessarily give them greater satisfaction, suggested Vishwanath Baba, a professor of Human Resources and Management at McMaster University. "These people turn to work to occupy their time and energy"⁹—as compensation for what is lacking in their lives, much as the drug addict employs substances.

At the core of every addiction is an emptiness based in abject fear. The addict dreads and abhors the present moment; she bends feverishly only towards the next time, the moment when her brain, infused with her drug of choice, will briefly experience itself as liberated from the burden of the past and the fear of the future—the two elements that make the present intolerable. Many of us resemble the drug addict in our ineffectual efforts to fill in the spiritual black hole, the void at the centre, where we have lost touch with our souls, our spirit, with those sources of meaning and value that are not contingent or fleeting. Our consumerist, acquisition-, action- and image-mad culture only serves to deepen the hole, leaving us emptier than before.

The constant, intrusive and meaningless mind-whirl that characterizes the way so many of us experience our silent moments is, itself, a form of addiction—and it serves the same purpose. "One of the main tasks of the mind is to fight or remove the emotional pain, which is one of the reasons for its incessant activity, but all it can ever achieve is to cover it up temporarily. In fact, the harder the mind struggles to get rid of the pain, the greater the pain."¹⁰ So writes Eckhart Tolle. Even our 24/7 self-exposure to noise, emails, cell phones, TV, Internet chats, media outlets, music downloads, videogames and non-stop internal and external chatter cannot succeed in drowning out the fearful voices within.

———

Not only do we avert our eyes from the hardcore drug addict to avoid seeing ourselves; we do so to avoid facing our share of responsibility.

As we have seen, injection drug use more often than not arises in people who were abused and neglected as young children. The addict, in other words, is not born but made. His addiction is the result of a situation that he had no influence in creating. His life expresses the history of the multigenerational family system of which he is a part, and his family exists as part of the broader culture and society. In society, as in Nature, each microcosmic unit reflects something of the whole. In the case of drug addiction, the sins of entire societies are visited unevenly on minority populations.

We know, for example, that a disproportionate number of prisoners incarcerated for drug-related crimes in the jails of the United States are African-American males. In 2002 45 per cent of the prisoners in U.S. jails were black, and according to the Department of Justice black males have about a one in three chance of being jailed at least once in their lives.[11] In federal prisons, an estimated 57 per cent of inmates have been convicted of drug-related crimes, and drug offenders represented the largest source of jail population growth between 1996 and 2002—increasing by 37 per cent.[12] The fate of black youth has much to tell us about the larger society in which their stories unfold. Similarly, there is an extraordinarily high ratio of Native Canadians among my Portland patients—and in Canada's drug-using population and prisons.

Dr. Robert Dupont, former U.S. drug czar, interprets such facts as flowing from what he calls the "tragic vulnerability" of traditional cultures to alcohol and drug problems. He describes the present susceptibility of Aboriginal minority populations to addiction as "one of the sad paradoxes of the world experience with alcohol and drug abuse."

> To see Native Americans suffer from the use of alcohol and other drugs, and even cigarettes, or to see similar suffering among Australian aborigines, is to face the painful reality that traditional cultures are not prepared to withstand exposure to modern drugs and to tolerant values governing drug-taking behaviors.[13]

There is, perhaps, a much more specific and robust cause for minority drug use than "tolerant values" toward drug taking. In fact, given the high incarceration rate of minority members, it's hard to see what these "tolerant values" even are.

As the stories of Serena, Celia and Angela in the first part of this book illustrate, many women who become injection drug users were severely abused in childhood—the vast majority, according to the research. Of those three women, two are Native. It is a fact that over the past several generations Native female children in Canada have been more likely to suffer sexual abuse in their families of origin than non-Natives. That this is so says nothing about the "innate" nature of Canadian Native peoples. Sexual abuse of young children among tribal peoples living in their natural habitats is virtually nonexistent, and so it was with North American Natives before European colonization. The current dismal statistics say everything about the relationship of Aboriginal societies to the dominant culture.

The precursor to addiction is *dislocation*, according to Bruce Alexander, professor of psychology at Simon Fraser University. By dislocation he means the loss of psychological, social and economic integration into family and culture; a sense of exclusion, isolation and powerlessness. "Only chronically and severely dislocated people are vulnerable to addiction," he writes.

> The historical correlation between severe dislocation and addiction is strong. Although alcohol consumption and drunkenness on festive occasions was widespread in Europe during the Middle Ages, and although a few people became "inebriates" or "drunkards," mass alcoholism was not a problem. However, alcoholism gradually spread with the beginnings of free markets after 1500, and eventually became a raging epidemic with the dominance of the free market society after 1800.[14]

Dr. Dupont agrees that in premodern societies, although substance use to the point of intoxication was permitted, "that use was infrequent and managed in families and communities . . . Stable communities in premodern times were the Golden Age for alcohol and drug use."[15]

With the rise of industrial societies came dislocation: the destruction of traditional relationships, extended family, clan, tribe and village. Vast economic and social changes tore asunder the ties that formerly connected people to those closest to them and to their communities. They displaced people from their homes and shredded the value systems that secured people's sense of belonging in the moral and spiritual universe. The same process is happening around the world as a result of globalization. China is a prime example. That country's breakneck-speed industrialization has made it an emerging economic superpower, but the accompanying social dislocation is likely to prove disastrous. Entire villages and towns are being depopulated to make room for megaprojects like the Three Gorges Dam. The pressures of urbanization are cutting millions of people adrift from their connections with land, tradition and community. The social and psychological results of massive dislocation are not only predictable; they're already obvious. China has had to set up a massive needle-exchange program in an attempt to prevent the spread of HIV and other infectious diseases among its rapidly burgeoning addict population. According to the Ministry of Health in Beijing, nearly half of China's estimated 650,000 people living with HIV/AIDS are drug users who contracted the disease by sharing needles.[16] There can be no doubt that the ravages of social breakdown—alienation, violence and addiction—will soon make vast and urgent claims on the attention and resources of Chinese authorities, academics and health professionals. In the rush to emulate the Western world's achievements, many countries are neglecting to learn from the disruptions, dysfunctions and diseases Western social models engender.*

Of all the groups affected by the forces of dislocation none have been worse hit than minority populations, such as the Australian Aborigines and North American Native peoples mentioned by Dr. Dupont, and the descendants of black slaves brought to North America. Among the latter, people were separated not only from their places of origin, their cultures and their communities, but often also from their immediate families. Long after the abolition of slavery, racial oppression and prejudice, along with economic deprivation, have continued to produce intolerable pressures on family life among many Afro-Americans—and the link to addiction is obvious. Equally obvious is the enticement of the drug trade to jobless and undereducated young black men excluded from the economic promises of the "American dream."

* Dr. Bruce Alexander's soon-to-be published next book is aptly titled *The Globalization of Addiction.*

The history of dispossession, dislocation, exploitation and direct abuse of Canada's Native peoples is also too well known to require much discussion. Tobacco and other potentially addictive substances, were available to North American Natives prior to the European invasions, even alcohol in what are now Mexico and the American Southwest—not to mention potentially addictive activities such as sex, eating and gambling. Yet, as Dr. Alexander points out, there is no mention by anthropologists of "anything that could be reasonably called addiction. . . . Where alcohol was readily available, it was used moderately, often ceremonially rather than addictively."

With the mass migration of Europeans to North America and the economic transformation of the continent came also the loss of freedom of mobility for Native peoples, the inexorable and still continuing despoliation and destruction of their homelands, the loss of their traditional livelihoods, the invalidation of their spiritual ways, persistent discrimination and abject poverty. Within living memory Native children were seized from their homes, alienated from their families and, for all intents and purposes, incarcerated in "civilizing" institutions where their lot was one of cultural suppression, emotional and physical maltreatment and, with distressing frequency, sexual abuse. It would be heartening to be able to say that our society has acknowledged its enormous historical, moral and economic debt to its Native citizens. Although that has occurred sporadically, the overall pattern continues to be economic dispossession, denial of historical rights and patronizing control. Canada, with our self-appointed "mission" to improve the health, education and well-being of Afghans, has not even come close to securing those same essentials for our First Nations citizens. The living situations, health conditions and social deprivation of many Canadian Natives are abysmal even by Third World standards. Under such circumstances, among tormented, dislocated and, most fundamentally, *disempowered* people, pain and suffering are transmitted from one traumatized generation to the next. It is no accident that both Serena and her mother live in the same Downtown Eastside hotel on Hastings; nor are they the only mother-daughter Native pairing among my patients. Of any group in North America, whether in the

U.S. or Canada, none can be said to be more psychologically and socially oppressed than Native women.[17]

Especially since working in the Downtown Eastside, I have often thought that if Canadian society ever apologized to our First Nations people for their dispossession and suffering as we have to Japanese Canadians for their internment during World War II, our contrition would need to be vast and our willingness to make restitution immensely generous. Perhaps that is why we have never accepted the responsibility.

—

Dislocation continues to be an ever-accelerating feature of modern living, owing to rapid economic and social changes that human culture and human relationships cannot swiftly adapt to. The disruption of family life and the erosion of stable communities afflict many segments of society. Even the nuclear family is under severe pressure with a high divorce rate and single-parent households or, in many cases, two parents having to work outside the home. For these endemic cultural and economic reasons many children today who are not abused and who come from loving homes have lost their primary emotional attachment with the nurturing adults in their lives, with results disastrous for their development. As children become increasingly less connected to adults, they rely more and more on each other—a wholesale cultural subversion of the natural order of things.

The natural order in all mammalian cultures, animal or human, is that the young stay under the wings of adults until they themselves reach adulthood. Immature creatures were never meant to bring one another to maturity. They were never meant to look to one another for primary nurturing, modelling, cue giving or mentoring. They are not equipped to act as one another's focus of orientation, to give one another a sense of direction or values. The predictable and widespread consequences of what my friend, psychologist Gordon Neufeld, has termed *peer orientation* are the increasing immaturity, alienation, violence and precocious sexualization of North American youth.

Another consequence is the entrenchment of addictive behaviours among young people. Research on both humans and animals has repeatedly demonstrated that extensive peer contact and the loss of adult attachments lead to a heightened propensity to addiction. Peer-reared monkeys, for example, are far more likely to consume alcohol than mother-reared ones.[18] "Peer affiliation," according to a review article in the journal *Drug and Alcohol Dependence,* "is possibly the strongest social factor in predicting the onset and early escalation of adolescent substance use."[19]

It is commonly thought that peer affiliation leads to drug use because kids set bad examples for each other. That's part of the picture, but a deeper reason is that under ordinary circumstances, adolescents who rely on their peers for emotional acceptance are more prone to being hurt, to experiencing the sting of each other's immature and therefore often insensitive ways of relating. They are far more stressed than children who are well connected to nurturing adults.

Kids are not cruel by nature, but they are immature. They taunt, tease and reject. Those who have lost their orientation to adults and look to the peer group instead find themselves having to shut down emotionally for sheer protection. As we have seen with children abused at home, emotional shutting down—what in a book* I co-wrote with Dr. Gordon Neufeld we call "the dangerous flight from feeling"—greatly increases the motivation to use drugs.

—

In short, the addiction process takes hold in people who have suffered dislocation and whose place in the normal human communal context has been disrupted: whether they've been abused or emotionally neglected; are inadequately attuned children or peer-oriented teens or members of subcultures historically subjected to exploitation.

To know the true nature of a society, it's not enough to point to its achievements, as leaders like to do. We also need to look at its shortcomings. What do we see, then, when we look at the drug ghetto of Vancouver's Downtown Eastside and similar enclaves in other urban

* *Hold On to Your Kids: Why Parents Need to Matter More Than Peers*

centres? We see the dirty underside of our economic and social culture, the reverse of the image we would like to cherish of a humane,
prosperous and egalitarian society. We see our failure to honour family
and community life or to protect children; we see our refusal to grant
justice to Aboriginal people and we see our vindictiveness toward
those who have already suffered more than most of us can imagine.
Rather than lifting our eyes to the dark mirror held in front of us, we
shut them to avoid the unsavoury image we see reflected there.

The Torah says that Aharon, the brother of Moses, was com-
manded to take two hairy goats and bring them before God. Upon
each, he was to place a lot—a marker. On one he was to place the
lot of the people's sins, "*to effect atonement upon it, to send it away
to Azazel into the wilderness.*" This was the scapegoat—who, cast
out, must escape to the desert.

The drug addict is today's scapegoat. Viewed honestly, much of our
culture is geared towards enticing us away from ourselves, into externally directed activity, into diverting the mind from ennui and distress. The hardcore addict surrenders her pretence about that. Her
life is all about escape. The rest of us can, with varying success, maintain our charade, but to do so, we banish her to the margins of society.

"Do not judge, and you will not be judged," a man of truth once
said:

> For the judgments you give will be the judgments you will get, and
> the amount you measure out is the amount you will be given. Why
> do you observe the splinter in your brother's eye and never notice
> the plank in your own? How dare you say to your brother, "Let me
> take the splinter out of your eye," when all the time there is a plank
> in your own? Take the plank out of your own eye first, and then you
> will see clearly enough to take the splinter out of your brother's eye.

In the following chapters we'll consider what our stance toward
addiction might be if we took Jesus' words to heart. We'll see that
his compassion integrates perfectly with what science has taught us
about addiction.

—

CHAPTER 24

Know Thine Enemy

Detective-Sergeant Paul Gillespie, head of Toronto's sex crimes unit, rescued children from the purveyors of Internet pornography. As the *Globe and Mail* reported on his retirement from police work, six years at that job had not inured him to the horrors he witnessed:

> Paul Gillespie still can't get used to the sounds of crying and pain in the graphic videos of children being raped and molested that he has seen all too often on the Web. "It's beyond horrible to listen to the soundtracks of these movies," said Canada's best-known child-porn cop . . . But it is the silent images of desolate children that tear the most at his heart. "They're not screaming, just accepting," he said of the infants captured in these pictures. "They have dead eyes. You can tell that their spirit is broken. That's their life."[1]

Dead eyes, broken spirits: in a phrase this compassionate man summed up the fate of the abused child. Yet there is a bitter irony in his words. The lives of abused children do not end when they are rescued—*if* they are rescued, as most never are. Many become teenagers with spirits not mended and reach adulthood with eyes still dead. Their fate continues to be a concern for the police and the courts, but by then they are no longer heartbreakingly sweet, no longer vulnerable looking. They lurk on the social periphery as hardened men with ravaged faces; as thieves, robbers, shoplifters; as done-up prostitutes selling backseat sex for drugs or petty cash; as streetcorner drug pushers or as small-time entrepreneurs distributing cocaine out of cheap hotel rooms. They are the hardcore injection users, and many will drift westward across Canada to the warmer climate and drug mecca of Vancouver's Downtown Eastside. Here, as in cities across North America, it is now the duty of Detective-Sergeant Gillespie's drug squad colleagues to keep a sharp eye on these people, to frisk them in back alleys, to confiscate their drug paraphernalia and to arrest them time and again.

Some of these former children are not pleasant to deal with. Scruffy and dirty, shifty and manipulative, they invite distaste. Fearful and contemptuous of authority at the same time, they evoke hostility. The police often handle them roughly. Cops are not necessarily predisposed to harshness, but a loss of humane interaction inevitably results whenever an entire group of people is de-legitimized while another group is granted virtually unrestrained physical authority over them. I've had a small taste of it, having been stopped by cops on my Hastings Street rounds—once for jaywalking and once for riding my bicycle on the sidewalk. An officer's tone shifts instantly from curt and contemptuous to polite when he realizes I'm not a Downtown Eastside resident. How utterly helpless I would feel, I have thought at such times, if I didn't have a respectable address on my driver's licence; if I lived in a restricted, ghettoized domain where a uniformed and armed force was the omnipresent power; if I depended on substances the police had to suppress and on activities they were obliged to prosecute; if I couldn't count on reliable friends and family to advocate for me if ever I got into trouble.

I have also witnessed officers treat my clients calmly and with kindness, but I know that's not the face they always turn toward the addict.

The Downtown Eastside addicts are acutely aware of their lack of power in any conflict with authority, be it legal or medical. "Who would believe me; I'm just a junkie" is the refrain I hear over and over again as patients complain of being beaten in jail or on the darkened streets or of being dismissed rudely by nurses or doctors at an emergency ward. Such experiences, for the addict, add more links to the chain of utter powerlessness that began in childhood.

With revolving-door regularity addicts are brought before the courts for crimes they commit to support their substance dependence. A few judges are mindful that addiction came upon these people as a defensive response to what they endured before their eyes went dead: heroin for the pain, cocaine to enliven dulled spirits. Some judges will speak to them with compassion, urge them to reform and offer them what narrow avenues of redemption our social and justice systems provide. Other judges appear to see them as society's evildoers and miscreants. Empathic judge or hanging judge, both are eventually compelled to send the addict-criminal to prison. Incarcerated in institutions where fear and violence often rule, many will re-experience exactly what they suffered early in their lives and ever since: helplessness and isolation. While on the positive side, jail at times gives people a much-needed break from their compulsive drug use, on release most of them will relapse into drug taking and, of necessity, into the illegal acts required to sustain those habits.

—

In any war there must be enemies. In the War on Drugs the enemies are most often children like the ones Detective-Sergeant Gillespie could not rescue or rescued too late. They are not the generals, of course, the masterminds or the profiteers. They are the foot soldiers, the ones who live in the trenches—and as in all wars, they are the ones who suffer and die. Or, they become what the military calls collateral damage.

The War on Drugs, from the Hastings-facing window of the Portland Hotel, is manifested in the pregnant Celia kneeling on the sidewalk, handcuffed wrists behind her back, eyes cast on the ground. There was no Detective-Sergeant Gillespie to protect her when, as a little girl, she was raped by her stepfather and subjected to the nocturnal spitting ritual, so in the War on Drugs she has become one of the enemy.

Also a foe in the War on Drugs is thirty-eight-year-old Shawn, who periodically disappears from my methadone practice. When he fails to show for his appointment, I know he's back in prison. He's a street dweller and petty thief, so his crimes never result in long jail terms. One time he was gone for nearly a year, but usually the absences last only weeks or months. Cocaine is his other habit apart from narcotics, and like many others, he unwittingly began to use this chemical as self-medication for his undiagnosed and untreated attention deficit hyperactivity disorder. His recollection of school life is typical for ADHD. "I was bored and restless waiting and watching the clock until I could get out of the classroom. I felt like I was in a jail cell. I could never pay attention."

In an attempt to help him establish a more stable life, his social worker recently sent Shawn to my office with a detailed medical disability application which, if approved, would get him off the street. It would be superfluous to tell Shawn's life story—the reader will have some sense of it by now—but it is instructive to see how the enemy describes himself. With his permission I reproduce here, precisely as he wrote them, the words Shawn scribbled at the beginning of the disability form:

> In My opinion My life as I no it to the truth. It started when I was about 11–12 yrs old and I was in the wrong crowd of people to associ-aiate with. Because of that my life as been in jail for approx 18 yrs out of 37. from being where I have been and seen what I have seen was a big problem and bad influence on my own life and for example at age of 18 seen a coulpe burttle murders happen within 7–8 yards as well people committing suaside. Plus I have now lived on Vancouver's worst streets. Skid row and using IV drugs heroin cocaine. Ive lived here homeless and in hotel rooms for 15 years minus all the jail time. I have Hepatitus C from IV use. P)luse Ive lost my ability to manage money because of addiction.
>
>   I grew with an alchol addiction from the he would Physicly Beat my Mom as was us kids.
>
>   Because I'm physically addicted to Methadone I'm very limited to what I can make extra money from, since all this has happened

Ive lost a lot of self esteem and get a mild paranoia from other peers.
witch I'm on medication for.

This a Breif opion of why I need Disability support.

Thank-You for you Time.

This man with severe ADHD and learning disabilities, post-traumatic stress disorder and deeply entrenched drug addiction; with no employment skills; with no history of successful human relationships—this is one of the culprits the police devote their time, skills and energy to investigating and arresting; about whose misdeeds prosecutors versed in the law gather evidence; whom socially conscious and poorly recompensed Legal Aid defenders assist; and whom learned judges admonish and repeatedly incarcerate. Such is the War on Drugs.

Another foe, now dead, was the Vietnamese refugee Raymond, who wasted away from AIDS, steadfastly refusing treatment for years as the disease corroded his immune system and his health. I never found out much about his life, but there are other addicts in his family and, as far as we could tell, much pain and disconnection. Raymond had been an engineer before he succumbed fully to his addiction. In the Downtown Eastside he survived by running a small time cocaine operation. Lisa, the child-like crack addict depicted in Chapter 15, had been his client. She, too, is one of the enemy and, as such, deserves to be known a little better. A glimpse into her world and her mind is given by a scrawled note she addressed to the dying Raymond. Once more, I reproduce the document exactly as written:

Mr. Raymond R:

I'm sorry, for been a pain on your butt. But i'm just a drug addict! who can not helpped it on knoking on your door to ask you for help. If I do it againg, and again it's because i keep my word to pay you and you know that right!

I apreciate what you do for me very much, that is the reason why I respect you and pay you exactly what you give me, sometimes you said I own you less and I tell you the truth by letting you know I own you more.

Raymond: You know, I don't still or sheet [steal or cheat] specialy to you whom has give me the chance to prove you that I did not use you or hurt you in any way. I haver had hard feelins agains you. Even do you though I stoll your money, I got hurt really bad I could even end up dead just because I was brock and a drug addict you acusme it's OK we all make mastakes, but why are you saying I don't pay you when I do.

You know last time you accusse me because you belive these girls, I hope this time you are accussing me in your own with out been told what to do, because you are smart intelegent enough to make your own decitions.

Lisa's semiliterate plea to her drug pusher for understanding could be turned toward a larger issue. I believe that if all of us as individuals and as a society were "smart, intelegent enough" to make our own decisions, we would not punish the addict or wage a war in which human beings like Celia, Lisa, Shawn and Raymond are treated as the enemy. We would seek peace.

As Lisa suggests, we all make mistakes. The War on Drugs is one of them, as we'll next see.

CHAPTER 25

A Failed War

After the onset of a war, when the patriotic fervour has faded to some degree, more sober considerations come to the fore. As this book goes to press, in Iraq there is no end in sight to extraordinary violence and the roll call of American casualties grows ever longer. In the United States, the Iraq war has become increasingly unpopular. A diminished number of people support either its stated purposes or the strategy and tactics by which it is being pursued. Similarly, what the Canadian government calls Canada's "mission" in Afghanistan is under critical scrutiny at home as military and civilian casualties mount in that faraway land.

The questions being raised about both conflicts are pertinent to any war and are equally relevant to the War on Drugs: Are the declared aims valid and attainable? Are the means employed likely to achieve the desired goals? What are the human and economic costs of carrying it out? Unlike the relatively recent interventions in Iraq and Afghanistan, the War on Drugs has been dragging on for many decades. Although the term was first coined in 1971 by Richard Nixon, its policies have been pursued with escalating force since the early years of the twentieth century. Were we to apply objective measures, we would rapidly abandon both the rhetoric and the practices of this war.

Were we to judge according to ethics and humane feeling, we would find the War abhorrent. "The single most conspicuous feature of wars is violence," writes Bruce Alexander in his book *Peaceful Measures: Canada's Way Out of the "War on Drugs"*:

> War mentality cleaves the world into noble allies and despicable enemies [and] justifies any measures necessary to prevail, including violence to innocent bystanders . . . In essence, war mentality suspends normal human compassion and intelligence.[1]

The want of compassion and intelligence that characterizes the War on Drugs is self-evident whether we look at its impact on my Downtown Eastside patients or its vast numbers of casualties internationally, its destructive environmental effects in Third World countries or its staggering economic and social costs.

For Canadians it is helpful and even necessary to consider closely the U.S. experience of the War on Drugs. Despite differences in political and social attitudes, our two countries have broad cultural similarities. The U.S. government aggressively promotes its view of drug addiction internationally and brings enormous pressure on other countries to fall in line with its own opinions. Even if we in Canada have resisted adopting U.S. practices wholesale, American influence has been exerted against the institution of less restrictive measures here. As we'll see in Chapter 28, U.S. interference makes it very difficult for other countries, including Canada, to establish enlightened drug policies.

It's beyond my purposes here to refute in detail the principles governing the U.S.-led War on Drugs or to document its global depredations. That information is readily available from, among others, high-level officials previously committed to prosecuting the War. One of them is Norm Stamper, former police chief of Seattle, who after his retirement, has become an advocate of decriminalizing drugs. Chief Stamper writes:

> Think of this war's *real* casualties: tens of thousands of otherwise innocent Americans incarcerated, many for 20 years, some for life; families ripped apart; drug traffickers and blameless bystanders shot dead on city streets . . . The United States has, through its war on drugs, fostered political instability, official corruption, and health and

environmental disasters around the globe.* In truth, the U.S.-sponsored international "War on Drugs" is a war on poor people, most of them subsistence farmers caught in a dangerous no-win situation.[2]

If the goal of the War on Drugs is to discourage or prevent drug use, it has failed. Among young people in North America drug use has reached unprecedented levels and enjoys unprecedented tolerance. According to figures quoted by Norm Stamper, the number of Americans who have used illegal drugs stands at 77 million. The U.S. Department of Justice reports that the number of prisoners has tripled, from 139 per 100,000 residents in 1980 to 476 per 100,000 in 2002, the vast majority being incarcerated after drug convictions. From 1980 to 1999 the annual number of Americans arrested for drug offences nearly tripled, from 580,900 to 1,532,200. "That's a lot of enemies," comments the ex–police chief.

If the War's purpose is to protect people and communities or to improve their quality of life, it fails disastrously. As the personal histories of Downtown Eastside addicts illustrate and as statistics show, the human costs are devastating. "One [result] which is especially cruel and will have a terrible impact on American life for many generations is the large increase in the number of women incarcerated for drug violations," U.S. District Court Judge John T. Curtin has pointed out.

> From 1980 to 1996, there has been a 400 percent increase in the number of women prisoners. Many of those jailed for drug violations were mules or assistants. I venture that none was a principal organizer. Many are the mothers of small children who will be left without maternal care, and most probably without any parental care at all . . . The engine of punitive punishment of mothers will haunt this nation for many years to come.[3]

If the War's aim is to end or even curtail the international drug trade, it has failed there, too. If it is to suppress the cultivation of

---

* Due, for example, to the spraying of pesticides on large tracts of agricultural land to raze hemp or coca or opium crops.

plants from which the major substances of abuse are derived: once again, abject failure. Truth, once again, is among the inevitable casualties of war. Official claims of victory in the War on Drugs have been no more reliable than similar announcements about the conflict in Iraq. As a *New York Times* correspondent reported from Afghanistan:

> A few weeks before I arrived in Helmand, John Walters, the director of the White House Office of National Drug Control Policy, told reporters that Afghan authorities were succeeding in reducing opium-poppy cultivation. Yet despite hundreds of millions of dollars being allocated by Congress to stop the trade, a United Nations report in September estimated that this year's crop was breaking all records—6,100 metric tons compared with 4,100 last year.[4]

Not even in its Latin American backyard had Washington's war been more successful. Colombia has remained the world's largest cocaine producer, supplying 90 per cent of the cocaine for the U.S. drug market, "despite receiving more than $5 billion in antinarcotics and counterinsurgency aid from the United States this decade, making it the largest recipient of American aid in the [southern] hemisphere," according to a report in the *New York Times*.[5]

Under conditions of extreme deprivation people will continue to grow crops that promise economic relief, and they will continue to trade in those crops and their products. The ultimate beneficiaries are neither the impoverished Afghan or Colombian peasant nor the streetcorner pusher in the U.S. ghetto or on Vancouver's Skid Row. The illegality of mind-altering substances enriches drug cartels, crime syndicates and their corrupt enablers among politicians, government officials, judges, lawyers and police officers around the world. If one set out deliberately to fashion a legal system designed to maximize and sustain the wealth of international drug criminals and their abettors, one could never dream up anything to improve upon the present one—except, perhaps, to add tobacco to the list of contraband substances. That way the traffickers and their allies could profit even more—although it's unimaginable that their legally respectable counterparts, tax-hungry governments and the nicotine pushers in tobacco company boardrooms, would ever allow that to happen.

According to Dr. George Povey, Professor of Health Care and Epidemiology at the University of British Columbia, in 1995 illegal drugs caused 805 Canadian deaths, alcohol 6,507 and tobacco 34,728. "So who's for a War on Tobacco?" he asks.[6]

A major study conducted on behalf of the British government in 2005 illustrated both the rich benefits that current drug legislation confers on major traffickers and the ludicrous impotence of law enforcement efforts against the drug trade. "The profit margins for major traffickers of heroin into Britain are so high they outstrip luxury goods companies such as Louis Vuitton and Gucci," reported the *Guardian*. "The traffickers enjoy such high profits that seizure rates of 60–80% are needed to have any serious impact on the flow of drugs into Britain but nothing greater than 20% has been achieved." Downing Street allowed only half the study's findings to be published, prompting an opposition spokesperson to argue, with reason, that "what this report shows and what the government is too paranoid to admit is that the 'war on drugs' is a disaster. We need an evidence-led debate about the way forward but if they withhold the evidence we can't have the debate."[7]

In North America the situation is no different. "The major reason why our society is awash in illicit drugs is the unbelievable profits that can be realized in their being manufactured and sold," writes Judge James P. Grey of the California Superior Court.[8] It is the same in Canada. Dr. Povey points out that "the billion Canadian bucks we throw at drug control each year have trivial effect upon supply but powerfully inflate market value. A kilo of heroin that costs $3,000 in Pakistan sells for $150,000 on our streets, which explains why a serious drug user needs $50,000 spare change yearly to stay cool."

The economic burden imposed by the War on Drugs is difficult to estimate, but most authorities agree that in the U.S. it's in the range of tens of billions of dollars annually. Gary Becker, Professor of Economics and Sociology at the University of Chicago's Graduate School of Business, has calculated $100 billion per year as a minimum figure:

These estimates do not include important intangible costs, such as
the destructive effects on many inner city neighborhoods, the use of
the American military to fight drug lords and farmers in Colombia
and other nations, or the corrupting influence of drugs on many
governments.[9]

How such expenses in support of a failed policy can be justified is
beyond imagining in a country where the poverty rate is increasing
and where in some areas the rising infant mortality rate is comparable to Third World figures. Although the War has not been prose-
cuted as ferociously in Canada, were our costs to be collated, they
would still be egregious at a time when health care, education and
social welfare conditions have all deteriorated owing to diminished
government funding.

An unintended but tragic consequence of the international campaign against narcotics is that through much of the underdeveloped
world, opiates are not available for soothing physical pain. Countless
human beings, from infancy to old age, live and die in pain. According
to the World Health Organization nearly five million people a year
with advanced cancer receive inadequate or no pain relief, along with
another 1.4 million with late-stage AIDS. The WHO has no statistics
for those suffering pain owing to a host of other causes, from injuries
to diseases of all sorts. The problem? An exaggerated fear of addiction.
"Pain relief hasn't been given as much attention as the war on drugs,"
David E. Joranson, director of the Pain Policy Study Group at the
University of Wisconsin's medical school, told the *New York Times*.[10]

Finally, if the purpose of the War is to deter substance use by
drug desperadoes such as the ones who inhabit Vancouver's
Downtown Eastside, the very idea of its success is laughable.

Drugs do not make the addict into a criminal; the law does.
When alcohol was prohibited, drinkers were breaking the law. If
cigarettes were illegal, there would be a huge underground market
for tobacco products. Gangs would form, criminal business empires
would flourish and smokers would be spending a large proportion
of their income on nicotine-containing substances. Add the health
ravages and medical and economic costs of nicotine addiction, the
hundreds of thousands of deaths it causes and the many family

tragedies it already creates—and then factor in the enormous costs of waging the War on Drugs on yet another front. The result would be a monumentally costly and futile effort. "We have been and will always be totally unsuccessful in our attempts to repeal the law of supply and demand," writes James P. Grey in his book *Why Our Drug Laws Have Failed.* "We might as well try to repeal the law of gravity."¹¹ As Judge Grey documents in his persuasive critique, subtitled *A Judicial Indictment of the War on Drugs,* most of the social harm related to drugs does not come from the effects of the substances themselves but from legal prohibitions against their use.

—

Quite apart from the multiple billions squandered on this futile war, the economic burdens of criminalization are incalculable, as we may glimpse from the daily pursuits of my own patients. Several have blown through large inheritances in short order—seventy thousand dollars over the course of a few weeks in the case of one woman, an inveterate cocaine and heroin addict now terminally ill, in her early fifties. Such windfalls are rare, leaving crime, panhandling and prostitution as the common sources of drug money. Drug dealing can range from the petty to the extensive, but in the Downtown Eastside there are few profiteers: most who engage in it do so only to fuel their own habits. "Two years ago I got back into dealing," one man told me recently. "I was making $19,000 a month. All gone . . . not a penny, except for the ten grand I gave to the mother of my little son. It went on for ten months, so I made $190,000 . . . and I walked away with ten thousand.

"It's a snap to spend that kind of money. Typically the hundred-dollar or three-hundred-dollar habits a day are mostly cocaine as opposed to heroin, 'cause heroin is so cheap. You can get a quarter gram of really, really good heroin for only thirty dollars and I don't care how bad your habit is, on thirty dollars' worth nobody needs to be sick.* But with cocaine, that's an easy three or five or seven hundred dollars a day.

* "Sick" here means to go through withdrawal.

"Now, when it comes to selling stolen goods, you're lucky if you get 10 per cent on the value. I've seen a two-thousand-dollar bicycle go for twenty-five dollars' worth of rock cocaine. So typically, if somebody is generating three hundred dollars a day, he's probably stealing three thousand dollars' worth of stuff. Yeah, you're lucky if you get 10 per cent."

In the privacy of my office many people are remarkably candid about how they find the cash to fund their drug habit. McDermitt, a forty-year-old with sunken eyes, gaunt features and a perpetual smirk on his face is even boastful as he tells me of his piratical exploits.

"What?" I say incredulously. "How much did you say?"

"That's what they estimated in court, that I stole two million, seven hundred thousand dollars over the course of two and a half years."

"That's just impossible."

"Well, that was their estimate . . ."

McDermitt does his thievery at the port of Vancouver, where container ships are moored. He and a buddy worked out a system for stealing goods from the ships without being picked up by security. Among other things, they steal cigarettes and get into "containers with expensive Asian clothing—long-sleeved silk shirts for men, women's fancy dresses."

Other ingenious schemes McDermitt has participated in involved stealing aluminum from construction sites and siphoning gasoline from big trucks. I ask him where he sells this stuff. He shrugs. "I used to deal with Larry, but they killed Larry. He got murdered. . . . He used to say, 'Fuck, McDermitt, at least cut these in half.' I get a bunch of fucking aluminum, I phone a wheelchair taxi, taxi pulls up . . . We put in three hundred pounds of aluminum. I usually make two hundred and ten dollars, minus thirty for the cab. That's a hundred and eighty bucks."

For many addicts crime becomes a necessary part of life—automatic, reflexive, to be taken for granted. One morning I marched up to a patient's room to retrieve an expensive leather coat. He'd stolen it half an hour earlier during a medical visit at a colleague's office. The doctor phoned me in an agitated state right after this man had left. "I just turned my back for a moment," he said. The patient was apologetic but not overly remorseful. "I couldn't help it," he pleaded. "It was lying on his chair. What could I do?"

"What could I do?" was also the defence of another patient, Mike, who pocketed my PalmPilot one day when I left him sitting in my office for no more than twenty seconds. It was during my early days at the Portland; I'd stepped into the next room to pick up a prescription pad. I naïvely believed that this man, who once made me a finely worked wood carving to express his gratitude, could be trusted. Perhaps *he* could be trusted, but his addiction could not. Five minutes after he left I noticed the empty space on my desk where the PalmPilot had been. I shut the office, reassured the waiting patients that I'd be back shortly and hurried down the block to Mike's hotel. It took a few sharp knocks before he opened the door.

"I want it back," I said.

"What?" he replied.

"Look, Mike, you have two options: you return my PalmPilot immediately or immediately I call the police." Mike slumped on his bed, a defeated look on his face.

"Okay, first thing tomorrow."

"No, first thing right now."

"I don't have it," Mike said.

"Then find it."

We walked down the stairs of the Sunrise Hotel together and entered the pawnshop around the corner. "I need that PalmPilot back," Mike announced to the owner. "It belongs to this guy."

The pawnbroker feigned shock. "What you mean?" he cried. Quite obviously, or so his body language implied, this was the first time ever that here, on the East Hastings drug and crime strip, anyone had tried to pass stolen goods at his establishment. "Why you no tell me it wasn't yours?" he said in a tone of reproach.

As the owner picked out my item from among a pile of electronic devices, Mike shuffled about, not seeming the least bit comfortable. "It was there on your desk," he explained as we left the store. "What could I do?"

There are thousands of destitute hardcore drug addicts in Vancouver's Downtown Eastside alone. Knowing that many of them have to steal, shoplift, scam and panhandle hundreds of dollars a day to sustain their habits, we can begin to compute the economic hit our society is taking in service of the arbitrary principle that people may poison themselves with alcohol or kill themselves with cigarette-derived toxins, but those whose drug of choice is a narcotic or a stimulant are to be considered criminals.

—

Undeterred by the miserable failure of its War on Drugs, the U.S. administration has taken upon itself to oppose decriminalization and harm reduction programs anywhere on the globe. In April 2006 the Mexican Senate approved a bill to decriminalize the possession of small amounts of marijuana, cocaine, heroin and other drugs for personal use.[12] The office of President Vicente Fox signalled his willingness to pass the bill into law. "We can't close our eyes to this reality," said Senator Jorge Zermeno of Fox's conservative National Action Party. "We cannot continue to fill our jails with people who have addictions." It took less than twenty-four hours of U.S. "advice" for the Mexican government to change its mind. The measure was sent back for "further study," which is to say, to its legislative grave.

Some political leaders in Ottawa welcome the hard-line mentality emanating from Washington. In December 2006, under the headline "Canada Looks to USA for Drug Policy Hints," the *Vancouver Sun* reported that Conservative cabinet ministers and their aides are consulting "keen" U.S. federal officials on a new national drug strategy, according to documents obtained by the paper. Neil Boyd, a criminologist at Simon Fraser University, commented that "the Harper government favours a U.S.-style approach to drug problems, which is to lock more people up." Rather than recognizing addiction as a health issue, said Dr. Boyd, this view sees it as "a criminal law problem of morality. That's very much at odds with what's going on in Europe and there's really no good evidence to suggest that it's going to be terribly useful."[13] The restrained and understated words of a carefully spoken academic.

In Washington State the King County Bar Association has acknowledged the devastation caused by prevailing drug policies. In 2001 it adopted a comprehensive statement asserting that the

War on Drugs is "fundamentally flawed and is associated with numerous negative societal consequences." Their summary of the War's disastrous effects reflects the consensus view of virtually all those, in North America and elsewhere, who have studied the question without ideological blinkers:

- the failure to reduce problematic drug use, particularly among children;
- dramatic increases in crime related to prohibited drugs, including economic crimes related to addiction and the fostering of efficient and violent criminal enterprises that have occupied the unregulated and immensely profitable commercial market made possible by drug prohibition;
- skyrocketing public costs arising from both increased drug abuse and increased crime;
- erosion of public health from the spread of disease, from the concealment and inadequate treatment of addiction and from undue restrictions on proper medical treatment of pain;
- the abridgement of civil rights through summary forfeitures of property, invasions of privacy and violations of due process;
- disproportionately adverse effects of drug law enforcement on the poor and persons of color; and
- the clogging of the courts and compromises in the effective administration of justice, as well as a loss of respect for the law.[14]

The War on Drugs fails, and is doomed to perpetual failure, because it is directed not against the root causes of drug addiction and of the international black market in drugs, but only against some drug producers, traffickers and users. More fundamentally, the War is doomed because neither the methods of war nor the war metaphor itself is appropriate to a complex social problem that calls for compassion, self-searching insight and factually researched scientific understanding.

The pertinent question is not why the War on Drugs is being lost, but why it continues to be waged in the face of all the evidence against it.

CHAPTER 26

Freedom of Choice and the Choice of Freedom

A core assumption in the War on Drugs is that the addict is free to make the choice *not* to be addicted and that harsh social or legal measures will deter him from pursuing his habit. It is not that easy. Contrary to Nancy Reagan's simplistic billboard messages, people cannot "just say no" in the face of addictive drives.

One arena in which freedom of choice operates is the social world—the world of interactions, opportunities, and relationships; another is the inner realm of the psyche. In the first arena, which is shaped by our materialistic culture, it is futile to pretend that we all have equal freedom: just ask the hardcore drug user, acutely aware of his position at the very bottom of the social hierarchy.

Steve, a forty-year-old addict, has spent eighteen years of his adult life in prison. As he sat in my office one morning recently, he was staring out the window or at the wall or the ceiling—anything but looking at me directly. He's angry, and he's afraid of his anger. Bitterness pours from his heart, first about being obliged to drink methadone every day under a pharmacist's supervision and then about many other features of his existence that he sees as being under the control of one authority or another—doctor, druggist, hotel staff, social worker. His frustration is not new: a sense of injustice colours the narrative of his entire life. "Freedom comes with a dollar sign attached," he says. "The poor sap who collects a welfare cheque to keep him from sleeping in the street gets walked all over. He has no freedom. I'm always being told what to do. It's like being back in jail; the only difference is that now and then I can get some pussy."

For all his self-pity, there is also truth in Steve's perception. Freedom in society is gauged by our success in getting what we want and conditioned by status and power, by race, class and gender. In the internal world of the psyche, however, freedom means something very different. It is the ability to opt for our long-term physical and spiritual well-being as opposed to our immediate urges. Absent that ability, any talk of "free will" or "choice" becomes nearly meaningless.

We recall Thomas De Quincey's reference to his opium habit as "the chain of abject slavery." The chains of addiction are internal and invisible. They fetter the mind first, the body second. We have seen that the addiction process commandeers powerful brain circuits and bends their activity towards maladaptive behaviours. We have also seen that in the addicted brain, the rational, impulse-regulating parts of the cortex are poorly developed even before the addiction takes hold, and they are further damaged by drug use. Thus the dilemma of freedom in addiction may be phrased this way: a person driven largely by unconscious forces and automatic brain mechanisms is only poorly able to exercise any meaningful freedom of choice.

A great deal of study has been devoted to the freedom-of-choice issue in the case of obsessive-compulsive disorder (OCD), a condition that has important features in common with addiction. We can learn a lot about psychic freedom from this research. Dr. Jeffrey Schwartz, Professor of Psychiatry at the UCLA School of Medicine, has devoted decades to studying OCD and has described his findings in two fascinating books.[ ] In OCD, certain circuits of the brain do not work normally. Several parts seem "locked" together—just as if a car's transmission was stuck so that turning on the engine automatically set the wheels into motion. In OCD, the neurological gears that would uncouple the engine of thought from the wheels of action are stuck. Completely irrational thoughts or beliefs trigger repeated behaviours that are useless and even harmful. The obsessive-compulsive person is intellectually aware that his impulse to, say, wash his hands for the hundredth time lacks reason, but he cannot stop himself. Owing to his stuck neuro-logical clutch, the idea of having to cleanse himself yet again leads automatically to hand washing. Dr. Schwartz and his colleagues at UCLA have demonstrated the mechanisms of this "brain lock," as he has called it, on brain scans.

OCD may be an extreme example of how the brain can dictate behaviour even against our will, but OCD sufferers are different from other people only in degree. Much of what we do arises from automatic programming that bypasses conscious awareness and may even run contrary to our intentions, as Dr. Schwartz points out:

> The passive side of mental life, which is generated solely and com-pletely by brain mechanisms, dominates the tone and tenor of our day-to-day, even our second-to-second experience. During the quo-tidian business of daily life, the brain does indeed operate very much as a machine does.[2]

Decisions that we may believe to be freely made can arise from unconscious emotional drives or subliminal beliefs. They can be dictated by brain mechanisms programmed early in childhood and determined by events of which we have no recollection. The stronger a person's automatic brain mechanisms and the weaker the parts of the brain that can impose conscious control, the less true freedom that person will be able to exercise in her life. In OCD, and in many other conditions, no matter how intelligent and well-meaning the individual, the malfunctioning brain circuitry may override rational judgment and intention. Almost any human being, when overwhelmed by stress or powerful emotions, will act or react not from intention but from mechanisms that are set off deep in the brain, rather than being generated in the conscious and volitional segments of the cortex. When acting from a driven or triggered state, we are not free.

I interviewed Dr. Schwartz by telephone late one Friday evening—a discussion on addiction that might have made an outside observer roll his eyes: two nighthawk, workaholic physicians talking shop, a classic case of "it takes one to know one." "When you get right down to the nuts and bolts of understanding what the brain is doing and the relationship between conscious experience and the brain," Dr. Schwartz said, "the data does not support the commonly held principle that you can just will yourself into one mental state or another.

"It's a subtle thing, freedom. It takes effort; it takes attention and focus to not act something like an automaton. Although we do have freedom, we exercise it only when we strive for awareness, when we are conscious not just of the *content* of the mind but also of the mind itself as a *process*."

When not governed by conscious awareness, our mind tends to run on automatic pilot. It is scarcely more "free" than a computer that performs preprogrammed tasks in response to a button being pushed. The distinction between automatic mechanism and conscious free will may be illustrated by the difference between punching a wall with your fist in a fit of reactive rage and mindfully saying to yourself, "I have so much anger in me, I really want to punch this wall right now"—or even more consciously, *"My mind tells me* I should punch the wall." The latter mind-states give you the option of not striking the wall, without which there is no choice and no freedom—just a fractured hand and a head full of regret. "Choice implies consciousness," Eckhart Tolle points out, "—a high degree of consciousness. Without it, you have no choice."[3]

We may say, then, that in the world of the psyche, freedom is a relative concept: *the power to choose exists only when our automatic mental mechanisms are subject to those brain systems that are able to maintain conscious awareness.* A person experiences greater or less freedom from one situation to the next, from one interaction to the next, from one moment to the next. Anyone whose automatic brain mechanisms habitually run in overdrive has diminished capacity for free decision making, especially if the parts of the brain that facilitate conscious choice are impaired or underdeveloped.

We have said that addiction itself is a continuum, at one end of which lives the intravenous user hopelessly hooked to his habit. Most humans exist somewhere on that line between enslavement to destructive habits at one end and total consciousness and nonattachment at the other. In exactly the same way, freedom of choice can be represented as a continuum. Realistically, very few people could ever be found operating at the positive extreme, truly conscious and consistently free.

In the mind-world of the psyche, as in the material world, some people have more freedom than others. It would be absurd to assert, for example, that in practical worldly matters such as choosing domicile or food, a street dweller has the same degree of freedom as, say, a Wall Street tycoon. On the other hand, in the realm of emotional freedom and conscious decision making a penniless hermit may enjoy much more latitude than a status-addicted millionaire who, still compensating for unconscious childhood hurts, is driven by an insatiable need to be feared or admired. The hardcore drug addict finds the worst of both worlds: low on the totem pole of psychological freedom, she is also at the base of the socioeconomic ladder. The rest of us perch more or less precariously, at whatever altitude, somewhere above her.

In many respects, the addict has as little freedom as the person with OCD. Once the impulse to use a substance arises, brain lock occurs. My patients tell me over and over again that they simply cannot resist the crack pipe or the "speedball" or the fix of heroin when it's offered to them or when they know it's available.* Neither can they refrain from using when they feel stressed or upset or lonely or restless or bored or excited. Even I, without any history of substance dependence, have immense difficulty resisting the mental pressure I experience when the urge to buy CDs begins to churn in my mind. Though I make resolution after resolution, promise after promise, in the end it seems easier just to give in, to get the struggle over with, to relieve the mental tension by running to Sikora's and handing over my money to the ruthless music traffickers who lurk there among the stacks of recordings. Although I know full well that I have a say in the matter, it often *feels* like I'm powerless. And if I can feel that powerless, a middle-class professional in middle age with a loving family and a life that (mostly) I love, how free are my Portland Hotel patients?

Once more, freedom is relative. I believe I have much more freedom than the hardcore drug users.

---

* Speedball: a combination of heroin and cocaine, prepared for injection

Both the obsessive-compulsive and the addict experience overwhelming tension until they succumb to their compulsive drive. When they finally do, they gain an immense, if momentary, sense of relief. Given this absence of psychic freedom, the addict might as well be an obsessive-compulsive—with one essential difference. *Unlike the addict, the person with OCD does not anticipate his compulsive activity with any pleasure.* Far from craving it as the addict does, she regards it as unpleasant and distressing.

It may seem at first glance that the addict is more culpable, since he "enjoys" his behaviour as compared with the OCD patient, who suffers from it. In reality, the addict's temporary enjoyment makes it all the more difficult for him to give up his habit, whereas the obsessive-compulsive would be only too glad to do so, if shown how. When it comes to choosing recovery, this momentary but highly enticing pleasure experience puts the addict at a disadvantage—even if what we call "pleasure" is, in addiction, little more than an evanescent sense of relief from mental distress or spiritual emptiness.

—

Of course, many addicts with forbidding early childhood histories and prolonged self-destructive chemical or behavioural habits have recovered and recreated themselves as conscious, effective and compassionate members of society. Their transformation is proof that we can never write off anyone as beyond the possibility of freedom. But in practice we are in no position to demand that all addicts *should* make that choice.

It is useful to study and consider what combination of self-knowledge, strength, supportive environment, good fortune and pure grace allows some people to escape the death grip of hardcore addiction. It is not helpful, however, to compare any one person with another. Just because one person succeeds doesn't mean that we're entitled to judge another for having failed. For all our similarities, from the moment of conception we are each shaped by our own unique makeup and set of life experiences. No two human brains look alike, not even those of identical twins. One person's pain cannot be compared with anyone else's, nor can we compare any two people's capacity to endure suffering. In addition to the visible factors, there are also many subtle, invisible ones that may positively influence our psychic strength and our capacity for choice: a kind word spoken long ago, a fortuitous circumstance, a new relationship, a flash of insight, a memory of love, a sudden opening to faith. People who have overcome severe addictions deserve to be celebrated and they have much to teach, but their example cannot be used to condemn others who have not been able follow in their footsteps.

It's even more nonsensical to judge addicts by arbitrary criteria derived from the experience of people with relatively normal lives. "If it is irrational and hypocritical to hold a minor to the same standard of behavioral control as a mature adult, it is equally unjust to hold a traumatized and neurologically impaired adult to the same standard as one not so afflicted," says brain researcher Martin Teicher.[4]

How much actual freedom to choose does any one human being possess? There's only one answer: *We cannot know.* We may have our particular beliefs, spiritual or otherwise, about this aspect of human nature—about how it is or how it should be. These beliefs may strengthen our commitment to helping others find freedom or they may become harmful dogma. Either way, in the end we all have to humble ourselves and admit to a degree of uncertainty. There is no way we can peer into a brain to measure a person's capacity for awareness and rational choice or to estimate how the relative balance of these brain-mind systems will operate when that person is stressed. There is no gauging the burden of emotional suffering weighing down one person's psyche against another's, and there is no way to know what hidden life-enhancing experiences one person may have enjoyed that another has been denied. That is why it's facile to demand that anyone should be able to "just say no" and to judge them as morally lacking if they can't.

Freedom of choice, understood from the perspective of brain development, is not a universal or fixed attribute but a statistical probability. In other words, given a certain set of life experiences a human being will have either lesser or greater probability of having freedom in the realm of the psyche. A warmly nurtured child is much more likely to develop emotional freedom than an abused and neglected child. "The brain forces us to become reflections of our personal histories," write two U.S. research psychiatrists. "Simply stated, children reflect the world in which they are raised."⁵ As we have seen, the *in utero* and early childhood experiences of hardcore addicts will likely diminish the possibility of freedom. The probability of these children attaining even a basic level of psychic freedom from automatic mechanisms and drives is correspondingly less— not completely absent but less.

If we cherish the human potential for transformation, the real issue becomes how to encourage and support the addict's motivation and capacity to choose freedom despite damaging beginnings and a lifelong history of painful events—how, in other words, to promote healthy brain development later in life when the conditions for it have been lacking from earliest childhood onward. We'll first look at how the experience of choice arises in the brain and, in particular, in the addicted brain.

—

In Chapter 16 I pointed out that the role of the cortex, the brain's executive part, is more to inhibit than to initiate. Impulses to act are generated in lower brain systems, but the job of the cortex is to censor some and permit others. As a prominent researcher expressed it, it's not a matter of free will but of "free won't."*

How much time elapses between impulse and action? Electrical studies of brain function show that it's about half a second. For most of that time we are not aware of what our brain is proposing to do. In other words, there is a lag period between the impulse arising as a physical signal in the brain and our becoming aware of it as a conscious urge. In a well-functioning cortex the interval between *awareness* of the impulse and the *activation* of the muscles that will carry out the impulse is only one-tenth to one-fifth of a second.⁶ Amazingly, it's only in this briefest of intervals that the cortex can suppress behaviour it judges to be inappropriate. That's the gap where, for example, we can stop ourselves from raising our hand in anger or saying something hurtful. In that sliver of time we

* Richard L. Gregory, Professor of Neuropsychology, University of Bristol

see ourselves about to perform the act and, if necessary, we can stand between ourselves and the behaviour in question.

Many people have watched themselves helplessly as they began to do something they knew would be unhelpful or self-defeating. That's the experience of brain lock: the clutch is stuck, so nothing can be done to stop the motor of "doing" from engaging. A failure of the brain to go into "neutral" may occur in any human being who is under physical strain, such as fatigue or hunger, or when they are emotionally stressed. In the brain of the addict the problem is worsened because her neurological circuits are impaired even under ordinary circumstances. This can be explained by what happens in the split second *before* the impulse emerges into awareness. In that fraction of a moment—which is still longer than the splinter of time devoted to conscious choice, when we can decide not to do something inappropriate—the brain carries out what is called "pre-attentive analysis." Pre-attentive analysis is the unconscious evaluation of what goals the brain circuits judge to be essential or irrelevant, valuable or worthless, desirable or unwanted. The cortex is primed to select actions that will achieve the goals set by this pre-attentive process.

And what is the brain of the addict likely to value? Recall that the brain is in large part the product of early influences and that the attachment-reward and incentive-motivation systems of the addicted brain were directed toward maladaptive habits when the child's needs for emotional nourishment were frustrated and denied. In the words of the seminal researcher Jaak Panksepp, "drug addictions wouldn't occur unless they were related to natural reward processes of some kind." Habits and the brain circuits that maintain them form around substances and behaviours that promise instant if only temporary satisfaction.

"Those habit structures are so incredibly robust, and once they form in the nervous system they will guide behaviour without free choice," Dr. Panksepp said in a personal interview. "Addicts become addicts because they develop these habit structures which become totally focused on non-traditional rewards, drug rewards. They get hooked and they can't break out of that psychological imprisonment."

Thus, the addict comes to make his choice with a brain that overvalues the addictive substance or behaviour and undervalues the healthy alternatives. Impulses favouring the addiction process arise. The cortex, whose job it is to censor inappropriate actions—to exercise the "free won't"—is hobbled. Brain lock sets in: the milliseconds that afford the possibility of "just saying no" flash by.

"The whole decision-making process is . . . it's not even really a process," a patient told one of my colleagues, an addiction physician in the Downtown Eastside. "You just decide to use. There is not a whole lot of thought going on there. You don't really . . . you don't really weigh the pros and cons, it's too overwhelming, right? You simply *do it,* with total disregard for anything else."[7]

As I write this chapter, on October 29, 2006, I'm paged from Vancouver Hospital. A patient of mine, whom I'll call Terence, has been discharged involuntarily. "He broke the contract," his nurse informs me, in an apologetic tone. Terence is a thirty-two-year-old heroin and cocaine addict with multiple medical problems, including HIV. I have known him for a few months. In speaking with him, one feels that every request is a manipulation, every word hides an agenda and every interaction serves some ulterior motive. I doubt he is aware of how he appears to others; to borrow from Nietzsche, he lies his way out of reality because he has been hurt by reality. The manipulation and dishonesty have been his automatic defences since childhood. He must be terrified that without them he will suffer deprivation.

Admitted to a medical ward last week for an infectious illness, two days later he was arrested at a nearby supermarket for shoplifting. The police took him back to hospital, where he signed an undertaking not to leave the unit and not to engage in any illegal behaviour. Today he stole a nurse's jacket, wallet and keys and disappeared for several hours. The jacket was retrieved; the money and keys were gone. The hospital saw no alternative but to discharge him, despite the fact that his infection had not been completely eradicated.

Terence's behaviour patterns do not change regardless of their disastrous consequences: over the years he has alienated every caregiver who has worked with him, has repeatedly sabotaged his medical treatment and his health, and has ensured that no facility in Vancouver other than the Portland Hotel will even consider having him as a resident. If we could peer into his brain at the moment he was about to lift the nurse's jacket from the ward office, I doubt we would see much activity in the segments that control impulse and generate conscious will; more likely the dopamine circuits of incentive, excitement and thrill would predominate. It's less a conscious decision to steal that led to Terence's expulsion from hospital than an inability *not* to, given the opportunity. No powerful "free won't" operates in his brain. Later he'll be filled with regret but at the next opportunity will re-enact exactly the same scenario. How much freedom does he really have?

The overvaluing of the addictive object, act, relationship or behaviour exists in all addictions, as does the brain lock phenomenon. In the substance addict it is fortified, as we have seen, by the effect of the drugs themselves on the brain. Drugs damage the parts of the brain—already impaired to begin with—that exercise conscious will. In a passage I partially quoted in Chapter 14, Dr. Nora Volkow, Director of the National Institute on Drug Abuse in the U.S., has written, "This aberrant behavior has traditionally been viewed as bad 'choices' that are made voluntarily by the addict. *However, recent studies have shown that repeated drug use leads to long-lasting changes in the brain that undermine voluntary control.*"[8]

The men and women I work with have had every possible negative consequence visited upon them. They have lost their jobs, their homes, their spouses, their children and their teeth; they have been jailed and beaten, abused and raped; they have suffered HIV infection and hepatitis and infections of the heart valves and of the backbone; they have had multiple pneumonias and abscesses and sores of every sort. They have seen close friends die young of overdose or disease. They are far from naïve about the seriousness of the matter and require no more convincing or coercing. And yet they will not, unless something transforms their perspective on life, abandon their compulsion to use drugs. We, as a society, cannot respond to their predicament with unenforceable laws, moral preaching and medical practices that do not employ the full range of possible options.

How, then, to create the circumstances in which the possibility of freedom can take root and flourish? That's the subject we turn to next.

—

CHAPTER 27

Imagining an Enlightened
Social Policy on Drugs

I'll start from the assumption that we want to redeem people
trapped in drug addiction—and that redemption can be something other than an addict's complete abstinence from addictive chemicals, a goal that's not always realistic. Under current
conditions it hardly ever is for most hardcore substance users,
although I believe our success rate could be much higher if we
abandoned our present intolerant and self-defeating social attitudes
toward addiction and the care of addicted people. Even in cases
where abstinence is not achieved, redemption would mean the
reintegration of the user into the larger community and the restora-
tion of his value as a person in his own eyes.

In the next pages, I'll outline what I believe would be a rational
and humane stance toward drug users, along with the policies
that would flow from it. I do not expect such ideas to be
embraced by society any time soon; an informed approach may
be, for now, no more than a dream. In a culture that projects its
darkest features onto the addict and makes addicted people into
scapegoats for its shortcomings, insight and knowledge are almost
entirely absent from public discourse concerning drug policies.
Moralizing displaces compassion and prejudice substitutes for
inquiry. The evidence accumulated by decades of scientific
research into the psychology of addiction, brain development,
child rearing and the social origins of addictive drives rarely enters

into the discussion of how to tackle the persisting problem of drug addiction. Indeed, as this book goes to press, the *Globe and Mail* reports that Canada's assault on drug addicts is about to escalate. According to the *Globe,* "the federal Conservative government [is preparing] to unveil a strategy that cracks down on illicit drug users," with harsher penalties for users of illicit substances. The mountain of evidence showing the worthlessness of this get-tough approch is, once more, ignored.[1]

The scarcity of scientific thought informing public debates on addiction is mirrored in the academic and medical arenas. In this era of sub-sub-specialization, each discipline appears to work in isolation from knowledge gathered by other researchers in closely related fields. We need far more integration of knowledge both in the professional realm and among laypeople.

Why does medical practice appear to be so opaque to the light of new findings? "I've thought about this a lot," child psychiatrist and researcher Dr. Bruce Perry said when I interviewed him, "because I've been involved in several public education campaigns. What we found is that the groups that have the greatest vested interest in the old beliefs are the last to absorb new content. As such, medicine has been the most resistant professional group to absorb and integrate the emerging findings about brain development and the importance of early childhood."

I don't believe that the "vested interests" of medical professionals are, in this case, consciously selfish or motivated by material considerations; they are the investment we have in maintaining that our way of thinking is right, that the principles and methods we have practised are sound and that approaches outside our emotional or intellectual comfort zones are not worth investigating. Institutions such as professional bodies, medical schools and scientific associations tend to be deeply conservative, even if in some ways they are at the forefront of bold exploration. They mistrust new paradigms and resist moving outside the boundaries of a narrowly defined science-ideology that separates mind from body, human beings from their lifetime environments.

Similarly, most political leaders and policymakers seem unaware of the abundance of facts and experience refuting the theory and practices of the War on Drugs or they lack the will to act on the evidence. In the worst-case scenario some may be too blinded by a moralistic and judgment-ridden ideology to act according to the Christian principles they profess. Hence the need to imagine a humane reality that we could create if we chose to honour what science, insight and the precepts of our ethical and spiritual traditions teach us.

"The current set of public beliefs and institutional beliefs about substance abuse are impediments to the application of high-quality successful intervention," says Dr. Perry. "The more we dehumanize and vilify substance abusers, the more it is impossible to put in place the kind of interventions that will help them."

In other words, we need to get outside the box. The system we have doesn't work—not for the addict and not for society. This system cannot be improved; it needs to be transformed.

I don't claim that what I will propose is without potential pitfalls, or that I could possibly have got all the details right. But for this discussion the details are not the issue. The issue is the relationship society creates between itself and its drug-addicted citizens; the fundamental question is whether or not we recognize these people as human beings who are legitimately part of the social fabric, deserving compassion and respect. "Action has meaning only in relationship," said the spiritual teacher Jiddu Krishnamurti, "and without understanding relationship, action on any level will only breed conflict. The understanding of relationship is infinitely more important than the search for any plan of action."[2] It's not the particulars of a social policy that matter most, but the relationship between those who influence policy and those who are affected by it.

People may well disagree with what is suggested in this chapter, but we cannot afford to ignore Krishnamurti's teaching on the precedence of relationship over action.

First, we need to take stock of ourselves and give up any hint of moral superiority and judgment toward the addict. Judging others clouds our eyes not only to their needs but to our own as well. Going back to the words of Jesus, *"first take the plank out of your own eye, and then you will see clearly to take the splinter out of your brother's eye."* We cannot help people when we put ourselves in a position of judgment. Addicts, all but the very few completely sociopathic ones, are deeply self-critical and harsh with themselves. They are keenly sensitive to judgmental tones in others and respond with withdrawal or defensive denial.

Second, any rational approach to the problem of addiction has to be grounded in an appreciation of the interactive psychology and brain physiology of addiction. "An understanding of emotions should not be separated from neuroscience," Dr. Jaak Panksepp told me. "If you don't recognize that the brain creates psychological responses, then neuroscience becomes a highly impoverished discipline. And that's where the battle is right now. Many neuroscientists believe that mental states are irrelevant for what the brain does. This is a Galileo-type battle and it will not be won very easily because you have generations and generations of scholars, even in psychology, who have swallowed hook, line and sinker the notion—the Skinnerian notion—that mentality is irrelevant in the control of behavior."*

Dr. Panksepp is not tilting at windmills. Narrow behaviourist thinking permeates political and social policy and medical practice, the childrearing advice dispensed by "parenting experts" and academic discourse. We keep trying to change people's behaviours without a full understanding of how and why those behaviours arise. "Inner causes are not the proper domain of psychology," writes Roy Wise, an expert on the psychology of addiction, and a prominent investigator in the National Institute on Drug Abuse in the U.S.A.[3] This statement seems astonishing, coming from a psychologist. In reality, there can be no understanding of human beings, let alone of addicted human beings, without looking at "inner causes," tricky as those causes can be to pin down at times. Behaviours, especially compulsive behaviours, are often the active representations of emotional states and of special kinds of brain functioning.

* B.F. Skinner of Indiana University is considered the founder of the hugely influential behaviourist school of psychology, which focuses only on behaviours, excluding "invisible" factors like emotions from its analysis of human conduct and relationships.

As we have seen, the dominant emotional states and the brain patterns of human beings are shaped by their early environment. Throughout their lifetimes, they are in dynamic interaction with various social and emotional milieus. If we are to help addicts, we must strive to change not them but their environments. These are the only things we *can* change. Transformation of the addict must come from within and the best we can do is to encourage it. Fortunately, there is much that we can do.

In the previous chapter I presented evidence that addictive habits, generally speaking, are too deeply entrenched in the brain of the hardcore substance user to be overcome by a simple act of will. As Jaak Panksepp put it: "Those habit structures are so incredibly robust, and once they are laid into a nervous system they will guide behaviour without free choice." My discussion with Professor Panksepp did not end there. We went on to consider what support addicts would need to overcome the powerful drives imprinted by their painful experiences. "The only way they can escape drug addictions is if their pain is alleviated, their emotions are brought back toward healthy balance, so they have a chance to think about it," Dr. Panksepp said, echoing both what brain research has told us about mental freedom and what human experience has confirmed. "Free choice only comes from thinking, it doesn't come from emotions. *It emerges from the capacity to think about your emotions.* When you're operating in the habit mode you are feeling, but those feelings are not being reflected upon. They are too powerful, they are too habitual. So, the treatment of addiction requires the island of relief where a need to soothe pain does not constantly drive a person's motivation. It requires a complex and supportive social environment."

How to create that island of relief is the core issue in projecting a humane policy toward addiction. The work of the Portland Hotel Society is an isolated, flawed but worthy attempt at offering the respite from anguish and anxiety that Dr. Panksepp suggests. Although the PHS has grown from an initial grant of $23,000 back in 1991 to a current annual operating budget of over $11 million— most of it for housing—the services it can provide are no more than a drop in the bucket compared with the needs of the community it serves in the Downtown Eastside.

—

Addicts are locked into addiction not only by their painful past and distressing present, but equally by their bleak view of the future. They cannot envision the real possibility of sobriety, of a life governed by values rather than by immediate survival needs and by desperation to escape physical and mental suffering. They are unable to develop compassion toward themselves and their bodies while they are regarded as outcasts, hunted as enemies and treated like human refuse.

As we have seen, a major factor in addiction that medical and social policies must take into account is stress. If we want to support people's potential for healthy transformation, we must cease to impose debilitating stress on their already burdened existence. Recall that uncertainty, isolation, loss of control and conflict are the major triggers for stress and that stress is the most predictable factor in maintaining addiction and triggering relapse. These are also precisely the conditions that the demonization of addiction and the War on Drugs (deliberately!) impose on hardcore substance users.

I have quoted a report in the *Journal of the American Medical Association,* which showed that a history of childhood abuse increases physiological stress reactivity for a lifetime, a reactivity "which is further enhanced when additional trauma is experienced in adulthood."[4] The addict is re-traumatized over and over again by ostracism, harassment, dire poverty, the spread of disease, the frantic hunt for a source of the substance of dependence, the violence of the underground drug world and harsh chastisement at the hands of the law—all inevitable consequences of the War on Drugs.

Studies on primates and other animals have also shown that low social status and being dominated enhance the risk of drug use, with negative effects on dopamine receptors. By contrast, after being housed with more subordinate animals, dominant monkeys had an *increase* of over 20 per cent of their dopamine receptors and less tendency to use cocaine.[5] The findings of stress research suggest that the issue is not control over others, but whether one is free to exercise control in one's own life. Yet the practices of the social welfare, legal and medical systems subject the addict to domination in many ways and deprive her of control, even if unwittingly.

In relegating the addict to the bottom of the social and moral scales and in our contemptuous rejection of her as a *person,* we have created the exact circumstances that are most likely to keep her trapped in pathological dependence on drugs. There is no island of relief, only oceanic despair.

"The War on Drugs is cultural schizophrenia," says Jaak Panksepp. I agree. The War on Drugs expresses a split mindset in two ways: we want to eradicate or limit addiction, yet our social policies are best suited to promote it, and we condemn the addict for qualities we dare not acknowledge in ourselves. Rather than exhort the addict to be other than the way she is, we need to find the strength to admit that we have greatly exacerbated her distress and perhaps our own. If we want to help people seek the possibility of transformation within themselves, we first have to transform our own view of our relationship to them.

—

That our current approach is a dead end has been acknowledged in Canada, in the U.S. and internationally by many people whose political and ideological starting point was not anywhere close to embracing the decriminalization of drugs. Today, November 17, 2006, as I'm writing this chapter, the *Globe and Mail* reports that the B.C. Progress Board, a blue-ribbon panel made up of businesspeople and academics appointed by the British Columbia government to offer advice on economic and social issues, has proposed that drugs either be decriminalized or that the War on Drugs be stepped up so as to completely eliminate the drug trade in this province. One or the other. The status quo is "clearly unacceptable if we seek truly to reduce the rates of crime and victimization in the province," the Progress Board stated.[6]

The panel warns, in the words of the *Globe* report, that "a crackdown on the drug trade would mean more police, tougher penalties for drug-related crimes and more jails to accommodate the dramatically increased demand for secure facilities." In effect,

the recommendations are a barely camouflaged call for decriminalization. The so-called other "option," the elimination of drug
trafficking and use, is no option at all—only a chimera that even
the most Draconian measures have failed to conjure into reality
anywhere in the world. Unless we are willing to see our society
metamorphose into a brutal police state, no coercive policy will
come close to even limiting drug use, let alone eliminating it.

Once we understand that the current assault on addicts creates
greater insecurity for everyone and severe hardship for users, once
we understand that stressing people chronically and mercilessly can
in no way promote their capacity for healthy transformation, it
becomes a straightforward matter to envision approaches that rely
not on moralizing but on science and humane values.

The indispensable foundation of a rational stance toward drug
addiction would be the decriminalization of all substance dependence and the provision of such substances to confirmed users under
safely controlled conditions. It's important to note that *decriminalization does not mean legalization*. Legalization would make manu-
facturing and selling drugs legal, acceptable commercial activities.
Decriminalization refers only to removing from the penal code the
possession of drugs for personal use. It would create the possibility
of medically supervised dispensing when necessary. The fear that
easier access to drugs would fuel addiction is unfounded: drugs, we
have seen, are not the cause of addiction. Despite the fact that
cannabis is openly available in Holland, for instance, Dutch per-
capita use of marijuana is half that in the United States. And no one
is advocating the open availability of hard drugs.

Decriminalization also does not mean that addicts will be able to
walk into any pharmacy to get a prescription of cocaine. Their drugs
of dependence should be dispensed under public authority and
under medical supervision, in pure form, not adulterated by
unscrupulous dealers. Addicts also ought to be offered the information, the facilities and the instruments they need to use drugs as
safely as possible. The health benefits of such an approach are self-
evident: greatly reduced risk of infection and disease transmission,
much less risk of overdose and, very importantly, comfortable and
regular access to medical care.

Not having to spend exorbitant amounts on drugs that, in themselves, are inexpensive to prepare, addicts would not be forced into crime, violence, prostitution or poverty to pay for their habits. They would not have to decide between eating or drug use, or to scrounge for food in garbage cans or pick cigarette butts out of sidewalk puddles. They would no longer need to suffer malnutrition.

I admit I am ambivalent about the decriminalization of certain drugs, particularly crystal meth, and I understand why some people would resist even discussing the possibility. But if it seems bizarre to suggest that such a potentially brain-toxic drug be legally administered to addicts, consider that the street products currently available are full of impurities, mixed with noxious chemicals that magnify the damage from the stimulant itself. By bringing the crystal meth addict into a therapeutic interaction with the health care system, we would be fostering the possibility of use and gradual detoxification and withdrawal under relatively safe circumstances—*relatively*, because there is no safe way to use crystal meth. Above all, such an approach would create a basis for gently shepherding the addict toward rehabilitation. It would provide an opportunity to create a healing relationship with users who are currently relegated to streets and back alleys. Further, if many users no longer had to turn to illicit drug labs and dealers for their substance, the underground economy of crystal meth would be deprived of much of its profit and allure. Not an ideal situation, but a vast mitigation of the present dismal scenario.

And, very much to the point, most young people who become hooked on crystal meth are self-medicating for other conditions: most commonly ADHD, but also depression, post-traumatic stress disorder or the effects of emotional and social dislocation. As we discussed in Chapter 3, some young street people who use crystal meth see it as a way of survival. If the necessary physical, psychological and social supports were provided, I believe it would not take long to diminish the appeal of methamphetamine and to wean the vast majority of stimulant addicts away from this harmful chemical.

Many people fear that decriminalization and the controlled dispensing of drugs will lead to widespread substance use among people who are now deterred from becoming addicts only by existing legal prohibitions. Like other tenets of the War on Drugs, this view

entirely lacks supporting evidence. Any data on the subject points
to the opposite prediction. For example, for many decades in the
United Kingdom, heroin has been dispensed, under legal supervision, to addicts. The same type of program has been offered on a
limited basis in other countries as well, and nowhere has it been
found that this measure served in any way to entice unaddicted
people into addiction. That is not surprising, given that addiction is
a response to life experience, not simply to a drug. People who do
not suffer the searing emotional pain that drives hardcore drug
addiction will rarely fall into dependency on chemicals, even if
these were more readily available—and, once more, public access
to habit-forming substances is not being proposed. The call for the
decriminalization of drugs for personal use does not imply legal
acceptance of drug dealing.

Criminalization and prevention are not identical—if anything,
the first undermines the other. Paradoxical though it may seem,
current drug laws against possession make drugs more readily available to potential new users than decriminalization would. Only the
War on Drugs creates the *raison d'être* of the international trafficking industry, most of whose wealth is based on satisfying the cravings of established drug addicts. Without the exorbitant profits
yielded by supplying to addicted users desperate for their substances, the illegal market would shrink to a fragment of its present
size. Further, much of the street-level front-line sales force of the
illicit drug trade consists of users raising money to support their
habit. With the decriminalization of possession for personal use and
the medically supervised distribution of drugs, the incentive to sell
to new "customers," including young kids, would largely evaporate.
Policing resources could then be concentrated on the remaining
large-scale traffickers—if any.

Addicts should not be coerced into treatment, since in the long
term coercion creates more problems than it solves. On the other
hand, for those addicts who opt for treatment, there must be a system of publicly funded recovery facilities with clean rooms, nutri-
tious food and access to outdoors and nature. Well-trained
professional staff need to provide medical care, counselling, skills
training and emotional support. Our current nonsystem is utterly

inadequate, with its patchwork of recovery homes run on private contracts and, here and there, a few upscale addiction treatment spas for the wealthy. No matter how committed their staff and how helpful their services may be, they are a drop in comparison to the ocean of vast need. In the absence of a coordinated rehabilitation system, the efforts of individual recovery homes are limited and occur in a vacuum, with no follow-up.

It may be thought that the cost of such a drug rehabilitation and treatment system would be exorbitant. No doubt the financial expenses would be great—but surely less than the funds now freely squandered on the War on Drugs, to say nothing of the savings from the cessation of drug-related criminal activity and the diminished burden on the health care system.

To expect an addict to give up her drug is like asking the average person to imagine living without all her social skills, support networks, emotional stability and sense of physical and psychological comfort. Those are the qualities that, in their illusory and evanescent way, drugs give the addict. People like Serena and Celia and the others whose portraits have appeared in this book perceive their drugs as their "rock and salvation." Thus, for all the valid reasons we have for wanting the addict to "just say no," we first need to offer her something to which she can say "yes." We must provide an island of relief. We have to demonstrate that esteem, acceptance, love and humane interaction are realities in this world, contrary to what she, the addict, has learned all her life. It is impossible to create that island for people unless they can feel secure that their substance dependency will be satisfied as long as they need it.

—

One of the greatest difficulties we human beings seem to have is to relinquish long-held ideas. Many of us are addicted to being right, even if facts do not support us. One fixed image we cling to, as iconic in today's culture as the devil was in previous ages, is that of the addict as an unsavoury and shadowy character, given to criminal activity. What we don't see is how we've contributed to making him a criminal.

There is nothing more intrinsically criminal in the average drug user than in the average cigarette smoker or alcohol addict. The drugs they inject or inhale do not themselves induce criminal activity by their pharmacological effect, except perhaps in the way that alcohol can also fuel a person's pent-up aggression and remove the mental inhibitions that thwart violence. Stimulant drugs may have that effect on some users, but narcotics like heroin do not; on the contrary, they tend to calm people down. It is withdrawal from opiates that makes people physically ill, irritable and more likely to act violently—mostly out of desperation to replenish their supply.

The criminality associated with addiction follows directly from the need to raise money to purchase drugs at prices that are artificially inflated owing to their illegality. The addict shoplifts, steals and robs because it's the only way she can obtain the funds to pay the dealer. History has demonstrated many times over that people will transgress laws and resist coercion when it comes to struggling for their basic needs—or what they perceive as such. Sam Sullivan, Vancouver's quadriplegic mayor, told a conference on drug addiction once that if wheelchairs were illegal, he would do anything to get one, no matter what laws he had to break. It was an apt comparison: the hardcore addict feels equally handicapped without his substances. As we have seen, many addicts who deal in drugs do so exclusively to finance their habit. There is no profit in it for them.

As with petty drug pushing, so with prostitution. As this book is being completed, the disturbing details of the serial murder case against pig farmer Robert Pickton are emerging in a British Columbia courtroom. If convicted, Pickton will be counted among the most prolific and most sadistic killers of women in North American history. I believe that as a society we are unwitting accomplices in the deaths of the Downtown Eastside women who allegedly became Pickton's victims because our criminalization of drug use drove those women into prostitution and into the underground street life that led to their deaths. If an evidence-based policy had been in operation in this country, these dozens of women—and their many counterparts elsewhere—might still be alive.

Society would have much to gain from decriminalization. On the immediate practical level, we would feel safer in our homes and on our streets and much less concerned about the danger of our cars being burgled. In cities like Vancouver such crimes are often committed for the sake of obtaining drug money. More significantly perhaps, by exorcising this menacing devil of our own creation, we would automatically give up a lot of unnecessary fear. We could all breathe more freely.

Many addicts could work at productive jobs if the imperative of seeking illegal drugs did not keep them constantly on the street. It's interesting to learn that before the War on Drugs mentality took hold in the early twentieth century, a prominent individual such as Dr. William Stewart Halsted, a pioneer of modern surgical practice, was an opiate addict for over forty years. During those decades he did stellar and innovative work at Johns Hopkins University, where he was one of the four founding physicians. He was the first, for example, to insist that members of his surgical team wear rubber gloves—a major advance in eradicating post-operative infections. Throughout his career, however, he never got by with less than 180 milligrams of morphine a day. "On this," said his colleague, the world-renowned Canadian physician Sir William Osler, "he could do his work comfortably and maintain his excellent vigor." As noted at the Common Sense for Drug Policy website:

> Halsted's story is revealing not only because it shows that with a morphine addiction the proper maintenance dose can be productive. It also illustrates the incredible power of the drug in question. Here was a man with almost unlimited resources—moral, physical, financial, medical—who tried everything he could think of and he was hooked until the day he died. Today we would send a man like that to prison. Instead he became the father of modern surgery.[7]

Most hardcore addicts could not function at such a high level, given the social and psychological adversity of their life histories. But surely, if their substance needs were met, they would have much greater opportunity to realize their potential to be creative and contributing members of society. At the very least, they would be a lesser burden. Decriminalization of drug use would establish the possibility of integrating addicts into the larger community, an essential step if they are to be rehabilitated in any large numbers.

—

In Chapter 1 I introduced Stan, a Native Canadian man, an addict and street dweller just out of jail. On chilly nights Stan should not be sleeping on stone steps under an archway in the Downtown Eastside. Without having to steal to support his drug habit, he would not have lived in prison the past eighteen months but in a recovery home or, if still needing to use, in a decent housing facility. He ought to be receiving remedial training for his learning disabilities and counselling to help him overcome the emotional defensiveness and impulsive reactivity that has so often landed him in trouble. Such support would help prepare him to join normal society.

Seeking insight into my First Nations patients, I spoke with psychiatrist Lewis Mehl-Madrona, author of *Coyote Medicine: Lessons from Native American Healing* and Associate Professor of Family Medicine and Psychiatry at the University of Saskatchewan. "People fall into these communities of substance, centred around drugs," Dr. Mehl-Madrona pointed out. "You can fall into communities around alcohol or cocaine and whatever. Everyone has a need to belong. Unless people have another community, an alternative community that provides them with more belonging, being wanted, and purpose, the so-called treatment always fails. What seems to work here for aboriginal people is to switch their allegiance to an alternative community, modern but honouring traditional values. As long as they can maintain their position in that non-using community, they are not using substances."

Lewis Mehl-Madrona's insights apply not only to Native people, but to all the marginalized addicts who, like Stan, haunt the streets and alleys in the vicinity of the Portland Hotel. They need to be invited into communities that can offer them acceptance, belonging and value. At least transitionally, such communities have to be founded and maintained with public support until, step by step, former users are fully able to join society at large. Those unable to give up their habits ought not to be ostracized, nor should their voices be excluded from social discourse. If we understood the sources of their dysfunction, we would want to reduce their suffering, whether or not they continue to use.

"Drug addiction has to be de-vilified," Bruce Perry said during our interview. "If we create environments that are safe and pre-dictable and relationally enriched, then all of the other factors involved in substance abuse and dependence will be so much eas-ier to dissolve away. Our challenge is to figure out how to create these environments.

"We really need . . . and I know it sounds kind of corny . . . we need to be very loving, very accepting, and very patient with people who have these problems. And if we are, they will have a much higher probability of getting better."

We need to absorb in our minds and guts the utter futility of what we are doing now. We need to wake to the reality that our present system actively generates misery for users and nonusers alike and places intolerable burdens on society. More of the same will only cause more of the same.

A 2007 study by physicians and researchers at the B.C. Centre for Excellence in HIV/AIDS stated that "the federal government continues to invest heavily in policies and practices that have been repeatedly shown in the scientific literature to be ineffective or harmful." According to a front-page report in the *Globe and Mail,* the study found that "law enforcement consumed by far the largest chunk (73 per cent) of the [national] drug strategy's annual $245 million budget, with no demonstrated impact on curbing the use of illegal drugs. At the same time, 14 per cent is spent on treat-ment, 7 per cent on research, and 3 per cent each for addiction prevention and harm reduction."[8]

"I'm paid to treat disease," said one of the authors, Dr. Thomas Kerr, "and I don't like what I'm seeing. Canada simply does not have an evidence-based drug strategy. There's way too much ideology and politics, and not enough science and principle."

On the same morning that this new study was reported, my last patient was Serena, the young Native woman from Kelowna whose life story is described in Chapter 4. She came late, panting into my office with a high fever and a strangulating cough. Her pneumonia had begun several days before that, when she woke up after one of Vancouver's heavy windstorms to find that the windows of her hotel room had been shattered during the night and the water in her sink was frozen solid.

In a commentary published in the *Globe*'s web edition I summarized Serena's history and explained that she deals drugs only to support her own cocaine habit. "Proper nutrition, shelter, the controlled provision of their substances of dependence, counselling, and compassionate caring are what most addicts need if we are to help wean them from their debilitating habits," I wrote.

The piece ignited a lively set of exchanges at the newspaper's website, indicating how deeply felt are the views of many people on the issue of drug addiction. I was encouraged by the discourse. Many participants seemed interested in basing social policies not on subjective emotional responses toward addicts, but on facts and compassionate principle. "This is an excellent discussion that shows the complexity of the issue and the lack of perfect solutions," wrote one of the contributors.

> Few harm-reductionists who know their stuff recommend a market-led free-for-all in drugs like heroin and cocaine and the amphetamine stimulants. But there is now an undisputable body of evidence that demonstrates that developing mechanisms to make safer forms of these drugs available to those with an intractable need brings enormous benefits to both the drug user and the society around them. Thus both Holland and Switzerland and parts of Germany have changed policies and seen an enormous drop in the levels of drug related crime. The average age of hard drug users is rising there, indicated that fewer young people are taking up such an activity. The real obscenity here is the shocking lack of funding for treatment and care and harm reduction initiatives that have been shown to work. The UK National Treatment Outcome Survey (known as NTROS) showed that for every 1 pound invested in treatment and care, 3 pounds came back in health care and enforcement savings. If such a return was available in the financial markets, we'd all rush to take advantage.

Would the decriminalization of drug use and the controlled distribution of drugs bring up a new set of problems? No doubt they would. Innumerable practical issues would need to be resolved, some extremely complicated, and there would be risks. Around drug addiction there are no easy, risk-free solutions to be found. But for every fresh difficulty there would be new benefits that would weigh far more in the balance. No foreseeable risk can to any degree resemble the tremendous harm currently being done.

—

CHAPTER 28

A Necessary Small Step:
Harm Reduction

—

Whatever the arguments in its favour, a rational, evidence-based and integrated drug policy is unlikely to emerge in the near future. With no enlightened social consensus on the horizon, we are left with the question—still an important one—of how to limit the harm suffered by the addict. In this chapter we'll explore the hotly debated and much misunderstood issue of harm reduction.

—

Nearly eight years ago, on my very first day as the Portland doctor, I was guided up to the top floor of the old hotel to meet a resident described as a "difficult patient." As the nurse and I entered his room, Claude, a man from Quebec in his late thirties, was kneeling on the floor, peering down into a mirror that lay horizontally on his bed. Grimacing, head tilted to one side, his prematurely greying hair falling over his temples, Claude pulled on the skin and muscles of his neck with his left hand while he attempted to inject a vein with some cloudy fluid from the syringe he held in his right. I watched as he poked himself in the neck once or twice without finding a blood vessel. "*Tabernac,*" came the well-known Québécois curse.

"You're asking for a brain abscess if you keep that up," I said, becoming alarmed at this inept display. "Let's see if we can't find you a safer spot to inject." Wrapping a rubber tourniquet from the nurse's bag around Claude's left arm, I asked him to pump his hand a few times. When a vein bulged below his elbow crease, I instructed him to insert the needle. He did, and as he pulled on the plunger blood surged back into the syringe. The nurse removed the rubber hose and our patient injected himself with whatever concoction he had prepared. We made him a gift of the tourniquet.

I had never imagined that my medical career would lead me to assist an addict's self-administration of an illicit psychoactive substance in a musty Downtown Eastside hotel. Even on the way up to his room I was not expecting to do anything of the sort; my intention was to discuss his HIV treatment. Under the circumstances, however, it was the best I could do for him. Without that help, Claude would have persisted in his attempts to inject a neck vein, a procedure with a high risk ratio. I had no realistic hope of dissuading him from self-injection, let alone of "curing" his long-established drug habit. The immediate goal was to reduce potential harm and, beyond that, to establish a relationship with Claude in which he could feel open and trusting enough to receive medical support and advice.

Such was my rapid immersion in harm reduction.

Claude died over two years ago from complications of HIV. He had been one of the Portland's long time residents, one whose highly original personality and sense of humour make him stand out among the ranks of the departed. He was not a "difficult patient" after all—only someone who liked to do things his way and did not readily trust authority. He was an accomplished artist. A small,

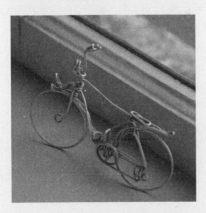

finely crafted aluminum-wire bicycle, a memento of his dexterity and creative skill, stands on the windowsill of my kitchen to this day, a gift from Claude. During his last four years, despite his medical treatment being compromised by his addiction, we did much to extend his life, to prevent symptoms and, in the end, to ease his physical and emotional distress.

What is harm reduction?

Harm reduction is often perceived as being inimical to the ultimate purpose of "curing" addiction—that is, of helping addicts transcend their habits and to heal. People regard it as "coddling" addicts, as enabling them to continue their destructive ways. It's also considered to be the opposite of abstinence, which many regard as the only legitimate goal of addiction treatment. Such a distinction is artificial. The issue in medical practice is always how best to help a patient. If a cure is possible *and* probable without doing greater harm, then cure is the objective. When it isn't—and in most chronic medical conditions cure is not the expected outcome—the physician's role is to help the patient with the symptoms and to reduce the harm done by the disease process. In rheumatoid arthritis, for example, one aims to prevent joint inflammation and bone destruction and, in all events, to reduce pain. In incurable cancers we aim to prolong life, if that can be achieved without a loss of life quality, and also to control symptoms. In other words, harm reduction means making the lives of afflicted human beings more bearable, more worth living. That is also the goal of harm reduction in the context of addiction.

Although hardcore drug addiction is much more than a disease, the harm reduction model is essential to its treatment. Given our lack of a systematic, evidence-based approach to addiction, in many cases it's futile to dream of a cure. So long as society ostracizes the addict and the legal system does everything it can to heighten the drug problem, the welfare and medical systems can aim only to mitigate some of its effects. Sad to say, in our context harm reduction means reducing not only the harm caused by the disease of addiction, but also the harm caused by the social assault on drug addicts.

We will look shortly at some harm reduction measures. First, however, we'll dispense with two prevalent arguments against harm reduction: that it squanders resources on undeserving people who are the authors of their own misfortune and that it justifies and enables addiction.

—

If our guiding principle is that a person who makes his own bed ought to lie in it, we should immediately dismantle much of our health care system. Many diseases and conditions arise from self-chosen habits or circumstances and could be prevented by more astute decisions. According to a recent study by British Columbia's health officer, the provincial government spends $1.8 billion dollars on diseases caused by unhealthy lifestyles.* The average per capita health care cost for those with no risk factors is "$1,003 compared with $2,086 per capita for those with three risk factors, including smoking, being overweight/obese and physically inactive."[1] All of these factors, we might say, represent "choices," and even after a heart attack, for instance, some patients will continue to bring these risks upon themselves. The same is true of people with chronic bronchitis who persist in smoking, skiers who brave moguls and steep slopes despite having sustained fractures and people who remain in a stressful marriage despite requiring treatment for depression or anxiety. No cardiologist, respiratory specialist, orthopaedic surgeon or psychiatrist would refuse treatment on the ground that the problem was "self-inflicted."

When it comes to drug addicts, some people believe we ought to apply different criteria. One afternoon in August 2006 I called a CBC radio program to discuss Insite, Vancouver's controversial supervised injection facility for drug users. Just before the moderator turned to me, he interviewed an RCMP officer. Dozens of addicts who have overdosed at Insite have been successfully resuscitated, the host pointed out. Lives have been saved that might otherwise have been lost. That's not necessarily a good thing, the Mountie spokesman explained. "It's well known that negative consequences are the only major deterrent to drug use. If you are saving people's lives, you are sending the message that it's safe to use drugs." This officer, on behalf of Canada's national law enforcement agency, seemed willing to let people die in the hope of teaching a lesson. He seemed unaware, or not to care, that in the 1990s Vancouver's

* If B.C. accounts for 10 per cent of Canada's population, the national figure would be about $20 billion annually; by extension, the comparable U.S. sum would be over $200 billion per year.

injection users had received an average of 147 such "lessons" every year in the form of overdose deaths, without any discernible deterrent effect.[2]

It would be encouraging to believe that such a dark perspective is confined to the minds of some police officers. Not quite so. At about this same time the *Globe and Mail* published an article on Insite that approvingly quoted Anthony Daniels, a retired British psychiatrist. "I suppose the argument for the safe injection site is it would reduce the number of deaths," he told *Globe* columnist Gary Mason. "But I don't see why we should reduce the number of deaths. It is not our responsibility to do so. It is the responsibility of the addicts themselves. If they want to inject themselves with heroin, it's a very bad choice. If people die from it, I don't feel any particular guilt because I don't feel any responsibility for it."[3]

It would have been instructive to know whether or not the psychiatrist and his faithful scribe at the *Globe* were willing to extend this principle to other groups, such as, say, smokers with lung cancer or emphysema, type A business executives who work themselves into a heart attack, battered women who remain loyal to an abusive partner or people injured in automobile accidents in full knowledge of the risks of driving. According to this same logic no smoker should be defibrillated and brought back to life after a heart attack and no one who drinks alcohol should receive a blood transfusion in the wake of intestinal bleeding. Anyone worried about the possibility of a myocardial infarction or a stroke ought to wear a large badge identifying him as a nonsmoker, nondrinker, regular exerciser and nonconsumer of trans fatty acids. Absent such a marker, no bystander should even dial 911 on their behalf.

Although we are all responsible for our lives, no human or medical principle dictates that we refuse to help others whose own decisions have brought trouble upon their heads—unless we believe that in trying to help them, we are perpetrating greater harm. That would perhaps be the case if harm reduction could be shown to enable substance abuse. But as we have seen, hardcore drug users do not wait to be "enabled," and there are few harsh consequences they haven't yet experienced. There is no evidence from anywhere in the world that harm reduction measures encourage drug use.

Denying addicts humane assistance multiplies their miseries without bringing them one inch closer to recovery.

—

There is also no contradiction between harm reduction and abstinence. The two objectives are incompatible only if we imagine that we can set the agenda for someone else's life regardless of what he or she may choose. We cannot. Short of extreme coercion there is absolutely nothing anyone can do to induce another to give up addiction, except—as discussed in the previous chapter—to provide the island of relief where contemplation and self-respect can, perhaps, take root. Those ready to choose abstinence should receive every possible support—much more support than we currently provide. But what of those who don't choose that path?

The impossibility of changing other people is not restricted to addictions. Try as we may to motivate another person to be different or to do this or not to do that, our attempts founder on a basic human trait: the drive for autonomy. "And one may choose what is contrary to one's own interests and sometimes one *positively* ought," wrote Fyodor Dostoevsky in *Notes from the Underground*. "What man wants is simply *independent* choice, whatever that independence may cost and wherever it may lead." The issue is not whether the addict would be better off without his habit—of course he would—but whether we are going to abandon him if he is unable to give it up. Are we willing to care for human beings who suffer because of their own persistent behaviours, mindful that these behaviours stem from early life misfortunes they had no hand in creating?

The harm reduction approach accepts that some people—many people—are too deeply enmeshed in substance dependence for any realistic "cure" under present circumstances. There is, for now, too much pain in their lives and too few internal and external resources available to them. In practising harm reduction we do not give up on abstinence—on the contrary, we may hope to encourage that possibility by helping people feel better, bringing them into therapeutic relationships with caregivers, offering them a sense of trust, removing judgment from our interactions with them and giving them a sense of acceptance. At the same time, we do not hold out abstinence as the Holy Grail and we do not make our valuation of addicts as worthwhile human beings dependent on their making choices that please us.

Harm reduction is as much an attitude and way of being as it is a set of policies and methods. Bruce Perry's words are worth recalling here: "We need to be very loving, very accepting and very patient with people who have these problems. And if we are, they will have a much higher probability of getting better."

Specific harm reduction practices depend on resources and need. One such practice is the prescription of methadone. These days I write regular methadone scripts for over one hundred patients. The drug is a synthetic narcotic that occupies opiate receptors on brain cells, blocking the access of heroin molecules to the same binding site. When ingested orally, it does not cause a "high" in chronic narcotic users, but for many addicts it prevents heroin craving and also withdrawal symptoms such as nervousness, pain, diarrhea and nausea.* It's long-acting, so a once-daily dose will see most people through twenty-four hours.

It is estimated that there are sixty thousand to ninety thousand illicit opioid abusers in Canada, but only about a quarter are receiving treatment.⁴ We offer methadone maintenance to addicts not to cure them of their narcotic dependence but to transfer that dependence to a narcotic that is legal, safe if ingested properly and which prevents them from having to prostitute themselves, steal and beg to avoid withdrawal. An addict chooses methadone when he tires of the endless daily scrounging for illicit narcotics and of the consequences of always having to dodge the law. None of my methadone patients would accept abstinence as an alternative to heroin use, and even with methadone the heroin craving remains irresistible for some.

There is no drug analogous to methadone to help with cocaine addiction. There have been some potentially encouraging trials with methylphenidate (Ritalin) and other stimulant preparations, and I have had some limited success in prescribing such medications to

---

* In nonaddicts methadone is a more potent analgesic than morphine, but addicts on methadone often become tolerant to its pain-killing effects.

decrease people's reliance on cocaine and crystal meth. For a few patients, the difference has been dramatic. I would like to see long-acting stimulants investigated more vigorously, despite their own addiction potential. It would be preferable, if possible, to have people dependent on an oral stimulant in a controlled dose rather than on smoked or injected cocaine or crystal meth.

Needle exchange is another harm reduction tactic: users bring in dirty syringes and needles and are given new ones. The spread of HIV and hepatitis C from one person to another occurs by way of body fluids, specifically blood or sexual secretions. Clean, unshared needles limit disease transmission, as does the use of condoms during intercourse. Clean needles also help prevent skin infections, abscesses and the spread of bacteria via the bloodstream. Even this simple measure is opposed by those who believe, once more, that somehow it "condones" or encourages addiction.

—

Not all addicts will accept methadone as a substitute (just as for some others whose drug of choice is morphine, neither methadone nor heroin will do). In such cases we can leave the addict to fend for herself in the underworld jungle or we can offer heroin or morphine unadulterated by who-knows-what impurities, to be self-injected in a clean environment, with uncontaminated needles. We are neither condoning nor encouraging addiction: the addiction exists and will continue to savage that person's life no matter what we believe. Our only choice is between compassion and indifference. By administering heroin in a controlled fashion we are attempting to minimize harm for the addict, with the social benefit of reducing crime, squalor and medical expenses.

The North American Opiate Medication Initiative (NAOMI) is a trial of controlled heroin administration in several cities, including Vancouver, where the project operates out of a corner storefront one block away from the Portland Hotel. A spokesperson in the office of John Walters, Director of the White House Office of National Drug Control Policy, called it "an inhumane medical experiment."[5]

There is another way to see it: the NAOMI trial is evaluating a method to lessen society's inhumanity toward drug addicts. The study's chief value may be to convince skeptics, since from the medical and social perspectives evidence is hardly required: we have decades of experience in Europe to draw on. In the United Kingdom opiate maintenance programs were administered from the 1920s to the 1970s but fell into disfavour under heavy U.S. opposition. Since then, despite the War on Drugs—or perhaps, in part, owing to it— the number of British opiate addicts has soared exponentially.[6]

One exception to the abandonment of heroin maintenance in the U.K. has been the Drug Dependency Service in the Merseyside area. All addicts registering with the program are offered treatment, including inpatient detoxification. Only about 10 per cent elect approaches leading to abstinence; the rest are prescribed narcotics in various forms, from the injectable to the inhaled. Among the results has been the second-lowest rate of HIV-positive drug users in all English regions, less than a quarter of the national average, as well as a reduction in criminal activity. "In 1991, the Merseyside police were the only force in the U.K. to register a decrease in crime rates."[7]

In the 1990s Switzerland, facing Europe's highest HIV infection rate from injection drug use, initiated a trial of either heroin maintenance or of methadone treatment supplemented with heroin. The findings were:

- fitness for work improved considerably: permanent employment more than doubled;
- patients' housing situations rapidly improved and stabilized (in particular, there was no homelessness);
- no fatal overdose due to prescribed substances;
- no notable disturbances in local neighbourhoods;
- significant economic benefits in terms of savings per patient-day, owing to marked reductions in legal and health costs; and
- a marked decrease in crime of all kinds, from shoplifting to drug dealing; overall offences down by 68 per cent.[8]

The Swiss achieved these effects, write two North American academic researchers,* "through a careful evaluation of prescribed heroin for over 1,000 of the country's most refractory, long-term heroin addicts—*targeting the most difficult of individuals who have had long-term difficulties with substance misuse and repeated failures with traditional abstinence based approaches to treatment.* The Swiss studies showed unequivocally that prescribing heroin produces substantial declines both in illicit drug use and in criminal activity for this most problematic group. In addition, they provided clear evidence of improved social reintegration, i.e. better housing, more gainful employment, fewer drug associates and more contact with previously estranged families and friends."[9]

The current NAOMI project's largest flaw is that the study's limitations curtail the time an addict can take part in it. Jenny, a twenty-nine-year-old Portland Hotel resident and sex trade worker was in my office a few weeks ago, asking to be reinstated on methadone. For a year she had been receiving heroin at the NAOMI site. Her health had improved and, contrary to previous times, during this period I had not had to treat her for infectious diseases. Now she presented with a red, swollen right leg and an abscess in her groin, where she had self-injected street heroin. The problem? Her scheduled participation at NAOMI had come to an end. Owing largely to U.S. opposition, heroin maintenance is unavailable in Canada outside this research project. "I would bet any amount of money the U.S. has exerted extreme pressure on Canada to abort this trial," Dr. Alex Wodak, a prominent Australian addiction physician said when NAOMI was just beginning.[10] Dr. Wodak, Director of the Alcohol and Drug Service at St. Vincent's Hospital in Sydney, was in a position to know. U.S. opposition had helped to abort an Australian heroin trial in 1997.

—

* Dr. Dan Small, a medical anthropologist at the University of British Columbia, and Dr. Ernest Drucker, an epidemiologist at the Albert Einstein College of Medicine, New York

We in Vancouver have also not been spared White House advice regarding Insite, the supervised injection site (SIS) administered by the Portland Hotel Society in conjunction with local health authorities. John Walters, the White House drug czar, has called this project state-assisted slow suicide.*

When you walk into the injection room at Insite on Hastings Street you see about a dozen cubicles, each with a sink, clean needles, a large mirror, lighting, towel and alcohol swabs for cleansing the skin. At first blink it's as if you'd entered the dressing room in an off-Broadway theatre. A nurse is present at all times, observing the addicts who occupy the cubicles and wrap clean tourniquets around their arms before they probe their own veins with syringe and needle. Next door is a "chill lounge," where coffee is served and where staff and counsellors engage addicts in conversation. There is also a treatment room at the facility and all the equipment and medications needed for resuscitating overdosed users. That equipment has not lain idle: in an eighteen-month period there were nearly five hundred overdoses at Insite but no deaths. The accepted assumption is that there is about a 5 per cent mortality rate without intervention, in which case twenty-five lives have been saved—to the likely disapproval of the Mounties and the British psychiatrist Dr. Daniels, who, we may guess, would also prefer to see addicts continue to inject themselves with puddle water, as was sometimes the case prior to Insite.

More than five thousand users are registered with Insite, of whom over six hundred visit on any given day. None of the fears generated before this facility began to operate in 2003 have been realized: it has not encouraged drug use or drug-related crime; it has not brought more dealers into the areas and it has not made the streets less safe. More than twenty studies published in the *Journal of the Canadian Medical Association,* the *British Medical Journal, Lancet,* the *New England Journal of Medicine* and other peer-reviewed journals have documented its benefits. The program:

* The White House drug czar was actually reported to have said "slow assisted state suicide," but we can assume this is what he meant.

- is attracting the highest-risk users—those more likely to be vulnerable to HIV infection and overdose, public drug use and unsafe syringe disposal;
- has reduced the number of people injecting in public and the amount of injection-related litter in the Downtown Eastside;
- has reduced hassles for local businesses;
- has reduced overall rates of needle sharing in the community;
- is not increasing rates of relapse among former drug users, nor is it a negative influence on those seeking to stop drug use;
- has led to increased enrolment in detoxification programs and addiction treatment; and
- has not drawn drug users from other areas into the neighbourhood.

As summed up in the *Canadian Medical Association Journal*, "Vancouver's safer injecting facility has been associated with an array of community and public health benefits without evidence of adverse impacts."[11] The city's current mayor and his three most recent predecessors, including the present premier of British Columbia—no liberal when it comes to social policy—support the continuation of Insite. Despite initial skepticism, so do local merchants and the Vancouver Police Department. Inspector Scott Thompson, head of youth services and drug policy coordinator for the VPD, rebuked the RCMP publicly for its opposition to Insite—a resistance that persisted despite internal RCMP studies vindicating the project. "We're the ones on the ground, and we support the public health objectives of reducing fatal overdoses and lessening the risk of HIV and AIDS among drug users," he said.[12] "The evidence in favour of Insite is so overwhelming," the *Vancouver Sun* noted in an editorial, "that police chiefs in Great Britain have backed a proposal to open supervised injection sites in that country."[13]

In September 2007, the services offered at Insite were enhanced by a detox centre in the same building, called Onsite. Here, addicts, both male and female, are supported through the process of withdrawal without being permitted to use drugs, and short-term housing is available for those wishing to leave domiciles where substance abuse is rampant. The detox floor has twelve rooms, each with its own bathroom, which provides unprecedented privacy, unknown at other local facilities. "It's very painful to withdraw and you really don't want to be around people and doing a lot of throwing up," a recovering heroin addict explained to a journalist.[14] I'm one of the two physicians currently providing medical care at this venue.

In September 2006, the three-year federal authorization for the supervised injection site was to run out. During its successful campaign in the previous election, the Conservative party had indicated its distaste for everything but abstinence-based drug programs. Now the government of Prime Minister Stephen Harper was flooded with requests from politicians, police and health authorities; citizens' groups; users' advocates and many individuals to permit Insite to continue. As a physician whose patients are served by the supervised injection site (SIS), I also penned a letter to Mr. Harper. "The SIS is a facility that attempts, in a modest but essential way, to reduce the harm attendant on the disease of dependence," I wrote.

> This is a difficult population to work with. Because of their uniformly tragic early childhood histories they do not well know how to take care of themselves and they do not readily seek help from health providers. The SIS is a link—for some their only link— between their street lives and the health care system and, for many, it is one of the first institutions they have encountered where they feel treated in a supportive, humane way. For the physically and emotionally wounded people they are, that is no small matter . . . The SIS is far from a full answer to the complex problem of drug addiction, but it is an innovative and necessary small step, a project Canada can be proud of, one that in time will be emulated in many jurisdictions around the world.

The government waited until a few days before the final deadline before announcing that they would renew authorization for Insite for a limited, year-and-a-half period, leaving its long-term future very much in limbo. They also cut off federal research money for the site. "Why would the government on the one hand announce that additional time is needed to study the potential success of the Vancouver safe injecting site and on the other hand eliminate the funding needed for such evaluations?" asked Dr. Mark Weinberg, Director of the McGill University AIDS Centre in Montreal.[15] At a press conference the federal health minister said there was insufficient evidence that the program reduces drug use and fights addiction.[16]

A harm reduction program does not "fight addiction"—whatever that means. It only reduces misery and prevents death and disease. The controversy has demonstrated that harm reduction may not be a medical or social question at all; the issue is not what's best for either the addicted person or for society. At heart, it's a matter of ideology. Inflamed phrases such as "inhumane medical experiment" and "state-assisted slow suicide" are spoken, it seems to me, in the language of people with a higher regard for their own convictions than for the facts.

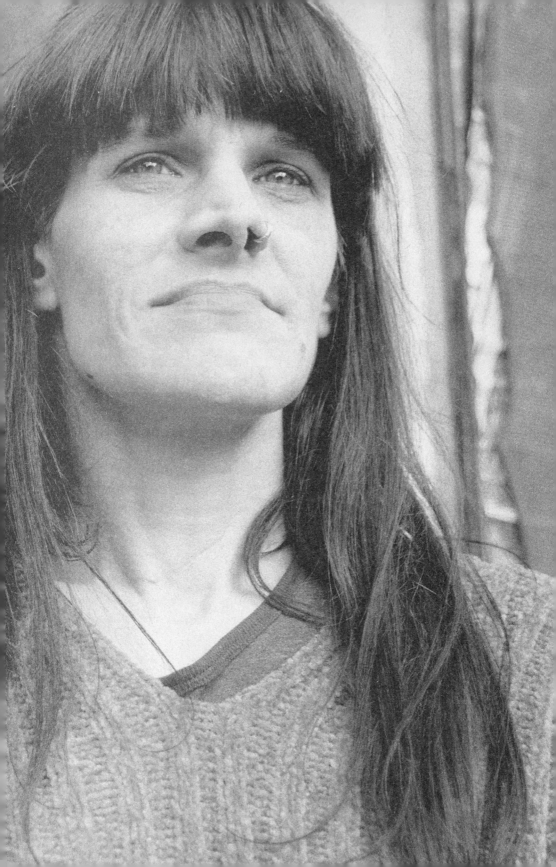

PART VII

—

The Ecology of Healing

The problem's not that the truth is harsh but that liberation from
ignorance is as painful as being born. Run after truth until you're
breathless. Accept the pain involved in re-creating yourself afresh.
These ideas will take a life to comprehend, a hard one interspersed
with drunken moments.

NAGUIB MAHFOUZ
Palace of Desire

—

CHAPTER 29

The Power of Compassionate Curiosity

*T*hese concluding chapters are intended to enhance the reader's understanding of the addicted mind and to support healing. They are not a guide for treating active substance dependence. Under the influence of brain-altering chemicals it's not possible for users to sustain the self-compassionate stance and conscious mental effort required to heal their addicted minds. The information and advice given here may complement, but cannot replace, treatment programs or self-help groups for addictions of any kind.

—

I had hoped to end this book on a triumphant note. I wanted, in this section on the self-healing of addiction, to describe how I overcame my addictive tendencies. Unfortunately, such a tale, while possibly uplifting and feel-good, would have to be filed in the fiction aisles.

For much of the writing of *Hungry Ghosts* I continued to relapse: bingeing, lying, shamed and hollow. Despite my earnest resolutions, I never returned to the Twelve-Step group, nor did I follow any other program consistently. I was like Dean, Canada's self-described "most famous junkie," who vowed at the beginning of the documentary *Fix* that by film's end he would clean up his act. He didn't and I didn't; or at least, in my case, not until recently—too recently to stand flak-jacketed on an aircraft carrier and shout, "Mission accomplished!" "Mission accepted" would be more accurate.

We teach what we most need to learn—and sometimes give what we most need to receive. It was impossible to study addiction without observing myself closely, and I can say truthfully that I have learned much through this exercise. No matter how hard I try, I have found out that I may never fully defeat my addiction-prone tendencies. And I've also learned that this is all right. Triumph and defeat: these are still metaphors of war. If, as the research shows, addictions arise near our emotional core, to defeat them we would have to wage a war against ourselves. And a war against parts of the self—even against nonadaptive, dysfunctional parts, can lead only to inner discord and more distress.

—

One day this winter, Nurse Kim and I met with a thirty-one-year-old woman, a heroin and cocaine addict I will call Clarissa. Clarissa has had three children taken away from her by child protection authorities and is now expecting again. She admits she is high on cocaine— not that she could conceal that fact, given her restless, agitated body movements; staccato speech and emotional reactivity. "But I'm like this even without the rock," she pleads—and she is, nearly, due to severe attention deficit hyperactivity disorder.

"I hate myself," she says. "I've known I've been pregnant for weeks, and I haven't stopped hooting. I've been fucking up, feeling sorry for myself and not thinking about the baby. . . ." Kim and I listen without interruption as Clarissa lurches from self-accusation to complaints about the staff to demands for food supplements and a new two-room apartment. In the midst of the tirade she stops speaking, sucks in a deep breath, buries her face in her palms and sobs, "I'm scared. I'm so very scared."

Clarissa sits on the sofa by the window, her tear-brimmed eyes skipping from nurse to doctor to the street scene outside. Her half-bare breasts, enlarged by the hormones of gestation, quiver in the push-up bra she wears to help attract potential customers. A few questions, and the distraught young woman's life story pours out—

the all-too-familiar, well-nigh formulaic Downtown Eastside life story. As ever, the tale is so toxic the sheer hearing of it leaves one benumbed.

Clarissa was sexually abused by her father from age one to four, and after that by a series of men until she was a teenager. By the time she was five years old, her mother was dead of an overdose. "My mom was a junkie even when she carried me in her belly," she says, "and now I'm doing it to my own kid."

Kim and I hear her out, give what counsel we can and take the necessary steps. First is a dating ultrasound. Clarissa's wishes are to terminate if the pregnancy is not past twelve weeks or to give up her drug use and move into a shelter for pregnant women if she is beyond the early-abortion stage. We support her intention to discontinue the cocaine but warn that putting the fetus through a narcotic withdrawal is not desirable: it would be better to replace the heroin with low-dose methadone for the duration of the pregnancy. I write a couple of notes for Clarissa's financial aid worker before Kim drives her to SheWay, the Downtown Eastside prenatal care clinic. "Just one bit of advice," I say, "if you think you can listen." Clarissa, on her way out of the office, turns to glance back at me. "I can listen," she says.

"What you said about hating yourself and feeling sorry for yourself. What if you were to replace your harsh judgments with some genuine curiosity about why you do what you do? What if you use drugs because you're afraid that you can't bear the pain without them? You have every reason to feel hurt after all you've been through. It's not a matter of 'fucking up.' You just haven't found any other way to cope. If your child had had the same experiences and ended up on drugs, would you accuse her so harshly?"

"No," Clarissa says. "I'd love her . . . I'd give her tough love."

"Forget the tough," I tell her. "All she'd need is your love. And so do you."

Clarissa, weeping again, asks if she can come back to talk to me. "Sure," I say, "but come back when you're not stoned. You can't absorb anything when you're high."

"That's what my counsellors always told me when I was a teenager," Clarissa protests, "not to come back when I'm stoned. But it's not true." I look at her for a few silent moments and relent. "Okay, come back whichever way you need to come back."

Clarissa is all smiles. "That's what I wanted to hear," she says.

—

When I'm reasonably balanced in my personal and spiritual life, I don't have difficulty finding compassion for my addicted patients. I'm curious about their life histories and self-perceptions and, for the most part, I'm able to avoid imposing judgments on them. As with Clarissa, my aim is to open their eyes to the possibility of a nonjudgmental, compassionate curiosity toward themselves.

Things are very different when it comes to my own self in the midst of an addicted phase. Suffused with corrosive shame, I attempt to hide the self-loathing from my own sight with feigned joviality or self-justifying combativeness, neither of which do the job near adequately. As with my drug-dependent, fellow hungry ghosts, this slush of pitiless, negative self-judgment only intensifies the desire for escape and oblivion. The spiral of addiction-shame-addiction keeps swirling on.

As Dr. Bruce Perry said about drug addicts, "we need to be very loving, very accepting, and very patient with people who have these problems." We also need to extend that same loving, accepting and patient attitude toward ourselves. And, as Dr. Jaak Panksepp has suggested, to deal successfully with addictions we have to bring emotions back into healthy balance; we have to give ourselves "a chance to think about it." When we're awash in a poisonous soup of self-recrimination and shame, we cannot think creatively.

Among the necessary initial moves toward sobriety is the directing of compassionate curiosity at oneself. Many teachings, from spiritual writings to psychological works, tell us that we need to look at ourselves this way. "In cultivating loving-kindness, we learn first to be honest, loving and compassionate towards ourselves," writes the American Buddhist nun Pema Chödrön. "Rather than nurturing self-denigration, we begin to cultivate a clear-seeing kindness." Chödrön also suggests it's a good idea to lighten up:

Being able to lighten up is the key to feeling at home with your body, mind and emotions, to feeling worthy of living on this planet . . . In addition to a sense of humor, a basic support for a joyful mind is curiosity, paying attention . . . Happiness is not required, but being curious without a heavy judgmental attitude helps. If you are judgmental, you can even be curious about that.[1]

Posed in a tone of compassionate curiosity, "Why?" is transformed from rigid accusation to an open-minded, even scientific question. Instead of hurling an accusatory brick at your own head (e.g., "I'm so stupid; when will I ever learn," etc.), the question "Why did I do this again, knowing full well the negative consequences?" can become the subject of a fruitful inquiry, a gentle investigation. Taking off the starched uniform of the interrogator, who is determined to try, convict, and punish, we adopt toward ourselves the attitude of the empathic friend, who simply wants to know what's going on with us. The acronym COAL has been proposed for this attitude of compassionate curiosity: curiosity, openness, acceptance and love: "Hmm. I wonder what drove me to do this again?"

The purpose is not to justify or rationalize but to understand. Justification is another form of judgment every bit as debilitating as condemnation. When we justify, we hope to win the judge's favour or to hoodwink her. Justification connives to absolve the self of responsibility; understanding helps us assume responsibility. When we don't have to defend ourselves against others or, what's more, against ourselves, we are open to seeing how things are. I become free to acknowledge the addiction the moment the fact of having behaved along addictive patterns no longer means that I'm a failure as a person, unworthy of respect, shallow and valueless. I can own it and see the many ways it sabotages my real goals in life.

Being cut off from our own natural self-compassion is one of the greatest impairments we can suffer. Along with our ability to feel our own pain go our best hopes for healing, dignity and love. What seems nonadaptive and self-harming in the present was, at some point in our lives, an adaptation to help us endure what we then had to go through. If people are addicted to self-soothing behaviours, it's only because in their formative years they did not receive the soothing they needed. Such understanding helps delete toxic self-judgment on the past and supports responsibility for the now.

Hence the need for compassionate self-inquiry.

—

If I examine my addictive behaviours without judgment and ask "Why" in the spirit of compassionate curiosity, what do I find? More to the point, *whom* do I find? What is the full truth of me? Is it that I'm a respected thirty-year veteran of medical practice, spouse and parent, counsellor, public speaker, activist and author? What about the anxious, insecure man who has often felt empty and incomplete and has looked to the outside to allay some insatiable hunger? As fellow addict and author Stephen Reid said during our conversation in the cafeteria of the William Head penitentiary: " . . . makes my teeth hurt, the work of pulling back from all those outside things and looking inside myself." In my case, the unconscious tension literally made my teeth hurt—so forcefully have I ground my teeth at night since childhood that by the end of my fifth decade most of them were whittled stubs with the pulp exposed.

Along with my positive qualities—intellectual confidence, strengths, passions and commitments—there has always lurked near the very core of me a churning, inchoate anxiety. Had I been able to be honest with myself and had I been prepared to accept vulnerability, I would have declared at many stages of my life, as Clarissa did: "I'm scared. I'm so very scared." My anxiety clothes itself in concerns about body image or financial security, doubts regarding loveability or the ability to love, self-disparagement and existential pessimism about life's meaning and purpose—or, on the other hand, it manifests itself as grandiosity, the need to be admired, to be seen as special. At bottom it is nameless and formless. I feel sure it was forged in my chest cavity somewhere between my lungs and heart long before I knew the names of things.

Do I have reasons to be anxious? By its very nature, chronic anxiety has nothing to do with "reasons." First it springs into being and much later, once we develop the ability to think, it recruits thoughts and explanations to serve it. In contrast to healthy anxiety (for which a better word is *fear*) felt in the face of danger—like the fear a gazelle might experience in the presence of a hungry lion or that a small child might feel when his parents are not in sight, chronic anxiety is not rooted in the experience of the moment. It precedes thought. We may believe we're anxious about this or that—body image, the state of the world, relationship issues, the weather— but no matter what story we weave around it, the anxiety *just is*. Like addiction itself, anxiety will always find a target, but exists independently of its targets. Only when we become aware of it does it wrap itself in identifiable colours. More often we repress it, bury it under ideas, identifications, deeds, beliefs and relationships. We build above it a mound of activities and attributes that we mistake for our true selves. We then expend our energies trying to convince the world that our self-made fiction is reality. As genuine as our strengths and achievements may be, they cannot but feel hollow until we acknowledge the anxiety they cover up.

Incompleteness is the baseline state of the addict. The addict believes—either with full awareness or unconsciously—that he is "not enough." As he is, he is inadequate to face life's demands or to present an acceptable face to the world. He is unable to tolerate his own emotions without artificial supports. He must escape the painful experience of the void within through any activity that fills his mind with even temporary purpose, be it work, gambling, shopping, eating or sexual seeking. In my first book, *Scattered Minds*, I depicted this perennial psychic hunger:

> The British psychiatrist R.D. Laing wrote somewhere that there are three things human beings are afraid of: death, other people, and their own minds. Terrified of my mind, I had always dreaded to spend a moment alone with it. There always had to be a book in my pocket as an emergency kit in case I was ever trapped waiting anywhere, even for one minute, be it a bank lineup or supermarket checkout counter. I was forever throwing my mind scraps to feed on, as to a ferocious and malevolent beast that would devour me the moment it was not chewing on something else.[2]

At that time I ascribed that state of perpetual dissatisfaction to attention deficit disorder. Although a salient mental feature of ADD, the drive to escape the moment is a common, nearly universal human characteristic. In the addicted brain it is magnified to the point of desperation. It becomes the overriding force in directing choices and behaviour.

"But I don't feel any desperation," some may say. "I just love whatever I'm doing so much that I never want to stop." Workaholics are prone to think that way, and I used to. "Where is all this pain and grief I'm supposed to feel in order to heal," I once challenged a therapist. "Try as I may, I can't force myself to feel anything. Feelings either come or they don't." I was so busy stimulating and soothing myself with ceaseless activity, working overtime to keep my brain spinning and gorging it with mind candy that I didn't leave even a small gap for any feeling to seep through.

My workaholism and compact disc shopping have been only the most consistent forms of escape my mind chooses when it's uncomfortable. There have been other behaviours just as compulsive and just as impulsive. I see now that the underlying anxiety and sense of emptiness have been pervasive. Emotionally they take the shape of chronic, low-grade depression and irritability. On the thought level, they manifest as cynicism—the negative side of the healthy skepticism and independent thinking I've always valued. Behaviourally they mask themselves as hypomanic energy or as lethargy, as the constant hankering for activity or for oblivion. When the ordinary, everyday escape mechanisms fail to satisfy, I plunge into my overtly addictive patterns. If I had greater pain and fewer resources, if I had been less fortunate in the circumstances of my nurturing environment, I might well have been impelled to turn to drugs.

Compassionate curiosity directed toward the self leads to the truth of things. Once I see my anxiety and recognize it for what it is, the need to escape dwindles. It is clear to me that the sense of threat and fear of abandonment that make up anxiety were, in my case, programmed in the Budapest ghetto in 1944. Why attempt to escape some old brain pattern laid down when I was a frightened infant during a terrible time in history? It's there and the circuits in which its wordless stories are embedded are indelibly a part of my brain. It doesn't need to go away—indeed, it won't go away, not completely. But I can transform my relationship to it, become more intimately related to it. I can even gain some mastery over it, which means noticing it without allowing it to control my moods or behaviours. Similarly, I don't have to take on the impossible task of erasing the addictive impulses that arose from early acquired brain patterns—but I can transform my relationship to them, as well. Essential to any such transformations is a letting-go of judgment and self-condemnation.

Psychiatrist and psychoanalyst Anthony Storr has written about the value of allowing buried emotions to emerge without fear:

> When a person is encouraged to get in touch with and express his deepest feelings in the secure knowledge that he will not be rejected, criticized, nor expected to be different, some kind of rearrangement or sorting-out process often occurs within the mind which brings with it a sense of peace; a sense that the depths of the well of truth have really been reached.[3]

—

What is the first step to take once self-compassion allows the truth to emerge? Inevitably, it's the Step One taught by Alcoholics Anonymous and other Twelve-Step programs. Twelve-Step methods are not for everyone, and they may not be the only route out of addiction, but the principles on which they are based are common to any successful program of recovery.

"We admitted we were powerless over alcohol; that our lives had become unmanageable" is the classic AA formulation. Mindful of the fundamental similarity of all addictions, one can broaden that to say, "I admit I am powerless over my addiction process." That is, "I fully acknowledge that my cravings and behaviours have been out of control and that my inability to regulate them has led to dysfunction and chaos in important areas of my life. I no longer deny their impact on myself or my coworkers or my loved ones, and I admit my failure to confront them honestly and consistently." (A friend of mine, Anne, who is a long-time member of AA, cautions against my reformulation of the "*we* admitted" to "I admit." "The first word is plural for a reason," she says. "If I'm an addict and if I'm left alone to my own resources, then I'm pretty much lost.")

I have been reluctant to take this step until recently, despite the fact that I've not had a problem admitting and describing my addictive tendencies either in private or in public. The difficulty has been threefold. First, since I pride myself on a strong intellect, I've resisted accepting that I'm powerless over any mental process. On the contrary, it is in the nature of the ego to turn anything to its advantage. Even the public disclosure of my addictive patterns has served to reassure me of my sincerity and honesty and "courage." Audiences greet such self-disclosure with nods, appreciative smiles and applause. But real courage does not lie in speaking about addiction; it resides in actively doing something about it—and that, until very recently, I have not been prepared to take on.

Second, in focusing on the most visible compulsive behaviours, such as CD shopping, book bingeing or workaholism, I could still permit myself to ignore how addictive patterns have permeated much of my functioning. Narrowing it down to a few "problematic" issues has allowed me to deny that the addiction process shows up in numerous aspects of my daily existence. There are many things I do well and many tasks I accomplish, I could assure myself, so there is no cause for me to admit a loss of control. In other words, I have not wanted to accept that, at times, my life is made unmanageable by my own behaviours. In the absence of compassionate curiosity, any such admission brings up too much shame.

Finally, whenever I have felt wooden or alienated in the intimate areas of life, I've seen myself as deprived, rather than owning the reality that I create the sense of deprivation internally. For example, I have blamed my wife, Rae, for not satisfying my expectations instead of taking responsibility for the burdens I impose on our relationship through poor self-regulation and lack of differentiation (my capacity to hold on to a sense of self while interacting with Rae and others). That leaves me free to use the addictions for self-soothing and to justify doing so by citing my "unmet" needs. In other words, the *consequences* of my own wilful refusal to be a mature, self-regulating adult became my *rationale* for pursuing addictive behaviours. As I write about this, the image of a whirling puppy snapping at its own tail comes to mind.

There is no moving forward without breaking through the wall of denial—or, in the case of such an obstinate and slippery mind as mine, breaking through several walls, whose existence I do not even want to acknowledge.

—

CHAPTER 30

The Internal Climate

—

God does not change people's lot until they first change what's in
their own hearts.
The Qur'an (13:11)

No organism in nature is separate from the system in which
it lives, functions and dies, and no natural process can be
understood in isolation from its physical and biological
context. From an *ecological* perspective, the addiction process
doesn't happen accidentally, nor is it preprogrammed by heredity. It
is a product of development in a certain context, and it continues to
be maintained by factors in the environment. The ecological view
sees addiction as a changeable and evolving dynamic that expresses
a lifelong interaction with a person's social and emotional surround-
ings and with his own internal psychological space.

Healing, then, must take into account the internal psychological climate—the beliefs, memories, mind-states and emotions that
feed addictive impulses and behaviours—as well as the external
milieu. In an ecological framework recovery from addiction does
not mean a "cure" for a disease but the creation of new resources,
internal and external, that can support different, healthy ways of
satisfying one's genuine needs. It also involves developing new
brain circuits that can facilitate more adaptive responses and
behaviours.

At first sight, the task of a troubled mind transforming itself may seem hopelessly daunting. "What an abyss of uncertainty," wrote the novelist Marcel Proust, "whenever the mind feels overtaken by itself, when it, the seeker, is at the same time the dark region through which it must go seeking." Or, as a patient in Dr. Jeffrey Schwartz's obsessive-compulsive disorder clinic in Los Angeles said, "What we are looking for is what we are looking with." As these observations suggest, it would be impossible to recover from addiction if a person's mental life were determined purely by automatic brain functions and underground emotional dynamics. Powerful as those are—and decisive as they can be for many people in many circumstances—they are not the only actors on the scene. Fortunately for human beings, the mind is more than the workings of our automatic brain mechanisms and, it turns out, the brain itself can develop throughout a lifetime.

Not only in childhood, but for our entire lives our brains remain use-dependent. For example, a part of the hippocampus—a brain structure important for memory—has been shown to be much larger than average in London cabbies. The size increase was correlated with the number of years they'd spent navigating through the dense traffic of the British capital.[1] In the words of neurologist and brain researcher Antonio Damasio, "the design of brain circuits continues to change. The circuits are not only receptive to the results of first experience, but [are] repeatedly pliable and modifiable by continued experience."[2]

So there are two ways of promoting healthy brain development, and both are essential to the healing of addiction: by changing the external environment and by modifying the internal one. "The mammalian brain appears to have the capacity to remain responsive to environmental enrichment well into advanced age," asserted Dr. Marian Diamond, a renowned brain researcher at the Department of Anatomy-Physiology at Berkeley.[3] In her laboratory, newborn to elderly rats were kept in varying degrees of social isolation, stimulation, and environmental and nutritional enrichment. Autopsies showed that the layers of the cortex in the brains of the environmentally favoured rats were thicker, their nerve cells larger, their branching more elaborate and their blood supply richer. Privileged rats well past midlife could still grow connecting branches almost twice as long as their "standard" cousins, after only thirty days of differential treatment. Dr. Diamond reported these results in her book *Enriching Heredity: The Impact of the Environment on the Anatomy of the Brain.** "At any age studied," she wrote, "we have shown anatomical effects due to enrichment or impoverishment."[4]

Most encouraging were Dr. Diamond's findings that even the brains of animals deprived before birth or damaged in infancy were able to compensate through structural changes in response to enriched living conditions. "Thus," she wrote, "we must not give up on people who begin life under unfavourable conditions. Environmental enrichment has the potential to enhance their brain development too, depending on the degree or severity of the insult."[5] Since Marian Diamond's pioneering studies the power of an enriched environment to induce positive brain development has been demonstrated repeatedly. For example, rats in a superior housing situation gained new brain connections and as much as a 20 per cent increase in the size of the cortex. In the words of the researchers, "an extraordinary change!"[6]

In humans, too, we can expect the adult brain to be beneficially influenced by the environment. The same has long been known to be true for almost any other organ or part of the body. Unused muscles atrophy, but if well exercised they grow in size and strength; blood supply to the heart is improved by exercise and healthy diet; our lung capacity increases with aerobic training. Elderly people who remain physically and intellectually active suffer much less decline in their mental functioning than their more passive contemporaries. "Contrary to dogma, the human brain does produce new nerve cells in adulthood," reported two neurobiologists in *Scientific American* in 1999.[7]

Early in life the responsiveness of the human brain to changing conditions, known as *neuroplasticity,* is so great that infants who suffer damage to one side of their brain around the time of birth, even

* And since then, in a nonacademic book for the general public, *Magic Trees of the Mind.*

if they lose an entire hemisphere, may compensate for the deficit. The other half develops so that these children grow up to have nearly symmetrical facial movements and only a mild or moderate limp. With age, plasticity declines, but it is never completely lost. Neurological adaptability in adulthood may be seen in the recovery many people make from a stroke. In a cerebrovascular accident, or stroke, brain tissue is destroyed, usually due to bleeding. Although nerve cells that have died will not come back to life, often the patient will once more be able to use a limb that was paralyzed by the stroke. New circuits have taken over and new connections have been made. In fact, this process has recently been harnessed in the rehabilitation of stroke victims, leading to remarkable advances.

The work of Dr. Jeffrey Schwartz and his colleagues at UCLA has shown that in the brains of people with obsessive-compulsive disorder, new circuitry can be successfully established that over-rides the ill-functioning circuits. Dr. Schwartz suggests—and I completely agree—that methods used at UCLA can be adapted to the healing of addictive compulsions. We will take a close look at them in the next chapter. "Now there is no question," Dr. Schwartz writes, "that the brain remodels itself throughout life, and that it retains the capacity to change itself as the result not only of passively experienced factors such as enriched environments, but also of changes in the ways we behave and the ways we think . . . Nor is there any question that every treatment that exploits the power of the mind to change the brain involves arduous effort—by patients afflicted by stroke or depression, by Tourette or OCD—to improve both their functional capacity and their brain function."[8] Arduous effort is also required on the part of any addict—all the more since her compulsions entice her to behaviours that, contrary to other distressing conditions, promise pleasure and reward.

The mind activity that can physically rewire malfunctioning brain circuits and alter our dysfunctional emotional and cerebral responses is conscious mental effort—what Dr. Schwartz calls *mental force*. If changing external circumstances can improve brain physiology, so can mental effort. "Intention and attention exert real, physical effects on the brain," Dr. Schwartz explains.[9] Not surprisingly, the brain area activated in studies looking at the effect of self-directed mental effort is the prefrontal cortex, the apex of the brain's emotional self-regulation system. It's also an area where, we have learned, the brains of addicts are impaired. The mental activity most critical to the development of emotional self-regulation has been called "dispassionate self-observation" by the authors of an important article on the interface of brain and mind, published in the *Philosophical Transactions of the Royal Society* (*Biological Sciences*) in 2005. "The way in which a person directs their attention (i.e. mindfully or unmindfully) will," they write, "affect both the experiential state of the person and the state of his/her brain."[10]

Mindful awareness involves directing our attention not only to the mental content of our thoughts, but also to the emotions and mind-states that inform those thoughts. It is being aware of the *processes* of our mind even as we work through its *materials*. Mindful awareness is the key to unlocking the automatic patterns that fetter the addicted brain and mind.

—

The dominant emotions suffusing all addictive behaviour are fear and resentment—an inseparable vaudeville team of unhappiness. One prompts and sets up the other: fear of the way things are and resentment that they are that way; fear of life and resentment that life is as difficult as it is; fear of unpleasant mind-states and resentment that unpleasant moods and thoughts persist; fear that we'll never feel all right and resentment that we cannot feel the way we want to; fear of the present and the future and resentment that we cannot control destiny. "Addiction is running from reality," a patient of mine once said, "the reality you have that something is stronger. Something that's greater than you. Instead of admitting it and saying that something scares me—this thing scares me, or I don't know how to do this, or I don't know how to live—instead of just saying that, you do drugs. So you coexist with the people that are nonexistent. People are just surviving but not living."

As long as the effects of the addictive substance or behaviour last, resentment and fear are temporarily suppressed, but afterwards the emotions always rebound with greater force than before. It's an endless cycle because the addicted life will unfailingly generate new sources to feed the energy of anxiety and resentment. In such a state, the philosopher and writer Friedrich Nietzsche remarked, "One cannot get rid of anything, one cannot get over anything, one cannot repel anything—everything hurts. Men and things obtrude too closely; experiences strike one too deeply; memory becomes a festering wound."[11]

How to break the cycle? "Everything has mind in the lead, has mind in the forefront, is made by the mind," the Buddha said. With our minds we create the world we live in. The teaching of Buddhism is that the way to deal with the mind is not to attempt to change it, but to become an impartial, compassionate observer of it. Traditional Buddhist psychology did not have our scientific knowledge about the development of the *brain*, whose activity generates most of what we understand as *mind*. It did recognize, however, that once mind structures are in place they determine our perceptions, behaviours and experiences. By consciously observing the workings of our mind, we are able gradually to let go of its habitual, programmed interpretations and automatic reactions. Reflection on the addicted brain, not wilful resistance to it, is the way to tame it. "The unreflecting mind is a poor roof," Buddha taught. "Passion, like the rain, floods the house. But if the roof is strong, there is shelter." Brain research is demonstrating that mindful awareness is able to release the grip of harmful thoughts and also to change positively the physiology of the brain circuits where those thoughts originate. The implications for the healing of addiction are far-reaching.

We can distinguish between two kinds of mind function: awareness (the dispassionate observer) and the jumble of automatic processes (conscious, semiconscious and subconscious) that dictate our emotional states, thoughts and much of our behaviour. One of the first scientists to recognize this distinction was the great Canadian neurosurgeon Wilder Penfield. "Although the content of consciousness depends in large measure on neuronal activity, awareness itself does not," Penfield wrote. "To me it seems more and more reasonable to suggest that the mind may be a distinct and different essence from the brain."

The automatic mind, the reactive product of brain circuits, constantly interprets the present in the light of past conditioning. In its psychological responses it has great difficulty telling past from present, especially whenever it is emotionally aroused. A trigger in the present will set off emotions that were programmed perhaps decades ago at a much more vulnerable time in the person's life. What seems like a reaction to some present circumstance is, in fact, a reliving of past emotional experience.

This subtle but pervasive process in the body, brain and nervous system has been called *implicit memory,* as compared to the explicit memory apparatus that recalls events, facts and circumstances. According to the psychologist and memory researcher Daniel Schacter, implicit memory is active "when people are influenced by past experience without any awareness that they are remembering . . . If we are unaware that something is influencing our behavior, there is little we can do to understand or counteract it. The subtle, virtually undetectable nature of implicit memory is one reason it can have powerful effects on our mental lives."[12] Whenever a person "overreacts"—that is, reacts in a way that seems inappropriately exaggerated to the situation at hand, we can be sure that implicit memory is at work. The reaction is not to the irritant in the present but to some buried hurt in the past. Many of us look back puzzled on some emotional explosion and ask ourselves, "What the heck was that about?" It was about implicit memory; we just didn't realize it at the time.

The other mind entity is what we can call the impartial observer. This mind of present-moment awareness stands outside the preprogrammed physiological determinants and is alive to the present. It works through the brain but is not limited to the brain. It may be dormant in many of us, but it is never completely absent. It transcends the automatic functioning of past-conditioned brain circuits. "In the end," wrote Penfield, "I conclude that there is no good evidence . . . that the brain alone can carry out the work that the mind does."[13]

—

Knowing oneself comes from attending with compassionate curiosity to what is happening within.

Methods for gaining self-knowledge and self-mastery through conscious awareness strengthen the mind's capacity to act as its own impartial observer. Among the simplest and most skilful of the meditative techniques taught in many spiritual traditions is the disciplined practice of what Buddhists call "bare attention." Nietzsche called Buddha "that profound physiologist" and his teachings less a religion than a "kind of hygiene." When the Buddha seeks to liberate the soul from resentment, Nietzsche wrote, "It is not morality that speaks thus; thus speaks physiology." Many of our automatic brain processes have to do with either wanting something or not wanting something else—very much the way a small child's mental life functions. We are forever desiring and longing, or judging and rejecting. Mental hygiene consists of noticing the ebb and flow of all those automatic grasping or rejecting impulses without being hooked by them. Bare attention is directed not only toward what's happening on the outside, but also to what's taking place on the inside.

"Be at least as interested in your reactions as in the person or situation that triggers them," Eckhart Tolle advises. In a mindful state one can choose to be aware of the ebb and flow of emotions and thought patterns instead of brooding on their content. Not "he did this to me and therefore I'm suffering" but "I notice that feelings of resentment and a desire for vengeance keep flooding my mind." Although bare attention was developed as a meditative practice, its use is not limited to formal meditation. It is the conscious attending to what occurs in the mind as it takes in physical or emotional stimuli from within and outside the body. "Bare Attention is the clear and single-minded awareness of what actually happens to us and in us at the successive moments of perception," write the authors of the *Philosophical Transactions* article. "It is called 'Bare' because it attends just to the bare facts of a perception as presented either through the five physical senses or through the mind *without reacting to them*."[14]

The addict seldom questions the reality of the unpleasant mood or feeling she wants to escape. She rarely examines the perspective from which her mind experiences and understands the world around her and from which she hears and sees the people in her life. She is in a constant state of reactivity—not to the world so much as to her own interpretations of it. The distressing internal state is not examined: the focus is entirely on the outside: What can I receive from the world that will make me feel okay, if only for a moment? Bare attention can show her that these moods and feelings have only the meaning and power that she gives them. Eventually she will realize that there is nothing to run away from. Situations might need to be changed, but there is no internal hell that one must escape by dulling or stimulating the mind.

Addicted people often say, "I don't know who I really am." If the addict has more than the usual difficulty in holding on to a healthy sense of self, it's because in the addicted brain the reaction patterns, emotions and thoughts that create a sense of self fluctuate so widely. Due to impaired regulation over easily triggered feelings of craving and distress, the addicted mind lacks consistency. The psychological oscillations and pendulum swings are greater than those that most people experience. Thought patterns and emotional states pursue each other with an exaggerated rapidity and across a broader range. It seems there is less to hold on to—in fact, the addictive behaviours and substances are one way of trying to impose some structure. Many addicts define themselves through their addictions and feel quite unmoored and lost without them. Substance-dependent people do this, but so do workaholics and other behaviour addicts. They fear giving up their addiction not only because of the temporary relief it offers, but also because they just cannot conceive who they might be without it.

Bare attention allows us to take an objective stand outside the ever-moving ebb and flow of thought, reaction and emotion and to reinforce the part of us that can observe, know and decide consciously. It allows us to observe the many individual "frames," as it were, that make up the self-created movies in our minds.

"The key to the transformational potential of bare attention lies in the deceptively simple injunction to separate out one's reactions from the core events themselves," writes psychiatrist and Buddhist meditation teacher Mark Epstein.

Much of the time, it turns out, everyday minds are in a state of reactivity. We take this for granted, we do not question our automatic identifications with our reactions, and we experience ourselves at the mercy of an often hostile or frustrating outer world or an over-whelming or frightening inner one. With bare attention, we move from this automatic identification with our fear or frustration to a vantage point from which the fear or frustration are attended to with the same dispassionate interest as anything else. There is enormous freedom to be gained from such a shift. Instead of running from dif-ficult emotions (or hanging on to enticing ones), the practitioner of bare attention becomes able to *contain* any reaction: making space for it, but not completely identifying with it . . . [15]

Given that addiction is all about running from difficult emotions or hanging on to enticing ones, bare attention has the potential to dissolve the very motivations that drive the addicted mind.

The advice I will give in the next chapter about reducing stress by dealing openly with emotions may seem to conflict with the concept of bare attention, in which we notice the evanescent and shifting nature of emotions. In reality, they both come down to attending carefully to what is happening in our minds, neither sup-pressing our feelings nor allowing them to rule us.

—

As we've already seen, painful early experiences program both the neurophysiology of addiction and the distressing psychological states that addiction promises to relieve. Yet human beings who are able to direct conscious attention toward their mental processes discover something surprising: it's not what happened in the past that creates our present misery but the way we have allowed past events to define how we see and experience ourselves in the present. A person can survive being beaten but cannot remain psychologically intact if he convinces himself that he was beaten because he is by nature blameworthy or because the world by its very nature is cruel. A child can overcome sexual violation, but she will be debilitated if she thinks that she somehow either deserved the abuse or brought it upon herself. She also cannot function as a self-respecting adult if she comes to believe that she is loveable or acceptable only for her sexuality. A neglected child may be helpless, but the damage comes if he acquires the defining belief that helplessness is his real and permanent state in the world. The greatest damage done by neglect, trauma or emotional loss is not the immediate pain they inflict but the long-term distortions they induce in the way a developing child will continue to interpret the world and her situation in it. All too often these ill-conditioned implicit beliefs become self-fulfilling prophecies in our lives. We create meanings from our unconscious interpretation of early events, and then we forge our present experiences from the meanings we've created. Unwittingly, we write the story of our future from narratives based on the past.

Although my mother likely saved my life by sending me away from the dangers of the Budapest ghetto before my first birthday, I experienced the event the only way an infant could: as abandonment. It left me with a permanent core sense that I must never be emotionally open and vulnerable. When Rae, my wife, says no to me or behaves in a way that upsets me, my automatic belief is that I'm being rejected or abandoned by the woman whose love I need, and my mechanical reaction is to detach emotionally, to withdraw. This is a common response of young children who experience emotional or physical separation from their parents. Addiction confers invulnerability because it allows us to soothe vulnerable emotions like pain or fear or the aching for love with behaviours, objects or substances whenever we choose. It's a way to avoid intimacy. Mindful awareness can bring into consciousness those hidden, past-based perspectives so that they no longer frame our worldview. "Choice begins the moment you disidentify from the mind and its conditioned patterns, the moment you become present," writes Eckhart Tolle. "Until you reach that point, you are unconscious." Once I notice my programmed, defensive impulse to withdraw from intimacy and understand its source, I have some choice whether or not to act it out. With even a modicum of sanity, why would I? In present awareness we are liberated from the past.

"Your worst enemy cannot hurt you as much as your own thoughts, when you haven't mastered them," said the Buddha. "But once mastered, no one can help you as much—not even your father and your mother."

I don't propose meditation and mindfulness as panaceas. It is futile to dream of corralling a group of active cocaine addicts or alcoholics into a meditation class. To pursue such practices, one requires mental resources, a commitment to emotional clarity, an access to teaching and some mental space in one's life. They are also difficult, especially at the beginning. But for people whose lives are blighted by addictions without being totally gripped by them, these practices can help light the way to wholeness.

When asked about my view of meditation my stock answer has been, "I have a profound relationship with meditation; I think about it every day." It's true. Every day for years I've heard the call of contemplative solitude, and nearly every day I've turned a deaf ear. I've run from mental discipline like Jonah escaping the call of God until he ends up in the putrid belly of the whale. My addiction-prone, ADD brain always wants to look to the outside to get away from itself. As a result, I tend to oscillate between excessive, multitasking busyness and a proclivity for "vegging out" in ways that leave me nonrested and dissatisfied. Meditation, with its demand for stillness and self-observation, has not been an activity I've joyfully embraced.

At a recent meditation retreat, however, I had a breakthrough: I realized that my expectations for meditation practice had been too harsh—on myself. I wanted to be "good" at it, I wanted spiritually uplifting things to happen, I wanted deep insights to arise. I now know it's a gentle process. One doesn't have to be good at meditation, achieve anything or look for any particular result. As with any skill, only practice leads to improvement—and improvement is not even the point. The only point is the practice. What I have found is that when I do practise meditation, I find more ease in my life. I'm calmer, more emotionally present, more compassionate to others and far less reactive to external triggers. In other words, I'm more of a self-regulating adult and less prone to self-soothing, addictive behaviours.

Mindfulness practice will not by itself cool the addiction-heated mind, but, addicted or not, it is an invaluable adjunct to whatever else we do. It's a way of working with the most immediate environment, the internal one. "Mindfulness changes the brain," psychiatrist and brain researcher Daniel Siegel points out: "Why would the way you pay attention in the present moment change your brain? How we pay attention promotes neural plasticity, the change of neural connections in response to experience."[16]

Mindfulness can be practised throughout the day, not only on the meditation cushion. There are many techniques for this but they all come down to paying close attention to one's experience of each moment, without seeking distraction. When I go for walks now, I no longer have earphones piping music into my head. I try to stay present to the physical, aural and visual sensations I experience, as well as noticing my mental processes and reactions. Sometimes I can keep this up for as long as thirty seconds at a time before my mind scurries off into La La Land. I call that progress.

—

CHAPTER 31

The Four Steps, Plus One

This chapter outlines a specific method that I view as promising for behavioural addictions—for example, shopping, gambling and eating compulsions—or for anyone wishing to disengage from maladaptive habits of thinking or acting. Its other value is that it sheds further light on the nature of the addicted brain and mind. These steps are not a comprehensive treatment for addiction, but can serve as an adjunct to Twelve-Step programs or to the approaches recommended in the preceding and following chapters. They will not work if done mechanically, but require regular practice with conscious awareness.

The ability of conscious attention to transform the automatic mind and its physiological substrates in the brain has been successfully applied at UCLA to the treatment of obsessive-compulsive disorder. As we have noted, OCD has a similarity to addiction in the driven nature of its behaviours. They are both impulse-control disorders. Deeper than that, they are both based in anxiety. The person with OCD believes that something catastrophic may happen if she doesn't perform a particular activity a precise number of times and in a particular way. The addict's behaviour or substance use is also meant to calm anxiety—an unease about life itself, or about a sense of insufficient self. And, we recall, OCD and addiction seem to share the phenomenon Dr. Jeffrey Schwartz has described as "brain lock"—the stuck neurological gears that cause thought to be acted out before the action can be stopped, because the brain's transmission mechanism cannot be put into "neutral." When the obsessive or addictive thought occurs, obsessive or addictive action follows. There are further parallels on the biochemical level, with disturbances in neurotransmitter systems involving serotonin, for example.

The method Dr. Schwartz and his colleagues have developed applies conscious attention in a systematic, four-step fashion. On brain scans they have shown that the locked circuitry of OCD undergoes a change after a relatively brief period of consistent and disciplined practice by obsessive-compulsive patients. The demonstrated "brain lock" opens up, and the person is freed from the nonsensical thoughts that formerly compelled her behaviour. Can the same four steps be applied to addiction? "I haven't worked extensively with addictions," Dr. Schwartz told me, "but given that addiction also involves problems with intrusive urges and repetitive behaviors, there is good reason to think that the four steps could be useful in its treatment."

What follows, then, with Dr. Schwartz's kind permission, is my adaptation of the four steps to the healing of addiction.* There is no clinical evidence to support this specific application, but there are excellent theoretical grounds for anticipating its value. The method is consistent with traditional Twelve-Step approaches, although it is not intended to replace them. Addiction physicians elsewhere have also expressed interest in adapting this technique to their work. If a personal testimony is of interest, I'm glad to offer mine: it has made a difference for me.

—

The program devised at the UCLA School of Medicine for the treatment of OCD is formally called the Four-Step Self-Treatment

---

* The UCLA four-step method is detailed in Dr. Schwartz's first book, *Brain Lock*. This slim volume, meant for the general reader, deals with OCD, but it does contain the suggestion that its recommendations may also be used in conditions characterized by the addiction process, including overeating, sexual addiction, pathological gambling and substance abuse.

Method. Needless to stay, it depends on a high level of motivation for its success. As I pointed out earlier, motivation is generally higher in the case of OCD, where, unlike in addiction, the patient's experience of her symptoms is intrinsically unpleasant. For the substance or behaviour addict there is at least an initial promise of delight that flows from the activation of the brain's incentive-motivation and attachment-reward circuits. The suffering is delayed, rather than immediate. There is no bypassing the first step suggested at the end of the previous chapter—that is, before we can usefully apply UCLA's four steps, we have to take the First Step of acknowledging the full impact of the addiction, and we have to resolve to confront its power over our mind.

The Four-Step program is based on the perspective that makes the best sense of disorders like OCD and addiction: that they are rooted in malfunctioning brain circuits and in implicit stories and beliefs that do not match reality. That, as we have seen, is the core problem in addiction because the development of the brain and the mind was negatively affected by adverse early circumstances. The first two steps place the maladaptive behaviours in their proper context of brain dysfunction. The third directs the brain to a more positive focus. With the time and mental space granted by the first three, the fourth step then reminds the addict of what motivates her to get over her habit. To support that process, I've added a fifth step that I have found helpful.

The four steps should be practised daily at least once, but also whenever an addictive impulse pulls you so strongly that you are tempted to act it out. Find a place to sit and write—preferably a quiet place—but even a bus stop will do if that's where you happen to be when the addictive urge arises. You'll want to keep a journal of this process, so carrying a small notebook with you is an excellent aid.

A warning about possible pitfalls. I have a tendency, typical in ADD, of beginning projects with enthusiasm and a sense of commitment, only to abandon them after some lapse or failure. "I've tried that," I'll then say, "but it doesn't work for me." That attitude is also typical of self-recovery practices in addiction, since, by definition, addiction is characterized by relapses. I have to get that there is no "it" to work or not work. "It" doesn't have to work. I am the one who has to work. And what is commitment? Commitment is sticking with something not because "it works" or because I enjoy it, but because I have an intention that overrides momentary feelings or opinions. So, too, with the Four-Step program. You don't have to feel or believe that it's working for you: you just have to do it and to understand that if you have lapsed, it doesn't mean that you have failed. It's an opportunity to begin anew.

Step 1: Re-label

In Step 1 you label the addictive thought or urge exactly for what it is, not mistaking it for reality. I may feel, for example, that I must leave off whatever I'm doing right now and go to the classical music store. The feeling takes on the quality of a need, of an imperative that must immediately be satisfied. Another person will say that she needs to have a chocolate bar immediately or needs to do this or that, depending on the object of the addiction. When we re-label, we give up the language of need. I say to myself: "I don't *need* to purchase anything now or to eat anything now; I'm only having an obsessive thought that I have such a need. It's not a real, objective need but a false belief. I may have a feeling of urgency, but there is actually nothing urgent going on."

Essential to the first step, as to all the steps, is conscious awareness. It is conscious intention and attention, not just rote repetition that will result in beneficial changes to brain patterns, thoughts and behaviours. Be fully aware of the sense of urgency that attends the impulse and keep labelling it as a manifestation of addiction, rather than any reality that you must act upon. "In Re-labelling," writes Dr. Schwartz, "you bring into play the Impartial Spectator, a concept that Adam Smith used as the central feature of his book *The Theory of Moral Sentiments*. He defined the Impartial Spectator as the capacity to stand outside yourself and watch yourself in action, which is essentially the same mental action as the ancient Buddhist concept of mindful awareness."[1]

The point of re-labelling is not to make the addictive urge disappear—it's not going to, at least not for a long time, since it was wired into the brain long ago. It is strengthened every time you give in to it and every time you try to suppress it forcibly. The point is to observe it with conscious attention without assigning the habitual meaning to it. It is no longer a "need," only a dysfunctional thought. Rest assured, the urge will come back—and again you will re-label it with determination and mindful awareness. "*Conscious attention must be paid,*" Jeffrey Schwartz emphasizes. "*Therein lies the key.* Physical changes in the brain depend for their creation on a mental state in the mind—the state called attention. Paying attention matters."[2]

Step 2: Re-attribute

"In Re-attribute you learn to place the blame squarely on your brain. This is my brain sending me a false message."[3] This step is designed to assign the re-labelled addictive urge to its proper source. In Step 1 you recognized that the compulsion to engage in the addictive behaviour does not express a real need or anything that "must" happen; it's only a belief. In Step 2 you state very clearly where that urge originated: in neurological circuits that were programmed into your brain long ago, when you were a child. It represents a dopamine or endorphin "hunger" on the part of brain systems that, early in your life, lacked the necessary conditions for their full development. It also represents emotional needs that went unsatisfied.

Re-attribution is directly linked with compassionate curiosity toward the self. Instead of blaming yourself for having addictive thoughts or desires, you calmly ask why these desires have exercised such a powerful hold over you. "Because they are deeply ingrained in my brain and because they are easily triggered whenever I'm stressed or fatigued or unhappy or bored." The addictive compulsion says nothing about you as a person. It is not a moral failure or a character weakness; it is just the effect of circumstances over which you had no control. What you do have some control over is how you respond to the compulsion in the present. You were not responsible for the stressful circumstances that shaped your brain and worldview, but you can take responsibility now.

Re-attribution helps you put the addictive drive into perspective: it's no more significant than, say, a momentary ringing in your ear. Just as there is no "bell" that causes the ringing, so there is no real need that the addictive urge will satisfy. It is only a thought, an attitude, a belief, a feeling arising from an automatic brain mechanism. You can observe it consciously, with attention. And you can let it go. There are better sources of dopamine or endorphins in the world, and more satisfying ways to have your needs for vitality and intimacy met.

Once more, don't allow yourself to be frustrated when what you have let go returns. It will—probably soon. When it does, you will re-label it and re-attribute it: "Hello, old brain circuits," you say. "I see you're still active. Well, so am I." If you change how you respond to those old circuits, you will eventually weaken them. They will persist for a long time—perhaps even all your life, but only as shadows of themselves. They will no longer have the weight, the gravitational pull or the appeal they once boasted. You will no longer be their marionette.

Step 3: Re-focus

In the Re-focus step you buy yourself time. Although the compulsion to open the bag of cookies or turn on the TV or drive to the store or the casino is powerful, its shelf life is not permanent. Being a mind-phantom, it will pass, and you have to give it time to pass. The key principle here, as Dr. Schwartz points out, is this: "*It's not how you feel that counts; it's what you do.*"

Rather than engage in the addictive activity, find something else to do. Your initial goal is modest: buy yourself just fifteen minutes. Choose something that you enjoy and that will keep you active: preferably something healthy and creative, but anything that will please you without causing greater harm. Instead of giving in to the siren call of the addiction, go for a walk. If you "need" to drive to the casino, turn on the TV. If you "need" to watch television, put on some music. If you "need" to buy music, get on your exercise bike. Whatever gets you through the night—or at least through the next fifteen minutes. "Early in therapy," advises Jeffrey Schwartz, "physical activity seems to be especially helpful. But the important thing is that whatever activity you choose, it must be something you enjoy doing."[4]

The purpose of Re-focus is to teach your brain that it doesn't have to obey the addictive call. It can exercise the "free won't." It can choose something else. Perhaps in the beginning you can't even hold out for fifteen minutes—fine. Make it five, and record it in a journal as a success. Next time, try for six minutes, or sixteen. This is not a hundred-metre dash but a solo marathon you are training for. Successes will come in increments.

As you perform the alternative activity, stay aware of what you are doing. You are doing something difficult. No matter how simple it may seem to others who do not have to live with your particular brain, you know that holding out for even a short period of time is an achievement. You are teaching your old brain new tricks. Unlike the case with old dogs, no one can tell you it can't be done.

Step 4: Re-value

This step should really be called De-value. Its purpose is to help you drive into your own thick skull just what has been the real impact of the addictive urge in your life: disaster. You know this already, and that is why you are engaged in these four steps. It's because of the negative impact that you've taken yourself by the scruff of the neck and delayed acting on the impulse while you've re-labelled and re-attributed it and while you have re-focused on some healthier activity. In this Re-value step you will remind yourself why you've gone to all this trouble. The more clearly you see how things are, the more liberated you will be.

We know that the addicted brain assigns a falsely high value to the addictive object, substance or behaviour, the process called *salience attribution*. The addicted mind has been fooled into making the object of your addiction the highest priority. Addiction has moved in and taken over your attachment-reward and incentive-motivation circuits. Where love and vitality should be, addiction roosts. The distorted brain circuits, including the orbitofrontal cortex, are making you believe that experiences that can come authentically only from genuine intimacy, creativity or honest endeavour will be yours for the taking through addiction. In the Re-value step you de-value the false gold. You assign to it its proper worth: less than nothing.

What has this addictive urge done for me? you will ask. It has caused me to spend money heedlessly or to stuff myself when I wasn't hungry or to be absent from the ones I love or to expend my energies on activities I later regretted. It has wasted my time. It has led me to lie and to cheat and to pretend—first to myself and then to everyone close to me. It has left me feeling ashamed and isolated. It promised joy and delivered bitterness. Such has been its real value to me; such has been the effect of my allowing some disordered brain circuits to run my life. The real "value" of my addictive compulsion has been that it has caused me to betray my true values and disregard my true goals.

Be conscious as you write out this fourth step—and do write it out, several times a day if necessary. Be specific: What has been the value of the urge in your relationship with your wife? your husband? your partner, your best friend, your children, your boss, your employees, your co-workers? What happened yesterday when you allowed the urge to rule you? What happened last week? What will happen today? Pay close attention to what you feel when you recall these events and when you foresee what's ahead if you persist in permitting the compulsion to overpower you. Be aware. That aware-ness will be your guardian.

Do all this without judging yourself. You are gathering informa-tion, not conducting a criminal trial against yourself. Jesus said: "If you bring forth what is within you, what you have will save you."* That is true in so many ways. Within you is knowledge of the real value of the impulses you have obeyed until now. To quote and par-aphrase Dr. Schwartz, the more consciously and *actively* you come to re-value the addictive drive in light of its pernicious influence on your life, "the more quickly and smoothly you can perform the Re-label, Re-attribute and Re-focus steps and the more steadily your brain's 'automatic transmission' function returns. Re-valuing helps you shift the behavioral gears!"[5]

---

* The Gospel of Thomas

—

Dr. Schwartz introduces what he calls the two A's: Anticipate and Accept. To *anticipate* is to know that the compulsive drive to engage in addictive behaviour will return. There is no final victory—every moment the urge is turned away is a triumph. What is certain is that with time the addictive drive will be drained of energy if you continue to apply the four steps and also take care of the internal and external environments in the ways suggested in these chapters. If there are times when it reappears with new force, there is no reason to be disappointed or shocked by that. And *accept* that the addiction exists not because of yourself, but in spite of yourself. You did not come into life asking to be programmed this way. It's not personal to you—millions of others with similar experiences have developed the same mechanisms. What is personal to you is how you respond to it in the present. Keep close to your impartial observer.

I take the liberty of suggesting a fifth step to be added to the Four-Step Self-Treatment Method, at least in the context of addiction. I call it Re-create.

Step 5: Re-create

Life, until now, has created you. You've been acting according to ingrained mechanisms wired into your brain before you had a choice in the matter, and it's out of those automatic mechanisms that you've created the life you now have. It is time to re-create: to choose a different life.

You have values. You have passions. You have intention, talent, capability. In your heart there is love, and you want to connect that with the love in the world, in the universe. As you re-label, re-attribute, re-focus and re-value, you are releasing patterns that have held you and that you have held on to. In place of a life blighted by your addictive need for acquisition, self-soothing, admiration, oblivion, meaningless activity, what is the life you really want? What do you choose to create?

Consider, too, what activities you can engage in to express the universal human need to be creative. Mindfully honouring our creativity helps us transcend the feeling of deficient emptiness that drives addiction. *Not* to express our creative needs is itself a source of stress. I permit myself here to quote from the final pages of *When the Body Says No,* my book on illness, stress and mind-body unity:

> For many years after becoming a doctor I was too caught up in my workaholism to pay attention to myself or to my deepest urges. In the rare moments I permitted any stillness, I noted a small fluttering at the pit of my belly, a barely perceptible disturbance. The faint whisper of a word would sound in my head: *writing.* At first I could not say whether it was heartburn or inspiration. The more I listened, the louder the message became: I needed to write, to express myself through written language not only so that others might hear me but so that I could hear myself.
>
> The gods, we are taught, created humankind in their own image. Everyone has an urge to create. Its expression may flow through many channels: through writing, art or music or through the inventiveness of work or in any number of ways unique to all of us, whether it be cooking, gardening or the art of social discourse. The point is to honour the urge. To do so is healing for ourselves and for others; not to do so deadens our bodies and our spirits. When I did not write, I suffocated in silence.
>
> "What is in us must out," wrote the great Canadian stress researcher, Dr. Hans Selye, "otherwise we may explode at the wrong places or become hopelessly hemmed in by frustrations. *The great art is to express our vitality through the particular channels and at the particular speed Nature foresaw for us.*"

Write down your values and intentions and, one more time, do so with conscious awareness. Envision yourself living with integrity, creative and present, being able to look people in the eye with compassion for them—and for yourself. The road to hell is not paved with good intentions. It is paved with lack of intention. Re-create. Are you afraid you will stumble? Of course you will: that's called being a human being. And then you will take the four steps—plus one—again.

CHAPTER 32

Sobriety and the External Milieu

—

What matters is not the features of our character or the drives and
instincts per se, but rather the stand we take toward them. And the
capacity to take such a stand is what makes us human beings

VICTOR FRANKL
The Will to Meaning

L ately, I have come to experience and appreciate the difference between abstinence and sobriety.

I've mentioned earlier that substance users cannot envi
sion a life without their drug of choice. Since their addictions
offer biochemical substitutes for love, connection, vitality and
joy, to ask them to desist from their habits is to demand that they
give up on the emotional experiences that make life worth living
for them. Anne, a forty-three-year-old Vancouver college instructor, had her last drink on March 17, 1991. She has been attending
AA ever since. "It became clear that I needed to stop drinking,"
she recalls. "On the other hand I just kept thinking, 'Oh, this
can't be possible because if I stop drinking how could I ever have
sex again? How could I ever socialize again? You know . . . how
could I ever sleep again? How could I ever do anything again . . . ?'
I couldn't imagine living without the alcohol. I thought it was
helping me. That's the nature of denial. One thinks that the addiction is actually enhancing one's life, bettering one's life, satisfying a basic need."

A behaviour addict like me faces a similar predicament. My addictions, be it purchasing music or the perpetual juggling of several projects in my professional life, serve to fill an emptiness. The idea of "just saying no" left me with a sense of loss. The intellectual awareness that in every way it would be "good for me" to get off the compulsive merry-go-round didn't mean much to the impatient emotional apparatus where my impulses and behaviours originated.

There are two ways of abstaining from a substance or behaviour: a positive and even joyful choice for something else that has a greater value for you or forcing yourself to stay away from something you crave and are spontaneously attracted to. This second type of abstinence, while it requires admirable fortitude and patience, can still be experienced in a negative way and contains a hidden danger. Human beings have an ingrained opposition to any sense of being forced, an automatic resistance to coercion that my friend Dr. Gordon Neufeld has called *counterwill*. It is triggered whenever a person feels controlled or pressured to do someone else's bidding—and we can generate counterwill even against pressure that we put on ourselves. The effects of counterwill appear in many human interactions. Although we see it most clearly in the automatic no-saying of immature children, we have likely witnessed it in ourselves and in other adults. As in the old folksong, "Mamma Don't Allow," nothing evokes resistance more effectively than someone forbidding us to do something, even when the prohibition comes from ourselves. The universal refrain is "We don' care what mamma don't allow, we're gonna keep on [doing whatever] anyhow. . . ."

The frustration and resistance induced by abstinence in one area often lead to the addiction process erupting somewhere else. "You've got to put the plug in the jug of your drug of choice," says Anne. "If you do that, you can work on yourself. Mind you, when I stopped drinking, I started eating like crazy and put on weight. I was also nastier to my kids than I had been when I was drinking." As long as a person has a need to self-soothe—or from the biochemical perspective, to trigger dopamine release in their brain—one addiction may automatically substitute for another. We have noted that many people begin to binge eat, for example, when they quit smoking cigarettes. "Of course, it was still better for me to overeat than to drink," Anne adds. "You might say that for me food was a form of harm reduction."

Given that my pursuits were never substance based, I could easily move from one compulsion to another without ever recognizing the underlying addiction process that fuelled them all. I found myself in a much more powerful position once I began to appreciate the nature of sobriety as distinct from mere abstinence. Now I could move toward something positive, something that gives me lightness, that doesn't feel like a duty and that allows for joy without artificial, external supports. For me personally, sobriety means being free of internal compulsion and living according to principles I believe in. Unlike abstinence, I don't experience it as a constraint but as liberation. I don't say I'm fully sober. I do say I recognize and value conscious awareness—another term for sobriety. It excites me more than the fool's gold of acquisition or ego stroking that I've spent much time and energy pursuing in the past.

In choosing sobriety we're not so much avoiding something harmful as envisioning ourselves living the life we value. What sobriety looks like will vary from person to person, but in all cases it has the individual, rather than the addictive compulsion, in the lead.

Ultimately, the goal of all Twelve-Step programs is not abstinence but sobriety. "What were my real needs that I thought alcohol satisfied?" says Anne. "Attachment, attunement, to be in a community, to be loved by people, to be able to give love, to have joy, to be able to be myself. AA, and what I have learned in AA, has more successfully, more adaptively fulfilled these basic needs."

I have said that creating an external environment that can support one's move towards conscious awareness is one essential feature of the recovery process. For many people, whether with substance addictions like alcoholism or behaviour addictions like gambling or sexual acting out, Twelve-Step programs are a crucial part of that healing environment. Their insights and methods go the very heart of the addiction process. Take, for example, the technique of an addict having a sponsor to contact whenever the addictive urge threatens to gain the upper hand—the desire to have a drink or to play cards at the casino. When the addict makes that call he recognizes his powerlessness over the compulsion, in other words, the relative weakness of the impulse-regulating parts of his cerebral cortex. Until those circuits develop some muscle of their own, the sponsor acts the regulator by talking the addict through his compulsion. Talking it out prevents acting it out.

Although not for everyone—nothing is for everyone—Twelve-Step programs provide the best available healing environment for many people. They're not without flaws and they may even take on an addictive quality themselves. Being human institutions, they may have, here and there, become forums for gossips or for people on the make. But they have saved more lives—emotionally and probably even physically—than the medical treatments of addiction. If I don't say more about them, it's only for lack of personal experience. They have been well described many times from many angles—historical, psychological, practical, personal, religious and spiritual. I've read illuminating Twelve-Step books written from Christian, Buddhist and Taoist perspectives.

Ultimately, I didn't choose a Twelve-Step program for myself. I have no reasons to give—it just didn't quite feel like a fit, despite my positive experience at the one meeting I did attend. And, I admit, I have difficulty committing to attending long-term programs of any kind. For all that, I have found the Twelve-Step principles and my discussions with Twelve-Step members most helpful. I encourage anyone dealing with any addiction to investigate Twelve-Step approaches, even if they have no interest in participating in group work.

—

Not long ago I was confronted by an example of just how thoroughly addictive attitudes have pervaded my life and how sharply they affect other people. It's no different for most addicts.

I am chronically and notoriously late—to work, to meetings, to family gatherings. I've been able to blame that propensity partly on ADD, because a deficient time sense is a well-known feature of attention deficit disorder. One Friday afternoon in mid-September of 2006 I was sitting in my car on Cortes Island, waiting for the ferry. Cortes is the home of Hollyhock, a spectacular oceanside gathering place and healing centre where many people come for programs and seminars or for rest and rejuvenation. I had just completed co-leading a five-day mind-body health workshop there. As I watched the ferry arrive, I was basking in the warm gratitude expressed by the participants, who, many of them said, had experienced transformational insights and an awakening of vitality. My head was filled with "What a good boy am I"–type thoughts. Then I opened the email on my PDA. The first was from Susan Craigie, the Portland health coordinator: a missive exploding with long-suppressed anger and frustration. For the week I'd been away, another doctor had filled in for me and she was actually on time every day. What a difference it was, Susan wrote, to have the physician show up punctually. "Kim and I didn't have to listen to all the abuse from the upset patients in the waiting room day after day—you're the one that's always late, and we have to take all the crap." She reminded me of the many promises I'd made to put an end to my tardiness and of my utter failure to keep them. "You're doing this only because they're junkies and you think you can get away with it. You excuse yourself by saying that you're too busy working on your addictions book, but you've been doing this for years, long before that book was a glint in your eye." The very words shook with rage as I read them on the little screen in my hand.

My initial reaction was anger—the addicted mind's way of resisting shame—but only for a moment. I soon allowed the feelings of shame to wash over me without either resisting them or letting them knock me down, and I felt grateful. Roman emperors, as they proceeded in triumphant procession with the war booty and captives driven before them amongst the cheering throngs, had a slave behind them on the chariot whose duty it was to whisper in their ear at regular intervals: "Sire, you are mortal." Life finds ways of delivering those messages just when we most need them. Susan had done me the favour of reminding me what my reality was in the absence of sobriety and integrity.

If I didn't file it as yet another ADD trait, my habitual lateness represented three factors that also express the addictive process: *lack of impulse control*—I'd just keep on doing whatever it was that caught my attention instead of making sure I was on time; *failure to consider future consequences*—"forgetting to remember the future," in the words of psychologist and ADD researcher Russell Barkley; and *lack of thought for the impact of my behaviour on other people*. It became crystal clear that the addiction process—and the world-view that accompanies it—had polluted my life on levels I had not ever considered.

Addiction is primarily about the self, about the unconscious, insecure self that at every moment considers only its own immediate desires—and believes that it must behave that way. In all cases the process arises from the unmet needs of the helpless young child for whom this constant self-obsession appears, to begin with, as a matter of survival. That he cannot rely on the nurturing environment becomes his core myth. No such environment even exists—or so he has come to believe in his bones and in his heart, which were parched by early loss.

The mind of the addict is beset by constant worry, soothed only by the addictive substance or activity. The hunger and the urgent drive to satisfy it are ever present, regardless of circumstances. My family has remarked that when I eat, unless I take particular care, my habit is to bend low over the plate and shovel the food into my mouth as if it's about to disappear. And yet only one time in my life have I starved or experienced deprivation: during my first year in the Jewish ghetto of Nazi-occupied Budapest. That was enough to program my brain with the image of an uncertain, unyielding and indifferent world. Once programmed, the addicted mind creates a world of emptiness where one must scratch and grab for every bit of nourishment and be ever vigilant for every opportunity to get more. The addict hasn't grown out of the stage of infancy that has been called the narcissistic phase, the period when the fledgling human being believes that everything happens because of her, to her and for her. Her own self-ish needs are her only point of reference. We move through stages of development when the needs we have in each are fully satisfied. Then the brain can let go. The addicted mind never lets go.

The teaching in Susan's letter came at a time when I was secure enough to receive it, when I would neither deny its truth nor be overwhelmed by the shame it triggered. I had just been teaching and demonstrating compassionate curiosity to the workshop particitrpants and, lo and behold, had absorbed some of it myself. Now, as

I applied it to my own behaviour, I saw the chronic lateness not as a character flaw to beat myself up about or as a "nuisance" I could just dismiss flippantly, but as another attempt by my addiction-prone mind to maintain its illusion of freedom and control. "Nobody tells me what to do and when." And, of course, it was a sign of my persistent refusal to be responsible—another hallmark of the addicted mind. Seeing it that way, I could let go of it.

As soon as I got home, I wrote back:

Thanks for your very clear message. There is little I can say in defence, since you're absolutely right. The only charge to which I don't plead guilty is that I behave this way because these patients are junkies. A quick phone call to my former nurse, Maria, would convince you that it was no better in my private practice. Which, however, is no excuse.

Among the many ways I could make myself late for work was to stop by at Sikora's in the morning or during lunch break. I was indulging my addictions instead of treating my addicted patients. My letter to Susan continued:

I've made so many promises in the past that it's meaningless to make another one. So, more practically: On Monday I'll be there at 9:30. I'll be bringing ten signed, undated cheques for $100.00 each, made out to the Portland Hotel Society. Any day I'm even one minute past 9:30, you date the cheque and deposit it. Should those ten run out, I'll bring in another ten.

Thanks again. I deeply regret the hassle and frustration I've caused you and the inconvenience to our clients.

That e-mail exchange took place in late September. As of May 2007, Susan has had to cash nine of the cheques. The atmosphere in the clinic has been transformed. I've had the pleasure of facing my clients without shame clouding my eyes and of working along-side colleagues who no longer have to compensate for my tardiness and to disguise their resentment. Sweet are the rewards of sobriety.

The prewritten cheques are not a form of self-punishment, but a way of building a structure that helps keep me sober. They would not be necessary if I possessed sufficient self-regulation; I would just show up on time. They serve me as the sponsor serves the Twelve-Step novice: when in the morning an urge arises to stay writing by my computer or to keep pedalling on my exercise bike, the thought of the lost income reminds me of my responsibilities and helps to regulate my insufficiently active prefrontal impulse-control brain circuits. Creating such structures is part of establishing an external environment that supports mental awareness and responsible behaviour. All addicts need them.

Another mental structure I've committed to is truth-speaking. Even before I completely stopped buying compact discs, for example, for months I did not lie about my purchases. Arriving home with a new musical acquisition, I would tell Rae about it. I had nothing to hide, my compassionate curiosity discovered. I hadn't killed anyone; I'd only bought a symphonic recording. Exposed to the light of day the addictive compulsion does not develop power and heft. I had much less of the urge to binge, and the occasional visit to the music store did not evoke a helpless desire to go back the same day or the next—another freedom I relished. Music without guilt—a revelation. My advice to anyone with addictive behaviours is to begin telling the truth. If you are not ready to drop the behaviour, then choose it openly. Tell your spouse or friends what you are doing; keep it in the daylight. At the very least, do not compound your inner shame by lying. Better you should look "bad" in the eyes of others than to sink further in your own estimation of yourself.

More recently I've committed to not buying another CD until at least March 2009. Rae has three signed, undated cheques, each for one thousand dollars, as my guarantee. It's now the beginning of October 2007 as I'm revising the manuscript for this book. So far, so good. Quite contrary to feeling frustrated about any thwarted desires, I have discovered a much more satisfying freedom in not allowing the addiction process to run my life. And I've found another, unlooked-for benefit: just as the addiction process permeates every area of your existence, so does sobriety. As you become less attached to your addiction, you also become calmer, less attached to other things that don't matter nearly as much as you used to believe. Your responses are less automatic, less rigid. Not having reason to be so harsh on yourself, you are not so inclined to find fault with others. Things don't always have to go your way for you to be able to enjoy life.

I am not suggesting that every addict should write cheques to their spouses or fellow workers. My particular method here is not for everyone, but every behaviour addict can find his own way to build some appropriate structures into his life. That's a matter of individual circumstance, choice and inventiveness. It's also obvious that many people with behaviour addictions face much greater challenges. But anyone who has successfully achieved sobriety knows that no evanescent pleasure can be compared with the peace that comes from living in integrity. Many people think of commitment as a limitation of possibilities. Rather than a limitation, it is a source of joy. When you are true to your word, you are in charge. Governing your life are your values and your intentions, not some mechanical compulsion arising from the past. That emancipation means much more than the illusory freedom of obeying any impulse that arises in the moment.

One important warning: if you want to find liberation in your commitments, your word needs to be freely given or not given at all. Don't make promises to reform out of a sense of duty or to appease someone else. If you don't know how to say *no* to other people's expectations, howsoever well meant or valid those may be, your *yes* has no authenticity. This is what I have learned.

—

Truth-speaking will also make you more aware of the impact of your behaviour on others—what the Twelve-Step programs call taking inventory: "We made a searching and fearless moral inventory of ourselves," reads AA's Step Four. "For the addict/alcoholic, there is no substitute for the moral inventory," writes meditation teacher, musician and recovering alcoholic Kevin Griffin in *One Breath at a Time: Buddhism and the Twelve Steps*:

> What's odd about the inventory is that, for me, it was an admission
> that I had power in the world, power to hurt others, which I'd never
> acknowledged. Besides denying my own responsibility, I'd also often

denied that my words or actions could have any effect on anyone. So, even though what was revealed was painful and destructive, just admitting that I had hurt others was empowering. In fact, inventory is a review of past karma. To pretend that our existence doesn't affect others is to deny karma, to deny that every action has a reaction, to pretend that cause and effect aren't constantly in play. *This careful parsing of our past forces us to become more cognizant of karma.* When we see how our actions hurt others—and ourselves—we become more careful about what we are doing in the present. When we see our destructive patterns of thought, speech, and behavior, we begin to change, to unravel these habits, to act in ways that won't require more inventory writing.[1]

"Something happened to me at the first AA meeting," recalls Anne, the Vancouver college instructor. "They read Step Ten—which is *repeatedly* take a moral inventory of yourself, on a daily basis.* It clicked and I could just feel this huge gestalt shift for me internally. And I thought, This is brilliant. I felt a sense of possibility, and sense of hope . . . It was the pragmatism of the approach that I liked. The idea was that through examining my conscience daily, even multiple times a day—a kind of naming the assets and the deficits—I could keep my guilt level really low. And that if one had self-acceptance and low guilt, it would be easier to stay away from painkillers—in my case, alcohol."

"Continued to take personal inventory and when we were wrong promptly admitted it," says Step Ten. By structuring such responsible but nonjudgmental self-examination into our routine, by owning the impact of our behaviours on others, we diminish our karmic burden. We are lighter and freer. We have less need to escape into addiction.

—

A part of creating external structures to support recovery is the avoidance of environments and environmental cues that trigger

---

* In other words, Step Ten is commitment to the regular, daily application of Step Four. For the Twelve Steps, see Appendix IV.

addictive thoughts and feelings. Those cues and environments vary from person to person, from addiction to addiction but for all addicts they are powerful in setting off addictive behaviour. Someone quitting smoking, for example, who associates cigarettes with a round of lager at the pub with friends needs to stay out of beer parlors. In my case, once the addictive drive to binge on compact discs comes to predominate, I find it hard to resist the shopping urge. However, I do not need to look up music reviews on the Internet—that's a choice I find easier to make. Nor do I have to listen to classical music constantly. When I take the dog for a walk I can now focus on just being in the present, mindful of my sensory experience of the moment. In other words, I can avoid keeping music ever in the forefront of my mind.

Establishing the healing environment also entails removing what is toxic—the stresses that enhance the addictive drive and trigger addictive cravings. Once more, we have to move beyond abstinence and view things from an ecological and sustainable perspective.

Isabella, a married mother of three young children, asked for my advice about addictive sexual acting out that she could neither give up nor choose openly in her life. She was compulsively adulterous. An energetic Guatemalan woman in her late twenties, she felt paralyzed by her inability to abstain from a preoccupation she felt ashamed of and saw as destructive to her family. Typically, she was profuse in her expressions of self-loathing. "Could it be," I said, "that your sexual acting out is serving a function in your life—that it's helping you to endure a situation that otherwise makes you quite unhappy? There may be stresses in your life that you haven't fully recognized and haven't confronted. Perhaps you're using your sexuality as a painkiller and temporary stress reliever."

My comment opened the floodgates of self-disclosure. While still in her teens Isabella developed a relationship with a man for whom she had never felt passion and whom she finally married out of a vague sense of guilt and responsibility. She came to perceive herself as controlled financially and restricted by him in her need for artistic self-expression. Having given up her own successful jewellery-design business after the birth of their second child, she felt dependent and resentful. She also suspected he might be attracted to men, although the two had never discussed his sexual preferences in a frank manner. In short, she was living under tremendous emotional strain. My advice was that unless she dealt with the stresses in her life, she would continue to be tempted by her addiction. At best, she could remain sexually abstinent but pay a price in depression or some other addiction. Indeed, she was already concerned about her marijuana use, which had gone from occasional to daily in the past six months.

Stress is salient in the ecology of addiction. Let's quickly review some of what we have learned about it, so that we can apply this knowledge to the ecology of recovery:

- Stressors are the external triggers for the physiological stress reaction, a maelstrom of hormonal secretions and nervous discharges that involve virtually every organ and system in the body.
- The most potent stressors are loss of control and uncertainty in important areas of life, whether personal or professional, economic or psychological.
- Stress interacts powerfully with the biology of addiction in the brain.
- Stresses like emotional isolation or the sense that we are dominated by others change our brains in ways that increase the need for external sources of dopamine—that is, they increase the risk of addiction.
- Stress is a major trigger for substance abuse and other addictive behaviours and the most predictable trigger for relapse.
- Stress hormones can themselves become addictive.

Addiction is often a misguided attempt to relieve stress, but misguided only in the long term. In the short term addictive substances and behaviours do act as stress relievers.

The ecological approach to recovery must, therefore, address the stresses in one's life. It's impossible to cool the circuitry of the addicted brain if we leave it heated by chronic stress.

In Isabella's case, as in most, the stressors were not simply objective circumstances but a rash of attitudes and perceptions that both evoked and magnified the stresses of her situation. Consider, for example, her inhibitions in dealing with her emotions of fear and resentment toward her husband. Where she believed he was "controlling," she had never asserted her desire for financial equality and partnership in the marriage. Where she doubted his sexual orientation, she had kept her concerns secret for fear of "rocking the boat." Where she craved freedom to pursue her art, she allowed herself to be held back by her fear that he would disapprove.

As the famed stress researcher Dr. Bruce McEwen has pointed out, a key determining factor triggering the stress response is *the way a person perceives a situation.*[2] We ourselves give events their meaning, depending on our personal histories, temperament, physical condition and state of mind at the moment we experience them. Thus the degree to which we're stressed may depend less on external circumstances than on how well we are able to take care of ourselves physically and emotionally. We may also take on chronic stresses because of ingrained beliefs of how we "ought" to be. Some people, for example, may find themselves unable to say no to work demands or the emotional expectations of their spouse, adult children or family of origin. Something has to give—and what gives, if not our physical health, is our mood or peace of mind. Addiction comes along as an "antidote."

To see addiction as the only problem is to leave intact the context that triggered the addiction in the first place.

For human beings most stressors are emotional ones. Anyone wanting to gain mastery over their addiction process must be ready, through counselling or some other means, to look honestly and clearly at the emotional stressors that trigger their addictive behaviours, whether these stressors arise at work, in their marriage or in some other aspect of their lives.

In our culture, the suppression of emotion is a major source of stress and therefore a major source of addictions. Science tells us that not even in rodents can the link between emotions and mental organization be ignored. In her Berkeley laboratory Dr. Marian Diamond found improvements in the problem-solving abilities of rats treated with tender, loving care, and this corresponded with the growth of richer connections in their cortex. "Thus," Dr. Diamond has written, "it is important to stimulate the portion of the brain that initiates emotional expression. Satisfying [one's] emotional needs is essential at any age."₃

Once more, the release of addiction's hold requires awareness: awareness of where we keep ourselves hobbled and stressed, where we ignore our emotions, restrict our expression of who we are, frustrate our innate human drive for creative and meaningful activity and deny our needs for connection and intimacy. In the ecology of gardening it is not enough to pull up the weeds. If we want something beautiful to grow, we have to create the conditions that will allow it to develop. The same is true in the ecology of the mind.

When truly sober, we look back compassionately at our addicted selves and, like the human boy Pinocchio gazing at his wooden toy self slumped on a chair, we shake our heads and say: "How foolish I was when I was a puppet."

—

CHAPTER 33

A Word to Families, Friends
and Caregivers

—

Purity and impurity belong to oneself. No one else can purify another.
BUDDHA
The Dhammapada

To live with an addict of any kind is frustrating, emotionally painful and often infuriating. Family, friends and spouse may feel they are dealing with a double personality: one sane and loveable, the other devious and uncaring. They believe the first is real and hope the second will go away. In truth, the second is the shadow side of the first and will no sooner leave than will a shadow abandon the object whose shape it traces on the ground—not unless the light comes from a different angle.

While it is natural for the loved ones of an addict to wish to reform him, it cannot be done. The counterwill-driven resistance to any sense of coercion will sabotage even the most well-meant endeavour by one human being to change another. There are many other factors, too, including the powerful underlying emotional currents and brain physiology from which addiction springs in the first place. The person attached to his addiction will respond to an attempt to separate him from his habit as a lover would to someone who disparages his beloved: with hostility. Any attempts to shame him will also trigger rage. Until a person is willing to take on the task of self-mastery, no one else will induce him to do so. "There are no techniques that will motivate people or make them autonomous," psychologist Edward Deci has written. "Motivation must come from within, not from techniques. It comes from their deciding they are ready to take responsibility for managing themselves."[1]

Contrary to a popular misconception, confrontational "tough love" interventions are likely to fail. A 1999 study compared confrontation with a method employing a nurturing attitude by the family. "More than twice as many families succeeded in getting their loved ones into treatment (64 percent) with the gentler approach than with standard intervention (30 percent). But no reality shows push the less dramatic method, and it is difficult to find clinicians who use it," science and health journalist Maia Szalawitz commented in the *New York Times*.[2]

Family, friends and partners of addicts sometimes have only one reasonable decision in front of them: either to choose to be with the addict as she is or to choose not to be with her. No one is obliged to put up with unreliability, dishonesty and emotional withdrawal— the ways of the addict. Unconditional acceptance of another person doesn't mean staying with them under all circumstances, at no matter what cost to oneself; that duty belongs only to the parents of a young child. Acceptance in the context of adult-to-adult relationships may mean simply acknowledging that the other is the way he or she is, not judging them and not corroding one's own soul with resentment that they are not different. Acceptance does not mean saintly self-sacrifice or tolerating an eternity of broken promises and hurtful eruptions of frustration and rage. Sometimes a person remains with an addicted partner for fear of the guilt they might experience otherwise. A therapist once said to me, "When it comes to a choice between feeling guilt or resentment, choose the guilt every time." It is wisdom I have passed on to many others since. If refusal to take on responsibility for another person's behaviours burdens you with guilt, while consenting to it leaves you eaten by resentment, opt for the guilt. Resentment is soul suicide.

Leaving the addict or staying in the relationship is a choice no person can make for anyone else, but to stay with him while resenting him, mentally rejecting him and punishing him emotionally, or even just subtly trying to manipulate him into "reform" is always the worst course. The belief that anyone "should" be any different than he or she is is toxic to oneself, to the other and to the relationship.

Although we may believe we are acting out of love, when we are critical of others or work very hard to change them, it's always about ourselves. "The alcoholic's wife is adding to the level of shame her husband experiences," says Anne, a veteran of AA. "In effect, she is saying to the addict, he is bad and she is good. Perhaps she is in denial about her addiction to certain attitudes, like self-righteousness, martyrdom or perfectionism. What if, on the other hand, the wife said to her husband: 'I'm feeling good today, honey. I only obsessed about your drinking once today. I'm really making progress on my addiction to self-righteousness. How are you feeling?' Wouldn't that be a loving way to approach each other rather than one person trying to control another's addiction? After all, if the developmental roots of the addiction process lie in insufficient attachment, recovery includes forming attachments. As with good parenting, real attachment relationships are based on truth. The truth is, a wife who thinks she does not have plenty of her own spiritual or psychological work to do, that is, one for whom another's behavior becomes the central determinant of her own emotional/spiritual condition, is not in touch with the truth."

Does this mean that friends, loved ones or co-workers can never speak to an addict about her choices? Far from it. It's only that if such an intervention is to have any hope of success—indeed, any hope of not *further* poisoning the situation—it needs to be put into action with love, in a pure way that is not adulterated with judgement, vindictiveness or a tone of rejection. It requires clarity of purpose: Is my aim here to set my limits and to express my needs, or am I trying to change the other person? You may find it necessary, say, to tell your spouse or adult child about the negative way their actions affect you—not in order to control or blame them, only to communicate what you will accept and what you cannot and will not live with. Once more, you are fully entitled to take the steps you find necessary for your own peace of mind. The issue is with what spirit you approach the interaction.

If you want to point the addict toward more fulfilling possibilities in his life, drop the self-righteousness. The conversation needs to be opened not as a demand, but as an invitation that may be refused. It is helpful to acknowledge that the person had reasons for "choosing" the addiction, that it held some value for him. "It was your way of surmounting some pain, or helping you through some difficulty. I can understand why you went in that direction."*

I'm not describing a technique here: it is not *what* we do that has the greatest impact, but *who* we are being as we do it. Loving parent or prosecutor? Friend or judge? Any person who wishes to make a difference in the life of the addict should first conduct a compassionate self-inquiry. They need to examine their own anxieties, agenda and motives. "Purity and impurity belong to oneself," the Buddha taught. "No one else can purify another." Before any intervention in the life of another, we need to ask ourselves: How am I doing in my own life? I may not have the addiction I'm trying to exorcise in my friend or son or co-worker, but how am I faring with my own compulsions? As I try to liberate this other, how free am I—do I, for example, have an insistent need to change him for the better? I want to awaken this person to their genuine possibilities, but am I on the path to fulfilling my own? These questions will help to keep us from projecting our unconscious anxieties and concerns onto the other—a burden the addict will instinctively reject. Nobody wants to perceive himself as someone's salvage project.

If it is crucial for addicts to proceed with a fearless moral inventory, it is no less useful for the ones close to them to do so. AlAnon, the self-help group for the relatives of alcoholics, points out that alcoholism is a family disease—all addictions are—and therefore the whole family needs healing. Addiction represents a family condition not just because the behaviours of the addict have an unhealthy impact on those around him, but more profoundly because something in the family dynamic has probably contributed—and continues to contribute—to the addict's acting out. While his behaviours are fully his responsibility, the more people around him can shoulder

---

* In learning how to talk to others without judgment and with compassionate understanding, the work of Marshall Rosenberg on nonviolent communication is invaluable. I highly recommend his DVDs, CDs and books, especially *Nonviolent Communication: A Language of Life*.

responsibility for their own attitudes and actions without blaming and shaming the addict, the greater is the likelihood that everyone will come to a place of freedom.

A tremendous step forward, albeit a very difficult one, is for people who are in relationship with the addict not to take his behaviours personally. This is one of the hardest challenges for human beings—and that is precisely why it's a core teaching in many wisdom traditions. The addict doesn't engage in his habits out of a desire to betray or hurt anyone else but to escape his own distress. It's a poor choice and an irresponsible one, but it is not directed at anyone else even if it does hurt others. A loving partner or friend may openly acknowledge his or her own pain around the behaviour, but the belief that somehow the addict's actions deliberately betray or wound them only compounds the suffering.

Strange as it may seem, the hardcore drug users I work with are still shocked and tormented by a fellow addict's all-too-predictable patterns. "I'm always there for Joyce, no matter what," says Hal, a heroin and jib user I quoted in Chapter 2. "But every time my cash runs out, she's off with someone else. She keeps borrowing money and I never see it again. It's for food, she says, but it always ends going up her arm. How can she keep doing this to me?"

"I hear you complaining," I reply, "that an addicted human being is behaving like an addicted human being. It feels bad, Hal, I know, but does it surprise you? Do you really believe she is doing it to *you*?"

"I guess not," Hal concedes. But it surprises him every time, and he takes it personally. In his heart he is still a child wishing that the world was different. He'll keep riding the alternately sad and elated merry-go-round of his relationship with Joyce as long as he remains unable to integrate and accept the hurt that his parents could not love him unselfishly, the way he needed to be loved, and that, as a result, he has never learned to accept himself.

—

The addict's childish behaviours and immature emotional patterns virtually invite people around him to take on the role of the stern parent. It's not a genuine invitation and anyone who accepts it, no matter how well intentioned, will soon find herself resisted. No relationship can survive in a healthy form when either partner puts himself or herself in a position of being opposed and resented.

Partners, friends and family are wise to refuse an addict's attempts to recruit them as guardians of his behaviour. Addicts will do this at times, as a way of shifting responsibility onto others. It's a thankless task for those who shoulder it and doomed to failure. In my medical school days I often escaped into television addiction, mindlessly flipping channels without enjoying anything I watched, wasting precious hours and keeping myself awake late into the night. I finally struck on the bright idea of putting a tiny lock into the hole in the prong of the television plug, preventing it from fitting into the socket. I entrusted the key to Rae. "Under no circumstances should you give me the key," I instructed her, "no matter how much I whine, cajole, promise, pester or beg." The inevitable outcome was that I would whine, cajole, promise, pester and beg until Rae capitulated. After a few episodes of this she threw the key at my feet. "Your problem," she said.

I was all the more amused to read Thomas De Quincey's account of how the poet Samuel Taylor Coleridge, his fellow opium user, attempted to impose regulation on his habit by similar means:

> It is notorious that in Bristol he went so far as to hire men—porters, hackney-coachmen, and others—to oppose by force his entrance into any druggist's shop. But, as the authority for stopping him was derived simply from himself, naturally these poor men found themselves in a metaphysical fix . . . And in this excruciating dilemma would occur such scenes as the following:
> "Oh, sir," would plead the suppliant porter—suppliant yet semi-imperative (for equally if he *did,* and he did *not,* show fight, the poor man's daily five shillings seemed endangered)—"really you must not; consider, sir, your wife and—"
> [*Coleridge*]—"Wife! What wife. I have no wife."
> *Porter*—"But really now, you must not sir. Didn't you say no longer ago than yesterday—"
> [*Coleridge*]—"Pooh, pooh! Yesterday is a long time ago. Are you aware, my man, that people are known to have dropped down dead for timely want of opium?"

Porter—"Ay, but you tell't me not to hearken—"

[*Coleridge*]—"Oh, nonsense. An emergency, a shocking emergency, has arisen—quite unlooked for. No matter what I told you in times long past. That which I *now* tell you, is—that if you don't remove that arm of yours from the doorway of this most respectable druggist, I shall have good ground of action against you for assault and battery."[3]

———

The practice of mindful awareness and emotional self-searching is helpful not only for the friends and families of addicted persons, but for everyone who deals with them on any level. It can power-fully enhance the work of health professionals, especially with hard-core drug addicts.

I still laugh when I recall the cocaine- and opiate-dependent Beverly's frank acknowledgment of how she sometimes sees me, her physician. It happened three years ago.

It's Monday morning. I'm in a good mood and Bev is my first patient. "I'm writing a book on addiction," I tell her. "I wonder if I could interview you for it."

Tears well into Beverly's eyes and trickle down over her face where pick marks give her the look of a smallpox survivor. "I would be honoured," she says, "but I'm surprised that you asked me. I imagined you thought of me only as a useless junkie."

"Truth to tell, Bev, some days I do look at you like that. On those days I want only to shut you up, give you a quick prescription and have you out of my office so I can get on with it and see the next junkie. I'm sure, when I'm like that, you must think I'm quite a jerk."

"Well," says Bev slyly, her weeping now turned to mirth, "I could think of worse words than that."

Though not completely surprising, Beverly's comment was a jolt—a useful one. Like many doctors, nurses and others who work with addicts, I can be unmindful of the part that my own attitudes, moods, demeanour and body language play in setting up the inter-action with these so-called "difficult patients." We see their behav-iour but not the messages we telegraph to them. We see their reactions but don't realize that we ourselves may be creating what they are reacting to—not so much by what we say but by who we are being in the process. It is a common enough failing for human beings to be aware of the "what" but not of the "who" or the "how."

In emergency rooms I have witnessed scenarios get completely out of hand to the point where security personnel are called to escort a hostile addict out of the hospital, and yet my observation was that the escalation could have been averted had some of the hospital staff not allowed themselves to become triggered. Once in the Portland staircase I intervened as an overzealous and tense ambulance attendant turned a relatively minor situation with a blood-covered patient into a full-blown confrontation. It was with some difficulty that I convinced him and the police, who had by then arrived, to take a few steps back so I could talk the enraged woman into a calmer state. It didn't take much: just some quiet words and unthreatening body language. At other times, as the reader has seen, I've instigated a negative interaction. Whether I am a soothing presence or one that generates tension depends not on the situation but on my own state of mind. I am responsible.

There's no question that hard-core addicts are a challenging population to work with, challenging because they trigger our judgments and anxieties and because they threaten the comfortable self-image we've worked so hard to establish for ourselves as cool, competent and powerful professionals. They stand quite outside the "nicely-nicely" ethic of respectable middle-class social interaction.

We have seen that addicts lack differentiation—the capacity to maintain emotional separateness from others. They absorb and take personally the emotional states of other people. Their diminished capacity for self-regulation leaves them easily overwhelmed by their automatic emotional mechanisms. They are prone to experience themselves as demeaned and abandoned by authority figures and caregivers, for reasons we have explored. When a busy physician or overworked nurse is short tempered and impatient with them, they interpret it as personal rejection. They react instinctively to the least tension or condescension on the part of caregivers. At the same time, it's only natural that health care workers are especially prone to be stressed and impatient in the harried environments of overfull emergency departments and understaffed hospital wards. Irritability begets defensive hostility, and hostility sets off more reactive anxiety and rage. Two human beings—one who is seeking help and another who is committed to helping—are soon at loggerheads, quite contrary to their own intentions.

There would be much less confrontation and more effective care, I am convinced, if medical and allied staff all took some mindfulness training and if we practised observing, with awareness and curiosity, our mind-states and our reactions to these unconventional people. We would spare ourselves a lot of tension and stress, and protect our patients from further psychological trauma, if we learned to take responsibility for what we bring to our encounters with them. Five minutes of mindful meditation in the middle of a shift in the context of an emergency ward may seem like an absurd luxury, but the time saved and the bruised and inflamed emotions prevented would be a rich payoff. We may not be responsible for another's addiction or the life history that preceded it, but many painful situations could be avoided if we recognized that we are responsible for the way we ourselves enter into the interaction. And that, to put it most simply, means dealing with our own stuff.

With mindful awareness we might still experience judgment arising, but we would accept that as our own problem. When feeling frustrated and angry in response to an uncooperative patient, we would recognize these emotions as our own and understand that we ourselves are fully responsible for how we deal with them. Then we don't have to act out that anger and frustration on a patient or use authoritarian means to defend our self-image from imagined insult.

If we want to open up a healing space for others, we first have to find it in ourselves.

—

"I can find only three kinds of business in the universe: mine, yours, and God's," says the self-work teacher Byron Katie in her book, *Loving What Is,* which deserves to be high on the reading list of anyone who is in a close relationship with an addict. "For me,"

Katie writes, "the word God means *reality*. Anything that's out of my control, your control, and everyone else's control—I call that God's business."

> Much of our stress comes from mentally living out of our own business. When I think, "You need to get a job, I want you to be happy, you should be on time, you need to take better care of yourself," I am in your business . . . I realized that every time in my life that I had felt hurt or lonely, I had been in someone else's business.
>
> If you are living your life and I am mentally living your life, who is here living mine? We're both over there. Being mentally in your business keeps me from being present in my own. I am separate from myself, wondering why my life doesn't work.4

Partners, friends and family, whether despondently or optimistically trying to pressure the addict to change, would do well to remember the immortal words of Yogi Berra: "If the people don't want to come to the ball game, there's nothing you can do to stop them."

—

CHAPTER 34

There Is Nothing Lost:
Addiction and the Spiritual Quest

—

All problems are psychological, but all solutions are spiritual.

THOMAS HORA, M.D.

A barrier for many people when it comes to Twelve Step work around addiction is Step Two, evoking a higher power: [We] *came to believe that a Power greater than ourselves could restore us to sanity.*

The resistance is natural if the Power is identified as the God by whom the child felt betrayed.

Recall the cry of the cocaine- and heroin-dependent Serena after the death of her grandmother. "You know what I think about God? Who is this God that keeps the bad people behind and takes away the good people?" I was familiar with the rage that poured from her. The same anger vibrated in my chest whenever as a child I saw or heard the word God. "What kind of God would let my grandparents be murdered in Auschwitz?" I used to ask, scornful of anyone who accepted the fairy tale of a good and all-powerful Lord. Like Serena, I thought it was the death of a grandparent that embittered me— but I see now that an even greater loss was the loss of faith within my heart.

Children do not understand metaphors. When they hear "God, our Father" they do not know that these words can stand for the love, unity and creative power innate in the universe. They picture an old man somewhere up above the clouds. To Serena, he may even resemble the grandfather who used to rape her.

"The depressed person is a radical, sullen atheist," wrote the French psychotherapist Julia Kristeva."[1] At heart the addict may be the most radical and sullen atheist of all—regardless of what her or his *formal* religious beliefs are. Early stress is a potent inducer of addiction not just because it impairs brain development and emotional growth, but also because it destroys a child's contact with her essential self and deprives her of faith in a nurturing universe. "I had no mother—God forgot me—and I fell," says a doomed young girl of fourteen in Robert Browning's play *A Blot on the 'Scutcheon*. Serena, in her deep depression, lives in cosmic isolation. Her core anguish is that her sense of trust and connection with the infinite within her and without has been severed. Given all she has suffered, the God they told her was all she needed could not hold her faith intact. For any young person, if the deity she hears about is not manifested in the actions of the people who make up her world, the God-word turns into hypocrisy. If she does retain an image of God, it's likely to be the vindictive moralizer who judges her mercilessly or the impotent sky phantom I rejected as a child.

We can see the Power in other ways. In the grip of his habit the addict experiences himself as no more than a puny ego that must scratch and grasp and scrounge for every miserable scrap of satisfaction. Honouring the greater power could simply come in the form of finally recognizing the impotence of that small ego, the utter incapacity of its ways to keep a person safe or calm or happy. "I don't believe in God," a Narcotics Anonymous member told me, "but at least with Step Two I've accepted that I'm not Her."

"When you know yourselves, then you will be known," Jesus told his followers, "and you will understand that you are children of the living father. But if you do not know yourselves, then you dwell in poverty and you are poverty."*

Even as they speak to eternity, the great teachers employ the

* The Gospel of Thomas

language of their particular time, place and culture. The real wisdom is not in the literal meaning but in the spirit of their words. So it is possible to think of "living father" as religious code for the source of life, a reality that exceeds the powers of language to express directly. I believe all of us human beings, whether we know it or not, are seeking our own divine nature. Divine in this context does not mean anything supernatural or necessarily religious, only the truth of our oneness with all that is, an ineffable sense of connectedness to other people and other beings and to each and every shard of matter or spark of energy in the entire universe. When we cease to remember that loving connection and lose touch with our deep yearning for it, we suffer. That is what Jesus meant by poverty. It's also what the contemporary spiritual teacher Eckhart Tolle sees as the fundamental source of human anxiety:

> Basically, all emotions are modifications of one primordial, undifferentiated emotion that has its origin in the loss of awareness of who you are beyond name and form. Because of its undifferentiated nature, it is hard to find a name that precisely describes this emotion. "Fear" comes close, but apart from a continuous sense of threat, it also includes a deep sense of abandonment and incompleteness. It may be best to use a term that is as undifferentiated as that basic emotion and simply call it "pain."[2]

Addiction floods in where self-knowledge—and therefore divine knowledge—are missing. To fill the unendurable void, we become attached to things of the world that cannot possibly compensate us for the loss of who we are.

> *If I forget, thee, O Jerusalem, let my right hand forget her cunning.*
> *If I do not remember thee, let my tongue cleave to the roof of my mouth;*
> *   if I prefer not Jerusalem above my chief joy.*

Is the Biblical psalmist merely vowing fealty to a geographical location in this sacred oath, to man-made buildings and houses of worship? I see another, universal meaning that makes much more sense to me: when I neglect that which is eternal within me,

I detach from the authentic source of my strength and lose my voice. That, I find, is how it goes in life.

In a state of spiritual poverty, we will be seduced by whatever it is that can make us insensate to our dread. That, ultimately, is the origin of the addiction process, since the very essence of that process is the drive to take in from the outside that which properly arises from within. If we "prefer not Jerusalem"—the "City of Peace" within— above our worldly delights, we fixate on external sources of pleasure or power or meaning. The sparser the innate joy that springs from being alive, the more fervently we seek joy's pale substitute, pleasure; the less our inner strength, the greater our craving for power; the feebler our awareness of truth, the more desperate our search for certainty outside of ourselves. The greater the dread, the more vigorous the gravitational pull of the addiction process.

Anything can serve as the object of the addiction process, including religions that promise salvation and freedom. The physical entity called Jerusalem has itself become a fetish for many people of several faiths, with bloodshed and hatred being the consequence. It is no accident that in all major religions the most rigidly fundamentalist elements take the harshest, most punitive line against addicted people. Could it be that they see their own weakness and fear—and false attachments—reflected in the dark mirror addiction holds up to them?

Misplaced attachment to what cannot satiate the soul is not an error exclusive to addicts, but the common condition of mankind. It is this ubiquitous mind-state that leads to suffering and calls prophets, spiritual masters and great teachers into our midst. Our designated "addicts" march at the head of a long procession from which few of us ever step away.

—

For many people, the higher power concept need not be concerned with a deity or anything expressly spiritual. It simply means rising above their self-regarding ego, committing to serve something greater than their own immediate desires. I recall what a speaker at the AA meeting I attended had said. "As you study the Big Book and you serve people and help the community, your heart softens. That's the greatest gift, a soft heart. I wouldn't have believed it."

Our material culture tries to explain even unselfishness as arising from selfish motives. It is often asserted, cynically, that people who act in kindly ways, without any benefit to themselves, are doing so only to feel good. Neuroscience does not support that view: the brain area that lights up as a person performs an altruistic act is not the circuitry activated by pleasure or by the anticipation of reward. According to a recent study, a key contributor to humane behaviour is the posterior superior temporal cortex (pSTC), a region at the back of the brain whose function includes awareness of other people's emotional states.[3] It seems that we are wired to be in tune with one another's needs, which is one of the roots of empathy. "Perhaps altruism did not grow out of a warm-glow feeling of doing good for others, but out of the simple recognition that that thing over there is a person that has intentions and goals. And therefore, I might want to treat them like I might want them to treat myself," said one of the researchers—Scott Huettel, Associate Professor of Psychology at Duke University Medical Center, in Durham, North Carolina. The golden rule may be inscribed in our brain circuits, not as a commandment but as an essential part of who we are.

There is a quality or drive innate in human beings that the Austrian psychiatrist Victor Frankl called our "search for meaning." Meaning is found in pursuits that go beyond the self. In our own hearts most of us know that we experience the greatest satisfaction not when we receive or acquire something but when we make an authentic contribution to the well-being of others or to the social good, or when we create something original and beautiful or just something that represents a labour of love. It is no coincidence that addictions arise mostly in cultures that subjugate communal goals, time-honoured tradition and individual creativity to mass production and the accumulation of wealth. Addiction is one of the outcomes of the "existential vacuum," the feeling of emptiness engendered when we place a supreme value on selfish attainments. "The drug scene," wrote Frankl, "is one aspect of a more general mass phenomenon, namely the feeling of meaninglessness resulting from the frustration of our existential needs which in turn has become a universal phenomenon in our industrial societies."₄ For "drug scene" we can also read: "the gambling scene . . . the eating scene . . . the overwork scene" and many other addictive pursuits.

Human beings, in other words, do not live by bread alone. The higher power, if we wish not to think of it as God or as anything that even remotely smacks of religion, can still be found if we look past ourselves and find some meaningful relationship with the universe outside the confines of our egotistic needs. Judy, interviewed in Chapter 8, continues to live in the Downtown Eastside and is on methadone maintenance for her heroin habit but no longer injects or smokes cocaine. She has found new meaning in providing a service to others, sex trade workers who are still using. She helps keep them safe and offers a kind word and a supportive presence.

We have seen that addiction arises out of dislocation. The absence of meaning is yet another dislocation that we human beings, spiritual creatures that we are, cannot well endure. Meaning has to be defined and found in a personal way by each of us, but as one of Dr. Frankl's Viennese colleagues, Dr. Alfried Längle, said in a recent Vancouver talk, "meaning arises only out of a dialogue with the world." By her daily acts of kindness, Judy keeps herself in a dialogue that helps her transcend addiction.

———

While often expressed as a rational rejection of traditional religious belief, much of people's resistance to the higher power concept is really the ego's resistance to conscience and to spiritual awareness, to the part of us that recognizes truth and wants to honour it. The grasping ego fears its own annihilation in bowing to something greater, whether to "God" or to the needs of others or even to one's own higher needs.

A patient of mine, a former leader (and, possibly, future leader) among his First Nation people, experienced that greater power— and himself as part of it—during a fast he conducted in prison. "This was my second time back in the federal system on a five-year sentence," he recalled. "And what brought me back there was my addiction to substances. While I was in the reception centre I had a really hard time with it, going back having to face all the things that I said I would never have to face again. I went to Edmonton Max, and it was there that I had the most revealing thing come to me in my fast.

"It was on the third day, when I lit my smudge . . . I was fanning, fanning it with my hands and the feather. The smoke and the energy . . . And I felt all the life force through my pores, and that's when I knew right there. Everything had a life. Alcohol. Everything . . . everything that came from mother earth. The leather . . . our clothes . . . what we eat and drink from the earth. Everything is alive. Everything comes alive and has a spirit. Alcohol and drugs have a spirit. When you don't understand that, they have tremendous strength. They will beat you. But it's powerful. It was here before you. Everything was here before you. That's another thing that came to me . . . all these things that are here . . . were here before you. And they're going to be here when I'm gone. So I'm not bringing nothing new to the table. The only thing new to the table is myself. I'm actually the learner. I'm the last in line to learn—to learn to live, to coexist with everything, to adapt to a bigger thing, to the landscape of my life."

"Each carries within himself the all," wrote Joseph Campbell, "therefore it may be sought and discovered within." According to this seminal American writer and lecturer, all heroic myths are prototypes of what is the greatest journey of all, the quest for spiritual truth inside the soul. There is only one story, Campbell showed, only one quest, one adventure, what he called "the monomyth." And there is only one hero, though he or she may appear at different times in different cultures in a thousand guises. The hero is the human being who dares descend into the darkest depths of the unconscious—to the very source of our creative power—and there confronts the monsters thrown up by the fright-stricken infant psyche. As the hero pursues the journey, the phantoms and dragons all vanish or lose power or even become allies.

The psyche of the addict is populated by demons more frightful than those many other people have to face, but if she undertakes the quest, she'll find they are no more real and no more powerful. The reward at journey's end, the treasure the hero has been seeking, is our essential nature. The aim, Campbell asserted, is "to realize that one is that essence; then one is free to wander as the essence in the world. Furthermore, the world too is of that essence. The essence of oneself and the essence of the world: these two are one."[5]

—

Trauma in the strict sense is not required for a young human being to suffer the loss of essence, the sense of oneness with all that is. Infants come into the world fully present and alive to every possibility, but they soon begin to shut down parts of themselves that their environment is unable to recognize or accept with love. As a consequence of that defensive shutdown, says the psychologist and spiritual teacher A.H. Almaas, one or more essential qualities such as love, joy, strength, courage or confidence may be suppressed. In its place, we experience a hole, a sense of empty deficiency. "People don't know that the hole, the sense of deficiency, is a symptom of a loss of something deeper, the loss of essence, which can be regained. They think the hole, the deficiency, is how they really are at the deepest level and that there is nothing beyond it. They think something is wrong with them, something is basically wrong."[6] Such thoughts are not necessarily conscious but may take the form of unconscious beliefs. In either case, we develop behaviour patterns and emotional coping mechanisms to cover up the emptiness, mistakenly believing that the resulting traits represent our true "personality." Indeed, what we call the personality is often a jumble of genuine traits and adopted coping styles that do not reflect our true self at all but the loss of it.

There are people who are not addicts in the strict sense, but only because their carefully constructed "personality" works well enough to keep them from the painful awareness of their emptiness. In such a case, they'll be addicted "only" to a false or incomplete self-image or to their position in the world or to some role into which they sink their energy or to certain ideas that give them a sense of meaning. The human being with a "personality" that is insufficient to paper over the inner void becomes an undisguised addict, compulsively pursuing behaviours whose negative impact is obvious to him or to those around him. The difference is only in the degree of addiction or, perhaps, in the degree of honesty around the deficient self.

Spiritual work and psychological work are both necessary to reclaim our true nature. Without psychological strength, spiritual practice can easily become another addictive distraction from reality. Conversely, shorn of a spiritual perspective we are prone to stay stuck in the limited realm of the grasping ego, even if it's a healthier and more balanced ego. Our soul-needs for meaning and connection remain unsatisfied. Therapy strives to make the deficient self stronger by uncovering the sources of a person's emotional pain and releasing the rigid defensive patterns built up against it. Spiritual exploration ploughs the same ground but is less concerned with "fixing" or improving things than with rediscovering what is whole and has not been absent, just obscured. As Edmund Spenser wrote, "For there is nothing lost but may be found, if sought."[7]

What form of spiritual seeking a person chooses is determined by place, culture, belief and personal inclination. On this question there can be no prescriptions; nor would I be the one to provide them. In retrospect I can see that the God rage I trembled with as a small child was the beginning of my movement toward enlightenment, a goal that I may yet be far from attaining. I may have the equivalent of several Mount Everests left to scale, or perhaps I have only to reach out with my little finger to rend the veil of illusion between my soul and the most sacred realities. I cannot know and it's useless to speculate. Being on the path is what's important and we each need to tread a path on our own, no matter how many may have walked it before us. "Be a lamp onto yourselves," the Buddha advised his followers, just as Jesus taught his disciples to seek the Kingdom of God within. I have found a way that feels right to me and I look to the teaching wherever I recognize it. The world has never lacked great spiritual guides, precepts and practices, but surely it has had a shortage of people willing to learn.

—

The ego's tragic flaw is to mistake form for substance, surface illusion for reality. As long as the ego rules, we are all like the Hebrews who wandered the desert on their way to the Promised Land, "a stiff-necked people." We keep rejecting truth, bow to the Golden Calf and scorn what would save us. As the present state of the planet indicates, we're not fast learners, we human beings. Each generation must absorb the same lessons over and over again, groping its blind way through the realm of the Hungry Ghosts. The truth is within, which is why outward-directed attempts to fill in the void created when we lose touch with it cannot bring us closer to the serenity we long for. Late in the fourth century Augustine, Bishop of Hippo in what is present-day Algeria, wrote in his *Confessions* a passage that could be read today at any Twelve-Step gathering:

> Unaware of my own needs, I resisted what would make me less needy . . . yet starvation did not make me hungry since my system rejected spiritual nourishment—I was not fed with it, and the more I starved, the more would nourishment make me queasy. My soul, sick and covered with sores, lunged outward instead, in a mad desire to scratch itself against some physical relief.[8]

Spiritual awakening is no more and no less than a human being claiming his or her own full humanity. People who find themselves have no need to turn to addiction, or to stay with it. Armed with compassion, we recognize that addiction was the answer—the best answer we could find at one time in our lives—to the problem of isolation from our true selves and from the rest of creation. It's also what keeps us gloomy, sad and angry. Not the world, not what's outside of us, but what we hold inside traps us. We may not be responsible for the world that created our minds, but we can take responsibility for the mind with which we create our world. The addicted mind can project only a universe of grasping and alienation. "I just knew my little world and what I wanted was what I revolved around," the newly abstinent cocaine user Judy once said. Many of us conduct our lives just in that way. It's for us to choose consciously what world and what future we wish to live in.

Once a student's eyes are open, instructors appear everywhere. Everything can teach us. Our most painful emotions point to our greatest possibilities, to where our authentic nature is hidden.

People whom we judge are our mirrors. People who judge us call forth our courage to respect our own truth. Compassion for ourselves supports our compassion for others. As we open to the truth within, we hold safe a space of healing for others. They may do the same for us.

Healing occurs in a sacred place located within us all: "When you know yourselves, then you will be known."

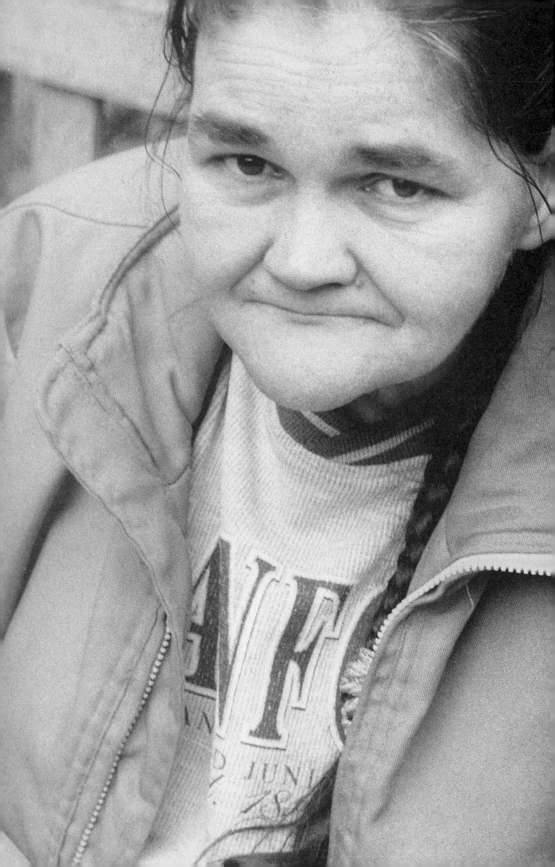

Memories and Miracles: An Epilogue

—

From hidden resources the miracle of survival renews itself with surprising force, as a geyser springs from underground waters through bare earth, shale and ice.

Standing by my desk one morning is Howard, leaning on a crutch to support his left leg. He is a burly, forty-year-old man whose adult life has been one prolonged jail sentence after another—twenty-two years in all. His childhood was a variation on a familiar theme.

Howard's heroin-addicted mother was forced to leave her reserve after she married a Caucasian; she disappeared forever shortly before her son's third birthday. He spent the next four years with his grandmother. "She gave me the most beautiful home," he says. "I carry her in my heart. She's the only reason why I'm still alive." The grandmother died young, and with her died the little boy's one earthly source of unconditional love and protection. Between his seventh year and his first prison term Howard's course took him from one foster home or institution to another, beaten or sexually abused wherever he went.

Howard tells his story during a methadone visit, the first since his recent brief hospitalization for a knee fracture and another weekend in prison for having missed a parole appointment. He wipes away tears as he mentions his grandmother and then says, "Enough," with an abrupt shift of tone from despondence to determination. "I have to give something back. I need to get off drugs. I didn't go through all that for no purpose. I could be dead in a year and nobody would know I was ever here. I must give something back. I learned a lot in jail, and if I can keep just one child from going down the same road . . ."

"You need help yourself first," I suggest.

"Yeah, I'll go for that now. My head always told me that I have to figure it out all myself. I can't."

Whether we see this man's history as defeat or triumph is a matter of perspective. He has risen through depths of despair most of the society that ostracizes him cannot begin to fathom, and there is still spirit in him that wants to contribute, to create meaning and to affirm life. I don't know if his future will see that spirit manifested in action, but its very existence is a miracle.

Later that morning little wizened Penny scampers into my office, followed by her hefty friend Beverly. Since the death of Penny's common-law husband, Brian, she and Beverly have been inseparable. I often see them together on Hastings: Penny shuffles her feet rapidly in small steps, her hunched back bent over her walker, and Bev ambles with heavy gait at her side. Today, as an unseasonable November snowfall drifts down from a leaden sky and blankets the street below, the two women can scarcely contain their excitement and their eagerness to share some glad tidings.

—

Brian's terminal liver cancer from hepatitis C was confirmed in the early summer of 2005, on the same day that I admitted Penny to St. Paul's Hospital with a spinal infection that would keep her on intravenous antibiotics for six months. It's a day I won't forget. The two of them lay in emergency a few beds apart. As I spoke with Brian, Penny's pain-driven, demented shrieking could be heard throughout the ward.

"I've had my CAT scan," Brian said. "You were right, they told me I have a few months to live. They're sending me to palliative care. When can I leave hospital?"

Beneath his sweat-beaded forehead matted with damp and tousled red hair, Brian's sunken eyes shone out from his gaunt, bearded face. He was emaciated from his silent battle with cancer. Not until his swollen liver bloated his belly and made it hard as a drum did he complain to me of pain. He asked, so I had to tell him that even "a few months" seemed overly optimistic to me.

"You want to be discharged as soon as your pain is under control?"

"Yeah, got things to do. Want to reconnect with my family."

"Where are they?"

"All over. I've got six kids—four living, two dead . . . I never told you about them? One died in a car accident; one got murdered. The fucker shot him over a lousy fifteen hundred dollars. I would've given him the money."

"Was it over drugs?"

"Yeah, that's what he was into. Wanted to be like the old man, I guess. I was in jail at the time. He was twenty-one."

"So the others, do you have any idea where they are?"

"Yeah, they shouldn't be that hard to find. Haven't spoken to any of them for twenty years, though . . . Penny, how is she, Doc?"

"I just saw her. As you can hear, she is in a lot of pain."

"She's going to make it, though?"

"She'll make it. The abscess in her spine could be affecting her brain now, but she'll make it. I'll look after her . . . Brian, are you as calm as you appear to be or are you pretending?"

"It's just another step, Doc. I came close a couple of times before. I've been shot at and stabbed and OD'd. I don't know . . . I'm not looking forward to it, I'll tell you that much. But I'm not afraid of it. If there's something there, there's something there. If there isn't, there isn't. We won't know till we get there. I prefer to believe there is."

A few weeks later Brian became the first of three patients in my practice to die of liver cancer within a period of four months. In his early fifties, he was the oldest. Stevie was the second; in her final days she used the subcutaneous infusion line inserted by the home nurses for pain relief purposes to inject herself with heroin. "I might as well go out singing," she said. I was okay with that—heroin is as good an analgesic as morphine. So Stevie went, skin and eyeballs bright yellow, shooting and smiling to the end. Several times a day she pulled the string on the mechanical, musical bear on her bed-side table and watched him cavort, wiggling his head, arms and butt to "Hey! Macarena."

On my rounds through the Downtown Eastside hotels I've seen that many of the women have large, soft teddy bears to hug. One sex trade worker keeps a collection of several hundred, stuffed in every corner of her tiny, dark room. The largest one is the size of a child. Stevie, with her characteristic exuberance, owned the only dancing bear.

Quiet, reclusive Cory was the third with hepatic cancer to go, just a few days after Stevie. "I've been partying too much and it's caught up with me," he said laconically on learning of his terminal illness. The time between Cory's diagnosis and death was little more than a week. He asked me to be present as he called his sister in Ireland to tell her he wouldn't be flying home to die. We used the speaker phone in my office. The sister spoke her questions with a musical, soft Irish lilt, answered by Cory's hoarse whisper.

"How you doin', baby. How are you, love. Are you okay, pet?"

"Bad news, Shany, bad news."

"Bad news, Cory. So when are you comin' home, pet? Tell the truth now."

"I'm not comin' home, Shany. Too much pain. I just decided yesterday. It's too painful. But I got good help here."

"Are you strong in yourself?"

"I'm okay that way."

"Cory, I want to come and hug and kiss you, pet. I want a hug."

"Yeah, me too, baby."

"I'll try to come very, very soon. We love you very, very much, Cory. And we're praying for you, Cory. I'll try to remember all the great times and how much you enjoyed your life. We have to remember all the good things. "

"Yeah, and I can get buried over there. You can bring me over there to get buried."

"Oh, yes, we'll bring you over here to bury you. We will, indeed, Cory. We will indeed, we'll bring you home, love. We really will bring you home, don't you be worried about that."

"No."

"I'll play good music for you, Cory. The best for you, Cory. We have great musicians and singers here in Derry."

"Yeah, play 'A Whiter Shade of Pale.'"

"What's that?"

I had intervened in the conversation only occasionally to clarify one clinical point or another. Now Cory, fatigued, motions me to the phone. "He would like you to play 'A Whiter Shade of Pale,'" I say.

"'A Whiter Shade of Pale.' I will do that for him."

"By Procol Harum," Cory croaks.

"I'll get that for you, Cory, and we have some lovely Irish music with some lovely instruments and we have all the great singers here during Mass on a Sunday in our cathedral, and I will bring them all down for you."

By now Cory was too uncomfortable to continue, either due to physical pain or emotional tension. He said his goodbyes to his sister and left the room. Shany and I went through the medical history and the dire prognosis. At that time she was still hoping to visit her brother.

"To tell you the truth," I said to Shany before our farewell, "after what you said about the singers in Derry, I'd like to be buried at your cathedral myself. Too bad I'm Jewish."

"Well, we could do a Jewish one for you, too. . . . Now what was that song he wanted again?"

"'A Whiter Shade of Pale' by Procol Harum." I spelled out the name of the group.

"I have to write it down, because my brain isn't working . . . I'll get on the ball with that for him. Oh, God, we're devastated. It's just torture. But I'm so happy to have spoken with you. I can hear the kindness. I can see he is in good hands."

"I can see how much he is loved over there, too."

"Yes, you have no idea how much he is loved. What a lovely boy he was . . . and then the addiction got the better of him."

That conversation took place on a Friday. Cory died in his room at the Portland Sunday evening. Many friends came to his wake, as did his ex-wife and son and daughter. Great stories were told. He is missed, gentle soul that he was. And the gap left by Stevie in everyone's hearts will not be filled. Her life, too, was a miracle. If, after all she had endured, it took drugs for her to be able to laugh and sing that life, who is to be her judge?

—

Nearly two years after his death, Penny continues to mourn Brian. "You always will," I tell her. The friendship with Beverly has been a godsend for Penny. Today, as I look at Bev's beaming face I note with surprise that the pick marks that chronically disfigure it have cleared—the relationship with Penny has done her a world of good, too.

"My son has called me," says Bev breathlessly. "He called me. He's going to drive here from Alberta and take me home for Christmas. And Penny's coming with me. He said it was okay to bring someone."

Beverly hasn't spoken with this son, a twenty-four-year-old who lives with his wife and two young children in a small Prairie town, for three years. She hasn't seen him for seven. "He wants his mom home for Christmas, can you believe it? I'll see my granddaughters."

Penny goes outside to have a smoke after hearing my assurance that all their medications will be arranged for the trip, including Beverly's HIV drugs and the methadone they both take.

"I was only worried about one thing," says Bev. "My former husband lives at my son's place. When he heard I was coming, he phoned and asked if I'd get back together with him. 'You crazy?' I said. 'What for? So I could be your doormat again? Your whipping post? Your punching bag? No thanks.' Penny will be with me. He won't do nothin' when someone else is around . . . I told my son she's my nurse."

"Don't do that," I suggest. "Don't lie. It will ruin your visit. You want to feel close with your son? Don't begin with a lie."

"You're right," Bev laughs. "But I'm so excited. My son wants his Mom home for Christmas. He's driving all the way here to get me . . . I know I'm crying. It's because I'm so happy. I never thought I'd be so happy ever again."

Beverly smiles through her tears and looks at me expectantly. She wants something. I note a slight twinge of resistance in my chest and quickly let it go. I remove the stethoscope from my neck and stand up as Beverly, too, rises from her chair. She sobs. We wrap our arms around each other in a wordless embrace.

—

On my way out through the downstairs lobby of the Portland I'm called into a side room, where Jerry lies panting on a bench by the wall. He clenches his right fist over his heart. Jerry is fifty-four, with coronary disease and a quadruple bypass. The cocaine he smokes regularly is not the best medicine for a man with a cardiac condition and a history of heart attacks. At present he is experiencing chest heaviness, with pain radiating down the left arm. He was discharged from the emergency ward last night with the same complaint—it's a flare-up of his angina. I examine him and send to a nearby pharmacy for nitroglycerin spray. As we await the courier's return, pregnant Clarissa rushes in and slumps down on the bench at Jerry's feet. She weeps and wails incoherently. Hopped on cocaine, she is emotionally overwrought following a loud verbal street altercation with her boyfriend, father of her child-to-be. I could hear them in the background even while I auscultated Jerry's heart sounds and lungs with my stethoscope.

Clarissa hasn't yet followed up on any of the prenatal care appointments we've arranged. The ultrasound showed she is seventeen weeks along, past the date for an early abortion. A late termination remains an option, but she's unlikely to choose that, having heard the infant's heartbeat during the ultrasound procedure. More precisely, she'll keep herself too wasted to decide anything. It will all just happen. We'd better prepare the staff for another Celia scenario, I say to myself. I comfort Clarissa briefly, until she is led away by another resident, who promises her "something to make you feel better." With her companion she walks toward the elevator, swaying in her high-heeled shoes, her jean-skirt leaving her bare thighs half-exposed. That's how she stood this morning on some street corner in the November chill.

Jerry's discomfort eases with the nitro, and I head for the exit once again. From behind his desk Sam, the senior staff worker, points to the entranceway between the hotel's outside gate and inner door. There stands Kenyon leaning on his cane, his body bent like a question mark. Blood dripping from his head forms a pattern of small, discrete droplets on the floor—a good sign; he's unlikely to have suffered a deep wound. "Three hundred assaults in four years," he keens, drawing out the vowels, his high-pitched voice now intensified by outrage and pain. "And this guy pushed me down 'cause I didn't have any tens or twenties when he robbed me. All I had was a dollar-fifty in change, so he ground my head into the cement . . . Three hundred assaults. You are my witness."

I recall that only last week Kenyon had requested an increase in his dose of imipramine, an antidepressant. "Because of my dreams," he said. "They make me cry."

"You're having bad dreams?"

"No, I'm having good dreams. I dream I'm back on the Prairies, with a home and a wife and children. Then I wake up to find I'm still here, in the Downtown Eastside. And I start to cry. I want more medication so I don't have to cry so much."

With gloved hand I part Kenyon's greying hair and discover a small, oozing scalp laceration. "It's okay," I tell him. "You don't need any stitches. You'll be all right." I give Sam the necessary instructions and step outside into the wind-blown, grey mid-afternoon.

On the Hastings Street sidewalk, under the tread of passersby the fresh-fallen snow has already turned to an icy slush.

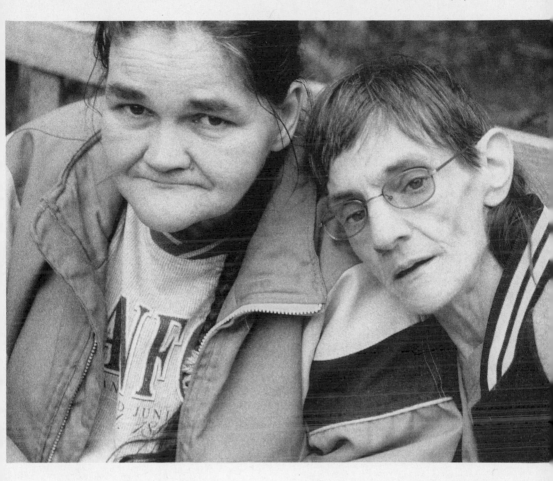

Postscript

Penny died on April 23, 2007, at St. Paul's Hospital, of a massive hemorrhage, owing to an inoperable rupture of her esophagus. She was fifty-two years old. "If I get out of this alive, I'll stop using coke," she told me a few days before her death—but she never did quit; almost to her last moments she begged people to smuggle cocaine to her hospital room.

"On her best friend Bev's advice, we will have cupcakes and grape soda following the service," said the announcement for her memorial event.

Adoption and Twin Study Fallacies

The weighted emphasis on genetic causation in medical literature, particularly when it comes to mental dysfunctions and addictions, is astonishing
given the shaky logic on which the supporting studies are based. As one
review stated:

> A critical analysis of the assumptions of any adoption or twin study, coupled
> with the succession of retractions of the genetic linkage studies indicates
> that the evidence for the genetic basis of mental illnesses is far from
> overwhelming.[1]

The two assumptions on which the heavily gene-based estimates in
addiction medicine rely are not sustainable if we examine them closely.
They are:

1. that studies of adopted children can distinguish genetic from environmental effects
2. that we can separate out genetic from environmental effects by
   looking at the similarities and differences between identical twins
   on the one hand, and fraternal twins on the other

A prominent researcher in the field of mental illness, including addiction, sums up this line of reasoning:

> Twin and adoption studies provide convincing evidence for significant
> genetic effects on virtually all major psychiatric disorders. *Therefore, genes
> that affect risk for these disorders must exist somewhere on the human genome.*[2]

The problem is insidiously circular: for someone to look at these studies and perceive convincing evidence of genetic causality, one already has to have accepted the idea that genes *cause*.

Why have geneticists chosen adoption studies as testing grounds for genetic effects? To understand this, imagine a regular (nonadoption) family situation, in which a child has been brought up in his family of biological origin. If a parent and child have the same disorder, that condition may, of course, have been passed on through genes. So far so good—but since it's obvious that children can be influenced by their parents in many other ways, the mere incidence of an ailment "running in the family" does not necessarily point to a genetic cause. For example, if one of my children went to medical school, it wouldn't necessarily establish that wanting to be a doctor is a hereditary disorder. As a leading behavioural geneticist points out, "because parents share family environment as well as heredity with their offspring, parent-offspring resemblance does not prove the existence of genetic influence."[3]

This is where adoption comes in. If a child is adopted, so the argument goes, he brings with him the genes he received from his parents but is now being raised in an entirely different environment. If he still manifests the same disorder that afflicted his birth father or mother, then that condition must be genetic. *If* we accept this logic and *then* look at the findings of adoption studies, an addiction like alcoholism will appear to be induced to a large degree by genetic inheritance—but that, upon inspection, is a rather enormous "if."

In Chapter 19 we saw how prenatal stresses affect the developing brain. To conclude from adoption studies that a predisposition to alcoholism "runs in the family" and must, therefore, be genetic is to ignore all this evidence of environmental effects before birth.

Then, not all adoptions take place immediately at birth. In the largest, most oft-quoted and perhaps most influential study "proving" a genetic cause for alcoholism, the adopted children stayed with their parent (or parents) of origin for up to three years; the mean age of adoption was eight months. This study, which compared the adopted children of alcoholic biological parents with those of nonalcoholic parents, concluded that the biological father's alcoholism had the greatest effect on the subsequent alcoholism of the male offspring.[4] Even if that is so, it doesn't necessarily indicate a genetic cause.

Given the long-term effects of prenatal stress and the dominant influence of the environment on brain development following birth, is it surprising that infants of alcoholic biological fathers would also have a greater propensity to drink? We know from the Adverse Childhood Experiences (ACE) Study that alcoholism is associated with many other traumatic circumstances—for example, either parent being alcoholic increases the chance of the mother being battered by a factor of thirteen.[5] When we consider what it's like for a woman to live with an alcoholic male partner—the insecurity she experiences through the pregnancy and beyond, and the abuse she may be subjected to—we can see that the stresses on such a woman, both before and after birth, would have been greater than the stresses on most other pregnant women. Furthermore, if a child spent the first months of his or her life—and possibly the first three years—under such circumstances, it would mean that by the time he was adopted, his attachment-reward, incentive-motivation and self-regulation systems would have been significantly impaired, along with his stress-response mechanisms. Such a study can tell us nothing about genetic effects. Similar objections, and a wide range of others, could be made—and have been made—to the other adoption studies.[6]

Twin studies are accepted to be the gold standard of genetic surveys of human populations. Many genetic researchers believe that we can separate the effects of genes from those of the environment by comparing identical with fraternal twin pairs. The underlying belief is that identical and fraternal twin pairs both share the same environment to the same degree. As a geneticist who has done many twin studies admits, "our twin models assume that the exposure to relevant environmental factors was similar in monozygotic and dizygotic* twins."[7] As we will now see, this is a completely unwarranted assumption.

Identical twins share the same genes; fraternal twins share some genes in common, but no more than any other pair of nonidentical siblings: about 50 per cent. A pair of identical twins, goes the argument, share not only genes but exactly the same environment—unless they are adopted by different families. Fraternal twins, being born at

---

* Monozygotic: same egg, same sperm, producing identical twins. Dizygotic: two different eggs and two different sperm, producing nonidentical twins.

the same time to the same parents, also share the same environment but not the same genes. Therefore, goes the logic, any differences between such kinds of pairs *must* be genetic. Indeed, in twin studies of addiction the similarities in findings—known in technical language as concordance—between identical twins are consistently high as compared with the concordance for fraternal twins. That is, identical twins are more likely to share an addiction than are fraternal twins. In alcoholism, for example, the concordance for identical twins is about twice the rate for fraternal twins: a result which, according to a review article, "is consistent with addictive genetic factors."[8]

But this finding is at least equally consistent with environmental factors. It's very obviously untrue that members of fraternal twin pairs share the environment to the same degree as identical twins. Far from it.

First, the fraternal twins are physiologically as different from each other as any pair of siblings. Whatever they experience, they will experience differently. If one, for example, is constitutionally highly sensitive, she will feel and absorb the effects of the same event more acutely than her "tougher" sibling, from early in the uterus and throughout childhood. Differences in temperament may also exist between identical twins, but not nearly to the same degree.

Second, recall that by far the most important aspect of the nurturing environment is the emotional interaction with the parent. Even with the best of love and good will, parents are much more likely to respond in the same way to identical twins than to nonidentical ones. For example, will a father or mother really look in the same way at nonidentical twins with different genders and temperaments? Will the parent use the same tone of voice or play in the same way with, say, a smaller female child than with her larger and more robust male sibling, or vice versa? On a deeper level, will the parents project the same fears, hopes and expectations on the children? Clearly not: each child represents something different to each parent and that means these two children do not grow up under identical conditions. They don't share the same formative environment—not in the home and not on the playground or in school where nonidentical twins are much more likely to have very different peers and experiences than identical twins. So the assumption that you can tell genetic from environmental effects by comparing identical with nonidentical twin pairs also collapses.

Identical twins share the environment much more extensively than any nonidentical pair possible can.*

That leaves one final line of defence for the genetically minded: twin studies in which identical twins are separated at birth and brought up in different families, neither family being the biological one. Surely here the similarities must be all genetic, the differences environmental. The two members of such a twin pair live in different families and are therefore exposed to different environments, while obviously, they continue to have the same genes. It follows that any similarities *must* be dictated by genes and any differences, by their rearing environment. So, at least, a genetic perspective would dictate. Thus the platinum standard of genetic studies is ostensibly provided by studies of identical twins who are adopted and brought up by different parents, in different families. We are back to adoption, and the genetic argument is no sounder here than it was before.

It's not the case that identical twins brought up by different adoptive parents did not share the same formative environment. They spent nine months in the same uterus, exposed to the same diet, same hormones and same "messenger" chemicals. At birth they were both separated from the birth mother—the very opposite of the natural agenda which has the mammalian infant immediately latch onto the mother's breast. By birth infants are sensitized to their mother's biorhythms, voice, heartbeat, energy. Being torn away from that familiar environment adds trauma to the profound but necessary shock of being expelled from the uterus.** We know from animal studies that early weaning can have an influence on later substance intake: rat pups weaned from their mothers at two weeks of age had, as adults, a greater propensity to drink alcohol than pups weaned just a week later, at three weeks of age.⁹ No wonder that adopted children are generally more vulnerable to various developmental disorders—for example, ADHD—that increase the risk for addiction. No wonder that many adults who were adopted as infants harbour a powerful

* In point of fact, not even identical twins necessarily have exactly the same environment. I have seen subtly but significantly different mothering given to a pair of identical twins.

** Twins also form a bond to each other, sharing the same womb. Separation from each other would also deal a significant, even if unconscious, blow.

and lifelong sense of rejection or that among adoptees the adolescent suicide risk is double that of nonadopted children.[10]

Finally, we have seen the pivotal necessity of a consistently present, emotionally available parenting caregiver for proper brain development. But in some studies the adoption does not happen immediately after birth—the infants may be in a hospital, cared for by nurses who work, at most, twelve-hour shifts and who come and go in the infant's life with bewildering irregularity. Other adoptees are cared for by foster parents, only to lose those familiar faces at the moment of adoption. Taking all these factors into account, the assumption of a nonshared formative environment is lopsided, to say the least. All in all, identical twins slated for adoption have shared major environmental influences *before* the adoption takes place.

There is one more important environmental factor at play here. The world is much more likely to respond in similar ways to identical twins— same gender, same inherited tendencies and identical physical features— than to fraternal twins, who may be of different gender and have very different looks and very different reactivity patterns. In other words, for identical twins the environmental factors are still more likely to be similar, even after adoption into different families.

Thus, adoption studies of identical twins can tell us much less about genetic effects than researchers have taken for granted.

Even the authors of another influential twin alcoholism study, who lean strongly toward genetic interpretations, wrote that "at this point we are not certain that *anything* is inherited."[11]

A Close Link: Attention Deficit Disorder and Addictions

The reader may have noticed that many of the patients I have described or quoted in this book have lifelong histories of attention deficit (hyperactivity) disorder, also known as ADHD (or ADD, if the hyperactivity trait is not present). It is common practice, although a bit confusing, to use the two acronyms interchangeably. For the sake of simplicity I'll employ ADHD as the defining term here, as long as we keep in mind that the hyperactivity may or may not be present. In addicted males especially, it often is.

Diagnosing ADHD in cocaine and amphetamine addicts is tricky, because the drugs themselves will drive physical and mental hyperactivity and disorganization. Under the influence of cocaine or crystal meth, a normally sedate person may resemble someone with severe ADHD. The other complicating factor is that, from adolescence onward, people with ADHD are at an elevated risk for addiction to cocaine and other stimulants. It becomes difficult to sort out what came first: addiction or ADHD. Having attention deficit disorder myself, I have an intuitive feel for recognizing the condition in others, but the diagnostic key is the history of ADHD symptoms since childhood, predating the drug use.

ADHD is a major predisposing factor for addiction, but it is frequently missed by physicians. I have been struck by how often addicted patients of mine with self-evident ADHD traits have eluded diagnosis throughout childhood and well into their adult years. Some others were diagnosed as children but never seem to have received consistent treatment. In very few cases have any of them been treated for the condition as adults. A Yale University study has shown that among cocaine users with ADHD, those who are treated only for their addiction but not for their predisposing ADHD don't do as well. In this Yale study as many as 35 per cent of cocaine users who presented for treatment met the diagnostic criteria for childhood ADHD.[1] In another study, as many as 40 per cent of adult alcoholics were found to have underlying attention deficit (hyperactivity) disorder.[2] People with ADHD are twice as likely as others to fall into substance abuse and nearly four times as likely as others to move from alcohol to other psychoactive drugs.[3] People with ADHD are also more likely to smoke, to gamble and to have any number of other addictive behaviours. Among crystal meth addicts a significant minority, 30 per cent or more, also have lifelong ADHD.[4]

The link between ADHD and a *predisposition* to addiction is obvious and, in fact, inevitable. The connection has little to do with genetics. ADHD is no more inherited genetically than addiction is, despite the widespread assumption among ADHD experts that it's "the most heritable of all mental disorders." The same facts that make twin and adoption studies largely irrelevant to the understanding of addiction also discredit the genetic theories regarding ADHD. There's no need to repeat them here. The basic point is that ADHD and addictive tendencies both arise out of stressful early childhood experience. Although there is likely some genetic *predisposition* toward ADHD, a predisposition is far from the same as a *predetermination*. Two children with similar predispositions will not automatically develop the same way—once more, the environment is decisive.

The brain developmental information regarding ADHD is presented in my book *Scattered Minds: A New Look at the Origins and Healing of Attention Deficit Disorder.** Scientific findings since then have only confirmed that pre- and post-natal stresses are the most important determinants of this condition. According to one recent study, for example, 22 per cent of ADHD symptoms in eight- and nine-year-old children can be directly linked to maternal anxiety during pregnancy.[5] Abused children are far more likely than others to be diagnosed with ADHD, and the same brain structures affected by childhood trauma are most consistently abnormal in scans of children with ADHD.[6]

---

* Published in the U.S. as *Scattered: How Attention Deficit Disorder Originates and What You Can Do About It*. Although the content is exactly the same, I regard the U.S. title as an unfortunate simplification, an example of pop-style can-do self-helpism.

My point is not that abuse is the cause of ADHD, although it certainly increases the risk for it, but that early childhood stress is the major factor—abuse being only an extreme form of childhood stress. It is the impact of early stress on the brain—maternal depression, for example—that creates vulnerability to ADHD and to addictions. Stresses or interruptions in the infant–mother relationship lead to permanent alterations in the dopamine systems of the mid-brain and prefontal cortex, disturbances that are implicated in both ADHD and in substance abuse and other addictions.[7] If the prevalence of ADHD and other childhood developmental problems is rising in our society, it is not because of "bad parenting," but because the burgeoning stresses on the parenting environment appear to increase with each successive generation. Parents, and mothers in particular, are getting less and less of the support they need during their children's early years. The issue is not one of individual parental failure, but rather of a social and cultural breakdown of cataclysmic proportions.

ADHD and addiction have much in common, both in their characteristics and in their neurobiology. They are both disorders of self-regulation. They both involve abnormal dopamine activity—in fact, the medications used to treat ADHD are stimulants like methylphenidate (Ritalin, Concerta) or amphetamines (Dexedrine, Adderall), whose method of action is to increase dopamine activity in important brain circuits.[8] The personality traits of people with ADHD and addiction are often identical: poor self-regulation, deficient impulse control, poor differentiation and a constant need to find distractions from distressing internal states. These distractions can be internal, as in tuning out, or external, as in the need to be stimulated by activities, food, other people or substances.

Thus people with ADHD are predisposed to self-medicate.

The implications are twofold. First, it is important to recognize ADHD and to treat it appropriately in childhood. As I point out in *Scattered Minds*, such treatment need not involve medication in every case, and in no case should medications be the only treatment. ADHD is not a disease, inherited or otherwise; it is primarily a problem of development. The key question is not how to control symptoms but how to help the child develop properly. That is the brunt of my argument in *Scattered Minds*, and I need not say more on it here. It is distressing to know, however, that most of the children diagnosed with ADHD are treated only with medication. Pharmacological treatment does have its place in treating both adults and children, but especially with the latter it should be used cautiously and rarely as the first-line approach. Nevertheless, the studies are clear that those children with ADHD who are not treated are at higher risk for later addictions than those who receive stimulants.[9] This makes sense, of course, since on one level all substance addictions are attempts to self-medicate. According to one study, 32 per cent of adolescents who began to use methamphetamine (crystal meth) between the ages of ten and fifteen did so for the drug's calming effect.[10] Even among rats, the most hyperactive are the ones most likely to self-administer stimulants.[11]

Second, when treating adults with any addiction, it is important to look for the possible coexistence of untreated ADHD. From my own personal experience and also from having worked with hundreds of ADHD adults even prior to taking on my current position in the Downtown Eastside, I know that addressing ADHD issues can be a great help to people struggling with addiction. Obversely, anyone treating adults or adolescents with ADHD must also look for addictive behaviours. It is not possible to treat ADHD successfully if we ignore addictions that may exacerbate the underlying disorder. This is so whether the person is addicted to substances or to one of several of the many behavorial addictions that our culture makes readily available and may even present in a glamorous light.

The Prevention of Addiction

A word about prevention, which is often teamed with harm reduction, treatment and law enforcement as one of the four pillars of social policy toward addiction. In practice, only the fourth—and least helpful— of these so-called four pillars receives unquestioned and generous financial support from governments.

The prevention of substance abuse needs to begin in the crib, and even before then, in the social recognition that nothing is more important for the future of our culture than the way children develop. There has to be much more support for pregnant women. Early prenatal visits should be an opportunity not only for blood tests, physical exams and nutritional advice, but also for a stress inventory in the woman's life. All possible resources should be mobilized to help her experience a pregnancy that is emotionally, physically and economically as stress-free as possible. Employers and governments need to appreciate the crucial importance of these gestational months to the infant's developmental well-being and, even more so, the crucial importance of the first months following birth and the first years. From any point of view—psychological, cultural or economic—that is the most cost effective approach. Children who are emotionally well nurtured and brought up in stable communities do not need to become addicts.

In my family practice days I often found myself in the ludicrous position of having to write letters explaining why it would be preferable, say, for a woman to stay at home a few months longer after the birth of her infant so that she can continue to breast feed. Our society has become so detached from this natural physiological and emotional parenting activity that it has to be justified on medical grounds. Rather than pressuring new parents—mothers or fathers—to return to work quickly, we should not spare resources to help them remain with their children for as long as possible, if that is their preference, during the crucial early developmental period. The financial savings to society would be enormous, not to mention the human benefits. If, on the other hand, early daycare is either unavoidable or happens to be the preferred option, we need to ensure that these facilities have the trained staff and the resources to provide not just physical care, but also emotional nourishment. That ought to be the case not only in daycare but throughout the child's education.

In the case of at-risk families, the benefits of early intervention in the form of supportive home nursing visits have been well established. Such programs need to be far more broadly available, given the many troubled families in our society.

When it comes to drug education, most governments appear to view prevention largely as a matter of informing people, especially young people, that drugs are bad for them. A worthy objective, certainly, but like all behavioural programs, this form of prevention is highly unlikely to make a significant impact. The reason is that the children who are at greatest risk are the least open to hearing the message, and even if they do hear it, they are the least capable of conforming to it. Intellectual knowledge, while important, is a poor competitor for deep-seated emotional and psychological drives. If this is true for many adults, it's even more so for children.

Children who have been abused by adults or are for any other reason alienated from adults, do not look to grownups for advice, modelling or information. And yet, as we have seen, these are the children most prone to substance use. We have witnessed the same problem with attempts to prevent or eliminate bullying: the dynamics of bullying or victimhood are rooted deep in a wounded child's psyche. This is why moral preaching and the plethora of antibullying programs have little or no impact on the growing bullying tendencies among youth. Programs aimed at changing or preventing behaviours always fail if they do not address the psychological dynamics that drive the behaviours in question.

If schools and other childrearing institutions are to engage in drug education with a view to prevention, they need first to create an emotionally supportive relationship between teachers and students in which the latter feel understood, accepted and respected. Only in such an atmosphere can the necessary information be transmitted effectively and only in such an atmosphere will young people develop enough trust to turn to adults with their problems and concerns.

All adults concerned with the care of young people need to remember that only healthy, nurturing relationships with adults will prevent kids from becoming lost in the peer world—a loss of orientation that leads rapidly to drug use.*

* See Chapter 23.

APPENDIX IV

The Twelve Steps

Although I have not been an active participant in Twelve-Step programs, I see great value in the process they prescribe and recognize their effectiveness in helping many people to live in sobriety—or at least in abstinence. As explained in Chapter 32, abstinence is the disciplined avoidance of an addictive substance or behaviour. Sobriety is developing a mind state focused not on staying away from something bad, but on living a life led by positive values and intentions. It means living in the present moment, neither driven by ghosts of the past nor lulled and tormented by fantasies and fears of the future.

The steps listed below are the classical ones suggested in the Big Book of Alcoholics Anonymous and they form the basis of all Twelve-Step programs. My comments are in italics.

1. We admitted we were powerless over alcohol [or narcotics or cocaine or eating or gambling and so on]—that our lives had become unmanageable.

Step One accepts the full negative impact of the addiction process in one's life. It's a triumph over the human tendency to deny. We recognize that our resolutions and strategies, however well meant, have not liberated us from the addiction process and all its mechanisms that are deeply ingrained in our brains, emotions and behaviours.

2. Came to believe that a Power greater than ourselves could restore us to sanity.

My understanding of the higher power concept is given in Chapter 34. It may, but does not necessarily, imply belief in a deity. It means heeding a higher truth than the immediate desires or terrors of the ego.

3. Made a decision to turn our will and our lives over to the care of God as we understood Him.

The word God could have a religious meaning for many people. For many others it means laying trust in the universal truths and higher values that reside at the spiritual core of human beings, but are feared and resisted by the grasping, anxious, past-conditioned ego.

4. Made a searching and fearless moral inventory of ourselves.

The idea here is not self-condemnation, but the preparation of a clean slate for a life of sobriety. We search our conscience to identify where and how we have betrayed ourselves or others, not to wallow in guilt but to leave ourselves unburdened in the present and to help clear our path to the future.

5. Admitted to God, to ourselves and to another human being the exact nature of our wrongs.

With compassion for ourselves, we fully acknowledge what we have found in Step Four. Communicating the information—to ourselves in the form of a journal, or to some other human being—makes our moral self-searching into a concrete reality. Shame for our actions is replaced by a sense of responsibility. We move from powerlessness to strength.

6. Were entirely ready to have God remove all these defects of character.

We accept that our missteps and our lack of integrity do not represent who we really are and commit to let go of these tendencies as they continue to arise in the future—for they surely will. In doing so, we look for inspiration and support to our own sense of the higher power, however we understand that.

7. Humbly asked Him to remove our shortcomings.

Our shortcomings are where we fall short of, and even lose sight of, our true potential. Thus in giving up the short-term rewards of addictive behaviours, we are choosing a vast enrichment of who we are. Humility is in order in place of pride, that desperate grandiosity of the ego.

8. Made a list of all persons we had harmed, and became willing to make amends to them all.

We are prepared to accept responsibility for each and every sin of commission or omission we have perpetrated on people in our lives. We do so not from shame, but out of commitment to our own growth and to the peace of mind of other human beings.

9. Made direct amends to such people wherever possible, except when to do so would injure them or others.

The phrase that's key to Step Nine is "became willing" from Step Eight. Step Nine is not about us, but about others. Its purpose is not to make us feel or look good, but to provide restitution where that's appropriate. With some people we have injured, this step will lead us to communicate full responsibility and remorse. Some others we may need, respectfully, to leave alone, depending on the circumstances and their particular feelings—even if that means accepting that they may continue to loathe us. Our fears of how we will look to others should neither drive this step nor inhibit it.

10. Continued to take personal inventory and when we were wrong promptly admitted it.

It goes without saying that this is Step Four in action. As human beings, most of us are far away from attaining perfect saintliness in all our behaviours and interactions, and therefore can afford to give up the process of moral self-inventory only when they lower us into the ground. Until then, we'll keep having to do the laundry.

11. Sought through prayer and meditation to improve our conscious contact with God as we understood Him, praying only for knowledge of His will for us and the power to carry that out.

This is not a demand for submission but a suggested path to freedom. Human life, I believe, is balanced on four pillars: physical health, emotional integration, intellectual awareness and spiritual practice. There are no prescriptions for the latter. "Be a lamp unto yourselves," said the Buddha. For myself, I have found that spiritual reading and contemplation and mindfulness meditation open portals to my soul. The language of prayer has not inspired me, although lately I've noticed that I'm finding myself more and more drawn towards it spontaneously. If we do pray, it's not for egoistic rewards and benefits but for the strength to follow where our higher power leads us.

12. Having had a spiritual awakening as the result of these steps, we tried to carry this message to others, and to practise these principles in all our affairs.

Carrying the message to others means manifesting the principles of integrity, truth, sobriety and compassion in our lives. It may call for providing support and leadership when appropriate and welcome, but does not mean proselytizing on behalf of any program, group or set of beliefs. It does not mean talking a lot and intruding with advice when uninvited. "Who hath ears, let him hear."

ENDNOTES

CHAPTER 1   THE ONLY HOME HE'S EVER HAD

1. Elliot Leyton, "Death on the Pig Farm: Take one," review of *The Pickton File*, by Stevie Cameron, *The Globe and Mail*, 16 June 2007, D3.

2. Anne Applebaum, *Gulag: A History* (New York: Anchor Books, 2004), 291.

CHAPTER 2   THE LETHAL HOLD OF DRUGS

1. Lorna Crozier and Patrick Lane, eds., *Addicted: Notes from the Belly of the Beast* (Vancouver: Greystone Books, 2001), 166.

CHAPTER 3   THE KEYS OF PARADISE

1. V.J. Felitti, "Adverse Childhood Experiences and Their Relationship to Adult Health, Well-being, and Social Functioning" (lecture at the Building Blocks for a Healthy Future Conference, Red Deer, Alberta, 24 May 2007).

2. J. Panksepp, "Social Support and Pain: How Does the Brain Feel the Ache of a Broken Heart?" *Journal of Cancer Pain and Symptom Palliation* 1(1) (2005): 29–65.

3. N.I. Eisenberger, "Does Rejection Hurt? An FMRI Study of Social Exclusion," *Science,* 10 October 2003, 290–92.

4. R. Shanta et al., "Childhood Abuse, Neglect and Household Dysfunction and the Risk of Illicit Drug Use: The Adverse Childhood Experiences Study," *Pediatrics* 111 (2003): 564–72.

5. Primo Levi, *The Drowned and the Saved,* trans. Raymond Rosenthal (New York: Vintage International, 1989), 158.

6. Ibid, 25.

7. Saul Bellow, *The Adventures of Augie March* (New York: Penguin Books, 1996), 1.

8. Peter Gay, *Freud: A Life for Our Time* (New York: W.W. Norton, 1998), 44.

CHAPTER 8   THERE'S GOT TO BE SOME LIGHT

1. Carl Rogers, *On Becoming a Person: A Therapist's View of Psychotherapy* (New York: Houghton Mifflin, 1995), 283.

CHAPTER 9   TAKES ONE TO KNOW ONE

1. Sakyong Mipham, *Turning the Mind into an Ally* (New York: Riverhead Books, 2003), 14.

2. Daniel Barenboim, *A Life in Music* (New York: Scribner's, 1991), 58.

3. Everett Fox, trans., *The Five Books of Moses* (New York: Shocken Books, 1995).

CHAPTER 11   WHAT IS ADDICTION?

1. D.K. Hall-Flavin and V.E. Hofmann, "Stimulants, Sedatives and Opiates," in *Neurological Therapeutics*, vol. 2, ed. J.H. Noseworthy (London and New York: Martin Dunitz, 2003), 1510–18.

2. N.S. Miller and M.S. Gold, "A Hypothesis for a Common Neurochemical Basis for Alcohol and Drug Disorders," *Psychiatric Clinics of North America* 16(1) (1993): 105–17.

3. F. Noble and B.P. Roques, "Inhibitors of Enkephalin Catabolism," chap. 5 in *Molecular Biology of Drug Addiction* (Totowa, NJ: Human Press, 2003), 61.

4. M.A. Bozarth and R.A. Wise, "Anatomically Distinct Opiate Receptor Fields Mediate Reward and Physical Dependence," *Science*, 4 May 1984, 516–17.

5. "Recovering Church: The 2005 Greenfield Lectures," St John the Baptist Episcopal Church, Portland, Oregon; http://www.st-john-the- baptist.org/ Greenfield_lectures.htm.

CHAPTER 12   FROM VIETNAM TO "RAT PARK"

1. G.M. Aronoff, "Opioids in Chronic Pain Management: Is There a Significant Risk of Addiction?" *Current Review of Pain* 4(2) (2000): 112–21.

2. A.D. Furlan, "Opioids for Chronic Noncancer Pain: A Meta-analysis of Effectiveness and Side Effects," *CMAJ* 174(11) (23 May 2006): 1589–94.

3. S.R. Ytterberg et al., "Codeine and Oxycodone Use in Patients with Chronic Rheumatic Disease Pain," *Arthritis and Rheumatism* 14(9) (September 1998): 1603–12.

4. L. Dodes, *The Heart of Addiction* (New York: HarperCollins, 2002), 73.

5. L. Robins et al., "Narcotic Use in Southeast Asia and Afterward," *Archives of General Psychiatry* 23 (1975): 955–61.

6. A.J.C. Warner and B.C. Kessler, "Comparative Epidemiology of Dependence on Tobacco, Alcohol, Controlled Substances, and Inhalants: Basic Findings from the National Comorbidity Survey," *Experimental and Clinical Psychopharmacology* 2 (1994): 244–68.

7. B. Alexander, "The Myth of Drug-Induced Addiction: Report to the Canadian

Senate," January 2001; http://www.parl.gc.ca/37/1/parlbus/commbus/senate/come-e/ille-e/presentation-e/alexender-e.htm.

8. Robins et al., "Narcotic Use in Southeast Asia," 955–61.

9. Peter McKnight, "The Meth Myth: Hooked on Hysteria, the Media Are Big on Anecdote and Short on Science in Dealing with the Latest 'Most Dangerous Drug,'" *The Vancouver Sun*, 25 September 2005, C5.

10. D. Morgan et al., "Social Dominance in Monkeys: Dopamine D2 Receptors and Cocaine Self-administration," *Neuroscience* 5(2) (2005): 169–74.

11. Alexander, "The Myth of Drug-Induced Addiction."

12. B. Alexander et al., "Effects of Early and Later Colony Housing on Oral Ingestion of Morphine in Rats," *Psychopharmacology Biochemistry and Behavior* 58 (1981): 175–79.

13. J. Panksepp et al., "Endogenous Opioids and Social Behavior," *Neuroscience and Biobehavioral Reviews* 4 (1980): 473–87.

14. I. N. Robins, "The Vietnam Drug User Returns," in *Special Action Office Monograph Series A (No. 2)* (Washington, DC: U.S. Government Printing Office).

CHAPTER 13   A DIFFERENT STATE OF THE BRAIN

1. Robert L. Dupont, *The Selfish Brain: Learning from Addiction* (Center City, MN: Hazelden, 2000), xxii.

2. C.P. O'Brien, "Research Advances in the Understanding and Treatment of Addiction," *The American Journal on Addiction* 12(836–847) (2003).

3. G. Bartzokis et al., "Brain Maturation May Be Arrested in Chronic Cocaine Addicts," *Biological Psychiatry* 5(8) (April 2002): 605–11

4. R.Z. Goldstein and N.D. Volkow, "Drug Addiction and Its Underlying Neurobiological Basis: Neuroimaging Evidence for the Involvement of the Frontal Cortex," *American Journal of Psychiatry* 159 (2002): 1642–52.

5. Charles A. Dackis, "Recent Advances in the Pharmacotherapy of Cocaine Dependence," *Current Psychiatry Reports* 6 (2004): 323–31.

6. T.E. Robinson and B. Kolb, "Structural Plasticity Associated with Exposure to Drugs of Abuse," *Neuropharmacology* 27 (2004): 33–56.

7. M.A. Nader et al., "PET Imaging of Dopamine D2 Receptors during Chronic Cocaine Self-administration in Monkeys," *Nature Neuroscience* 8 (9 August 2006).

8. N.D. Volkow et al., "Relationship between Subjective Effects of Cocaine and Dopamine Transporter Occupancy," *Nature* 386(6627) (April 1997): 827–30.

9. G.F. Koob, "Drugs of Abuse: Anatomy, Pharmacology and Function of Reward Pathways," *Trends in Pharmacological Science* 13(5) (May 1992): 177–84.

10. Dr. Richard Rawson, Associate Director of the Integrated Substance Abuse

Program, University of California at Los Angeles, Teleconference, 26 April 2006. Available from U.S. Consulate, Vancouver, BC.

11. P.W. Kalivas, "Recent Understanding in the Mechanisms of Addiction," *Current Psychiatry Reports* 6 (2004): 347–51.

CHAPTER 14   THROUGH A NEEDLE, A WARM SOFT HUG

1. J. Panksepp et al., "The Role of Brain Emotional Systems in Addictions: A Neuro-evolutionary Perspective and New 'Self-Report' Animal Model," *Addiction* 97 (2002): 459–69.

2. B. Kieffer and F. Simonin, "Molecular Mechanisms of Opioid Dependence by Using Knockout Mice," in *Molecular Biology of Drug Addiction*, ed. R. Moldano (Totowa, NJ: Human Press, 2003), 12.

3. Thomas De Quincey, *Confessions of an English Opium Eater* (Ware, Hertfordshire: Wordsworth Classics, 1994), 143 and 146.

4. A. Moles, "Deficit in Attachment Behavior in Mice Lacking the Mu-opioid Receptor Gene," *Science*, 25 June 2004, 1983–86.

5. Panksepp et al., "The Role of Brain Emotional Systems," 459–69.

6. J.-K. Zubieta, "Regulation of Human Affective Responses by Anterior Cingulate and Limbic μ-Opioid Neurotransmission," *Archives of General Psychiatry* 60 (2003): 1145–53.

7. J.K. Zubieta et al., "Placebo Effects Mediated by Endogenous Opioid Activity on Mu-opioid Receptors," *Journal of Neuroscience* 25(34) (24 August 2005): 7754–62.

8. J. Panksepp, *Affective Neuroscience: The Foundations of Human and Animal Emotions* (New York: Oxford University Press, 1998), 250.

9. Ibid, 256.

10. A.N. Schore, *Affect Regulation and the Origin of the Self* (Hillsdale, NJ: Lawrence Erlbaum Associates, 1994), 142–43.

11. N.I. Eisenberger, "Does Rejection Hurt? An FMRI Study of Social Exclusion," *Science*, 10 October 2003, 290–92

12. Schore, *Affect Regulation*, 378.

13. J. Hennig et al., "Biopsychological Changes after Bungee Jumping: Beta-Endorphin Immunoreactivity as a Mediator of Euphoria?" *Neuropsychobiology* 29(1) (1994): 28–32.

14. B. Bencherif et al., "Mu-opioid Receptor Binding Measured by [11C]carfentanil Positron Emission Tomography Is Related to Craving and Mood in Alcohol Dependence," *Biological Psychiatry* 55(3) (1 February 2004): 255–62.

15. D.A. Gorelick et al., "Imaging Brain Mu-opioid Receptors in Abstinent Cocaine Users: Time Course and Relation to Cocaine Craving," *Biological Psychiatry* 57(12) (15 June 2005): 1573–82.
16. N.S. Miller and M.S. Gold, "A Hypothesis for a Common Neurochemical Basis for Alcohol and Drug Disorders," *Psychiatric Clinics of North America* 169(1) (1993): 105–17.

CHAPTER 15 COCAINE, DOPAMINE AND CANDY BARS
1. C.E. Moan and R.G. Heath, "Septal Stimulation for the Initiation of Heterosexual Activity in a Homosexual Male," *Journal of Behavior Therapy and Experimental Psychiatry* 3 (1972): 23–30.
2. N.D. Volkow et al., "Role of Dopamine in Drug Reinforcement and Addiction in Humans: Results from Imaging Studies," *Behavioral Pharmacology* 13 (2002): 355–66.
3. N.D. Volkow et al., "Low Level of Brain Dopamine D2 Receptors in Methamphetamine Abusers: Association with Metabolism in the Orbitofrontal Cortex," *American Journal of Psychiatry* 158(12) (December 2001): 2015–21.
4. Eliot L. Gardner, "Brain-Reward Mechanisms," chap. 5, section II in *Substance Abuse: A Comprehensive Textbook,* by Joyce H. Lowinson et al. (Philadelphia: Lippincott, Williams & Wilkins, 2005), 71.
5. D.W. Self, "Regulation of Drug-Taking and -Seeking Behaviors by Neuroadaptations in the Mesolimbic Dopamine System," *Neuropharmacology* 47 (2005): 252–55.
6. J. Panksepp et al., "The Role of Brain Emotional Systems in Addictions: A Neuro-Evolutionary Perspective and New 'Self-Report' Animal Model," *Addiction* 97 (2002): 459–69.

CHAPTER 16 LIKE A CHILD NOT RELEASED
1. N.D. Volkow and T.-K. Li, "Drug Addiction: The Neurobiology of Behaviour Gone Awry," *Neuroscience* 5 (December 2004): 963–70.
2. Joseph LeDoux, *The Emotional Brain: The Mysterious Underpinnings of Emotional Life* (New York: Simon & Schuster, 1996), 165.
3. Jeffrey M. Schwartz with Sharon Begley, *The Mind and the Brain: Neuroplasticity and the Power of Mental Force* (New York: HarperCollins, 2002), 312.
4. S. Pellis et al., "The Role of the Cortex in Play Fighting by Rats: Developmental and Evolutionary Implications," *Brain, Behavior and Evolution* 39 (1992): 270–84, quoted in Gordon M. Burghardt, "Play: Attributes and Neural Substrates," in

Handbook of Behavioral Neurobiology, vol, 13, ed. E. Blass (New York: Plenum Publishers, 2001), 388.

5. E.D. London et al., "Orbitofrontal Cortex and Human Drug Abuse: Functional Imaging," *Cerebral Cortex* 10(3) (March 2000): 334–42; *see also* R.Z. Goldstein and N.D. Volkow, "Drug Addiction and Its Underlying Neurobiological Basis: Neuroimaging Evidence for the Involvement of the Frontal Cortex," *American Journal of Psychiatry* 159 (2002): 1642–52.

6. A.N. Schore, "Structure-Function Relationships of the Orbitofrontal Cortex," chap. 4 in *Affect Regulation and the Origin of the Self* (Hillsdale, NJ: Lawrence Erlbaum Associates, 1994), 34–61.

7. Goldstein and Volkow, "Drug Addiction and Its Underlying Neurobiological Basis."

8. London et al., "Orbitofrontal Cortex."

9. G. Dom et al., "Substance Use Disorders and the Orbitofrontal Cortex: Systematic Review of Behavioural Decision-Making and Neuroimaging Studies," *The British Journal of Psychiatry* 187 (2005): 209–20.

10. London et al., "Orbitofrontal Cortex."

11. Ibid.

12. Goldstein and Volkow, "Drug Addiction and Its Underlying Neurobiological Basis."

13. N.D. Volkow et al., "Low Level of Brain Dopamine D2 Receptors in Methamphetamine Abusers: Association with Metabolism in the Orbitofrontal Cortex," *American Journal of Psychiatry* 158(12) (December 2001): 2015–21.

14. Goldstein and Volkow, "Drug Addiction and Its Underlying Neurobiological Basis."

15. G. Bartzokis et al., *"Brain Maturation May Be Arrested in Chronic Cocaine Addicts,"* *Biological Psychiatry* 51(8) (April 2002): 605–11; Goldstein and Volkow, "Drug Addiction and Its Underlying Neurobiological Basis."

CHAPTER 17   THEIR BRAINS NEVER HAD A CHANCE

1. To name four seminal works: *Affect Regulation and the Origin of the Self: The Neurobiology of Emotional Development*, by Allan Schore; *Affective Neuroscience: The Foundations of Human and Animal Emotions*, by Jaak Panksepp; *The Developing Mind: Toward a Neurobiology of Interpersonal Experience*, by Daniel Siegel, and *Human Behavior and the Developing Brain*, edited by Kurt W. Dawson and Geraldine Fischer.

2. Antonio Damasio, *Descartes' Error: Emotion, Reason, and the Human Brain* (New York: G.P. Putnam & Sons, 1994), 255.

3. V.J. Felitti, "Ursprünge des Suchtverhaltens—Evidenzen aus einer Studie zu belaststenden Kindheitserfahrungen" ("The Origins of Addiction: Evidence from the Adverse Childhood Experiences Study"), *Praxis der Kinderpsychologie under Kinderpsychiatrie* 52 (2003): 547–59.

4. B. Perry and R. Pollard, "Homeostasis, Stress, Trauma and Adaptation: A Neurodevelopmental View of Childhood Trauma," *Child and Adolescent Clinics of North America* 7(1) (January 1998): 33–51. Citing data from R. Shore, *Rethinking the Brain: New Insights into Early Development* (New York: Families and Work Institute, 1997).

5. Kurt W. Dawson and Geraldine Fischer, eds., *Human Behavior and the Developing Brain* (New York: The Guildford Press, 1994), 9.

6. B.D. Perry et al., "Childhood Trauma, the Neurobiology of Adaptation, and 'Use-dependent' Development of the Brain: How 'States' Become 'Traits,'" *Infant Mental Health Journal* 16(4) (1995): 271–91.

7. R. Kotulak, *Inside the Brain: Revolutionary Discoveries of How the Mind Works* (Kansas City: Andrews and McMeel, 1996).

8. D. Siegel, *The Developing Mind: Toward a Neurobiology of Interpersonal Experience* (New York: The Guildford Press, 1999), 85.

9. Ibid, 67 and 85.

10. Dawson and Fischer, *Human Behavior*, 367.

11. M.R. Gunnar and B. Donzella, "Social Regulation of the Cortisol Levels in Early Human Development," *Psychoneuroendocrinology* 27(1–2) (January-February 2002): 199–220.

12. R. Joseph, "Environmental Influences on Neural Plasticity, the Limbic System, Emotional Development and Attachment: A Review," *Child Psychiatry and Human Development* 29(3) (Spring 1999): 189–208.

CHAPTER 18   TRAUMA, STRESS AND THE BIOLOGY OF ADDICTION

1. A.N. Schore, *Affect Regulation and the Origin of the Self* (Hillsdale, NJ: Lawrence Erlbaum Associates, 1994), 142.

2. S.L. Dubovsky, *Mind Body Deceptions: The Psychosomatics of Everyday Life* (New York: W.W. Norton, 1997), 193.

3. G. Blanc et al., "Response to Stress of Mesocortico-Frontal Dopaminergic Neurons in Rats after Long-Term Isolation," *Nature* 284 (20 March 1980): 265–67.

4. M.J. Meaney et al., "Environmental Regulation of the Development of Mesolimbic Dopamine Systems: A Neurobiological Mechanism for Vulnerability to Drug Abuse?" *Psychoneuroendocrinology* 27 (2002): 127–38.

5. Harold H. Gordon, "Early Environmental Stress and Biological Vulnerability to Drug Abuse," *Psychoneuroendocrinology* 27 (2002): 115–26.

6. C. Caldji et al., "Maternal Care During Infancy Regulates the Development of Neural Systems Mediating the Expression of Fearfulness in the Rat," *Neurobiology* 95(9) (28 April 1998): 5335–40.

7. J.D. Higley and M. Linnoila, "Low Central Nervous System Serotonergic Activity Is Traitlike and Correlates with Impulsive Behavior," *Annals of the New York Academy of Science* 836 (29 December 1997): 39.

8. A.S. Clarke et al., "Rearing Experience and Biogenic Amine Activity in Infant Rhesus Monkeys," *Biological Psychiatry* 40(5) (1 September 1996): 338–52; *see also* J.D. Higley et al., "Nonhuman Primate Model of Alcohol Abuse: Effects of Early Experience, Personality, and Stress on Alcohol Consumption," *Proceedings of the National Academy of Sciences* USA 88 (August 1991): 7261–65.

9. M.H. Teicher, "Wounds That Time Won't Heal: The Neurobiology of Child Abuse," *Cerebrum: The Dana Forum on Brain Science* 2(4) (fall 2000).

10. A. de Mello A et al., "Update on Stress and Depression: The Role of the Hypothalamic-Pituitary-Adrenal (HPA) Axis," *Revista Brasileiva de Psiquiatria* 25(4) (October 2003); *see also* G.W. Kraemer et al., "A Longitudinal Study of the Effect of Different Social Rearing Conditions on Cerebrospinal Fluid Norepinephrine and Biogenic Amine Metabolites in Rhesus Monkeys," *Neuropsychopharmacology* 2(3) (September 1989): 175–89.

11. Teicher, "Wounds That Time Won't Heal."

12. B. Perry and R. Pollard, "Homeostasis, Stress, Trauma and Adaptation: A Neurodevelopmental View of Childhood Trauma," *Child and Adolescent Clinics of North America* 7(1) (January 1998): 33–51.

13. G.W. Kraemer et al., "Strangers in a Strange Land: A Psychobiological Study of Infant Monkeys Before and After Separation from Real or Inanimate Mothers," *Child Development* 62(3) (June 1991): 548–66.

14. L.A. Pohorecky, "Interaction of Ethanol and Stress: Research with Experimental Animals:—An Update," *Alcohol & Alcoholism* 25(2/3) (1990): 263–76.

15. S.R. Dube et al., "Childhood Abuse, Neglect, and Household Dysfunction and the Risk of Illicit Drug Use: The Adverse Childhood Experiences Study," *Pediatrics* 111 (2003): 564–72.

16. Harold W. Gordon, "Early Environmental Stress and Biological Vulnerability to Drug Abuse," *Psychoneuroendocrinology* 271(2) (January-February 2002): 115–26. Special Issue: Stress and Drug Abuse.

17. S.R. Dube et al., "Adverse Childhood Experiences and the Association with Ever Using Alchohol and Initiating Alcohol Use During Adolescence," *Journal of Adolescent Health* 38 (2006).

18. C.M. Anderson et al., "Abnormal T2 Relaxation Time in the Cerebellar Vermis of Adults Sexually Abused in Childhood: Potential Role of the Vermis in Stress-Enhanced Risk for Drug Abuse," *Psychoneuroendocrinology* 27 (2002): 231–44.

19. Teicher, "Wounds That Time Won't Heal."

20. M.D. De Bellis et al., "Developmental Traumatology Part I: Biological Stress Systems," *Biological Psychiatry* 45 (1999): 1271–84.

21. M. Vythilingam et al., "Childhood Trauma Associated with Smaller Hippocampal Volume in Women with Major Depression," *American Journal of Psychiatry* 159: 2072–80.

22. Teicher, "Wounds That Time Won't Heal."

23. E.M. Sternberg, moderator, "The Stress Response and the Regulation of Inflammatory Disease," *Annals of Internal Medicine* 17(10) (15 November 1992), 855.

24. A. Kusnecov and B.S. Rabin, "Stressor-Induced Alterations of Immune Function: Mechanisms and Issues," *International Archives of Allergy and Immunology* 105 (1994), 108.

25. Hans Selye, *The Stress of Life,* rev. ed. (New York: MacGraw-Hill, 1978), 4.

26. Dr. Bruce Perry, interview by author.

27. M.D. De Bellis et al., "Hypothalamic-Pituitary-Adrenal Axis Dysregulation in Sexually Abused Girls," *Journal of Clinical Endocrinology and Metabolism* 78 (1994). 249–55.

28. M.J. Essex et al., "Maternal Stress Beginning in Infancy May Sensitize Children to Later Stress Exposure: Effects on Cortisol and Behavior," *Biological Psychiatry* 52(8) (15 October 2002): 773.

29. C. Heim et al., "Pituitary-Adrenal and Autonomic Responses to Stress in Women after Sexual and Physical Abuse in Childhood," *JAMA* 284(5) (2 August 2000): 592–97.

30. C.A. Pedersen, "Biological Aspects of Social Bonding and the Roots of Human Violence," *Ann N Y Acad Sci* 1036 (December 2004): 106–27.

31. Eliot L. Gardner, "Brain-Reward Mechanisms," chap. 5, section II in *Substance Abuse,* by Lowinson et al., 72.

32. K.T. Brady and S.C. Sonne, "The Role of Stress in Alcohol Use, Alcoholism Treatment, and Relapse," *Alcohol Research and Health* 23(4) (1999): 263–71.

33. P.V. Piazza and M. Le Moal, "Pathophysiological Basis of Vulnerability to Drug Abuse: Role of an Interaction Between Stress, Glucocorticoids, and Dopaminergic Neurons," *Annual Review of Pharmacology and Toxocology* 36 (1996): 359–78.

34. M. Papp et al., "Parallel Changes in Dopamine D2 Receptor Binding in Limbic Forebrain Associated with Chronic Mild Stress-Induced Anhedonia and Its Reversal by Imipramine," *Psychopharmacology* 115 (1994): 441–46.

35. S. Levine and H. Ursin, "What Is Stress?" in *Stress, Neurobiology and Neuroendocrinology,* ed. M.R. Brown, G.F. Koob, and C. Rivier (New York: Marcel Dekker 1991), 3–21.

36. Harold H. Gordon, "Early Environmental Stress and Biological Vulnerability to Drug Abuse," *Psychoneuroendocrinology* 27 (2002): 115–26.

37. Blanc, "Response to Stress of Mesocortico-Frontal Dopaminergic Neurons in Rats," 265–67.

38. S. Schenk et al., "Cocaine Self-Administration in Rats Influenced by Environmental Conditions: Implications for the Etiology of Drug Abuse," *Neuroscience Letters* 81 (1987): 227–31.

39. A. Jacobson, "Physical and Sexual Assault Histories Among Psychiatric Outpatients," *American Journal of Psychiatry* 146 (1989): 755–58.

40. L.M. Williams, "Recall of Childhood Trauma: A Prospective Study of Women's Memories of Child Sexual Abuse," *Journal of Consulting and Clinical Psychology* 62: 1167–76.

CHAPTER 19   IT'S NOT IN THE GENES

1. *Time,* 30 April 1990; http://www.time.com/time/magazine/article/0,9171,969965,00.html.

2. K. Blum et al., "Reward Deficiency Syndrome," *American Scientist,* 1 March 1996, 132–46.

3. K. Blum, "Allelic Association of Human Dopamine D2 Receptor Gene in Alcoholism," *JAMA* 263(15) (18 April 1990): 2055–60.

4. J. Gelernter and H. Kranzler, "D2 Dopamine Receptor Gene (DRD2) Allele and Haplotype Frequencies and Control Subjects: No Association with Phenotype or Severity of Phenotype," *Neurospsychopharmacology* 20(6) (1999): 642–49.

5. L. Dodes, *The Heart of Addiction* (New York: HarperCollins, 2002), 81.

6. R.E. Tarter and M. Vanyukov, "Alcoholism, a Developmental Disorder," *Journal of Consulting and Clinical Psychology,* Vol. 62, No. 6 (1994): 1096–1107.

7. M.A. Enoch and D. Goldman, "The Genetics of Alcoholism and Alcohol Abuse," *Current Psychiatry Reports* 3 (2002): 144–51.

8. K.S. Kendler and C.A. Prescott, "Cannabis Use, Abuse and Dependence in a Population-Based Sample of Female Twins," *American Journal of Psychiatry* 155 (1998): 1016–22.

9. S.W. Lin and R.M. Anthenelli: "Genetic Factors in the Risk for Substance Use Disorders," chap. 4 in *Substance Abuse: A Comprehensive Textbook,* by Joyce H. Lowinson et al. (Philadelphia: Lippincott Williams & Wilkins, 2005), 39.

10. K.S. Kendler and C.A. Prescott, "Cocaine Use, Abuse and Dependence in a Population Sample of Female Twins," *British Journal of Psychiatry* 173 (1998): 345–50.

11. J.S. Alper and J. Beckwith, "Genetic Fatalism and Social Policy: The Implications of Behavior Genetics Research," *Yale Journal of Biology and Medicine* 66(6) (November-December 1993): 511–24.

12. "The number of synaptic contacts in the human cerebral cortex is staggeringly high," writes Peter Huttenlocher, a neuroscientist at the University of Chicago. "It is clear that this large number cannot be determined by a genetic program, in which each synapse has an exact assigned location. More likely, only the general outlines of basic connectivity are genetically determined." (In Kurt W. Dawson and Geraldine Fischer, eds., *Human Behavior and the Developing Brain* [New York: The Guildford Press, 1994], 138.)

13. Jeffrey M. Schwartz and Sharon Begley, *The Mind and the Brain: Neuroplasticity and the Power of Mental Force* (New York: ReganBooks, 2002), 112.

14. B. Lipton, *The Biology of Belief* (Santa Rosa, CA: Elite Books, 2005), 86.

15. M.J. Meaney, "Maternal Care, Gene Expression, and the Transmission of Individual Differences in Stress Reactivity Across Generations," *Annual Review of Neuroscience* 24 (2001): 1161–92.

16. C.M. Colvis et al., "Epigenetic Mechanisms and Gene Networks in the Nervous System," *The Journal of Neuroscience* 25(45) (9 November 2005), 10379–89.

17. C.S. Barr, "Serotonin Transporter Gene Variation Is Associated with Alcohol Sensitivity in Rhesus Macaques Exposed to Early-Life Stress," *Alcoholism: Clinical and Experimental Research* 27(5) (May 2003): 812–17.

18. M. Weinstock et al., "Prenatal Stress Effects on Functional Development of the Offspring," chap. 21 in *Progress in Brain Research,* vol. 73, *Biochemical Basis of Functional Neuroteratology,* ed. G.J. Boer (New York: Elsevier, 1988): 319–30.

19. P. Zelkowitz and A. Papageorgiou, "Maternal Anxiety: An Emerging Prognostic Factor in Neonatology," *Acta Paediatr* 94(12) (December 2005): 1771–76; C. Sondergaard et al., "Psychosocial Distress During Pregnancy and the Risk of Infantile Colic: A Follow-Up Study," *Acta Paediatr* 92(7) (July 2003): 811–16. These are only two examples. The list of animal and human studies on this topic easily extends into the hundreds.

20. http://news.bbc.co.uk/2/hi/health/6298909.stm.

21. J.R. Seckl, "Prenatal Glucocorticoids and Long-Term Programming," *European Journal of Endocrinology* 151(Suppl 3) (2004): U49–U62, quoted in R. Yehuda et al., "Transgenerational Effects of Posttraumatic Stress Disorder in Babies of Mothers Exposed to the World Trade Center Attacks During Pregnancy," *The Journal of Clinical Endocrinology & Metabolism* 90(7): 4115–18.

22. R. Yehuda et al., "Transgenerational Effects of Posttraumatic Stress Disorder in Babies of Mothers Exposed to the World Trade Center Attacks During Pregnancy," *The Journal of Clinical Endocrinology & Metabolism* 90(7): 4115–18.

23. K.H. DeTurck and L.A. Pohorecky, "Ethanol Sensitivity in Rats: Effect of Prenatal Stress," *Physiological Behavior* 40 (1987): 407–10; L.A. Pohorecky, "Interaction of Ethanol and Stress: Research with Experimental Animals—An Update," *Alcohol & Alcoholism* 25(2/3) (1990): 263–76.

24. *The New Yorker,* 26 June 2006, 76.

CHAPTER 20 "A VOID I'LL DO ANYTHING TO AVOID"

1 Maurice Walsh, trans., *The Long Discourses of the Buddha: A Translation of the Digha Nikaya* (Boston: Wisdom Publications, 1995), 70.

2. A. Goodman, "Sexual Addiction: Nosology, Diagnosis, Etiology and Treatment," chap. 30 in *Substance Abuse: A Comprehensive Textbook,* by Joyce H. Lowinson et al. (Philadelphia: Lippincott Williams & Wilkins, 2005), 516.

3. M.A. Enoch and D. Goldman, "The Genetics of Alcoholism and Alcohol Abuse," *Current Psychiatry Reports* 3 (2002): 144–51.

4. M.S. Gold and N.S. Miller, "A Hypothesis for a Common Neurochemical Basis for Alcohol and Drug Disorders," *Psychiatric Clinics of North America* 16(1) (1993): 105–17.

5. M.N. Potenza, "The Neurobiology of Pathological Gambling," *Seminars in Clinical Neuropsychiatry* 6(3) (July 2001): 217–26.

6. G. Meyer et al., "Neuroendocrine Response to Casino Gambling in Problem Gamblers," *Psychoneuroendocrinology* 29(10) (29 November 2004): 1272–80.

7. *The Vancouver Sun,* 11 July 2006, 1.

8. H.C. Breiter, "Functional Imaging of Neural Responses to Expectancy and Experience of Monetary Gains and Losses," *Neuron* 30(2) (2001): 619–39.

9. M.J. Koepp et al., "Evidence for Striatal Dopamine Release During a Video Game," *Nature* 393(6682) (21 May 1998): 266–68.

10. G. J. Wang, "The Role of Dopamine in Motivation for Food in Humans: Implications for Obesity," *Expert Opinion on Therapeutic Targets* 6(5) (October 2002): 601–9.

11. C. Colantuoni et al., Excessive Sugar Intake Alters Binding to Dopamine and Mu-opioid Receptors in the Brain," *NeuroReport* 12 (2001): 3549–52; "Evidence That Intermittent, Excessive Sugar Intake Causes Endogenous Opioid Dependence," *Obesity Research* 20 (2002): 478–88.

12. A. Drenowski et al., "Nalaxone, an Opiate Blocker, Reduces the Consumption of Sweet High-Fat Foods in Obese and Lean Female Binge-eaters," *American Journal of Clinical Nutrition* 61 (1995): 1206–12.

13. Ibid.

14. M.S. Gold and J. Star, *Eating Disorders*, chap. 27 in *Substance Abuse*, by Lowinson et al., 470.

15. M. Alonso-Alonso and A. Pascual-Leone, "The Right Brain Hypothesis for Obesity," *JAMA* 297(16) (25 April 2007): 1819–22.

16. M. Deppe et. al. "Nonlinear responses within the medial prefrontal cortex reveal when specific implicit information influences economic decision making." *Journal of Neuroimaging*, 15(2) (April 2005):171–82.

17. "Study Finds Shopping Bypasses Rational Thought," *The Vancouver Sun*, November 8, 2003.

18. Goodman, "Sexual Addiction," 507.

19. M.N. Potenza, "The Neurobiology of Pathological Gambling."

CHAPTER 21 TOO MUCH TIME ON EXTERNAL THINGS

1. Lorna Crozier and Patrick Lane, eds., *Addicted: Notes from the Belly of the Beast* (Vancouver: Graystone Books, 2001), 166.

2. Crozier and Lane, *Notes from the Belly of the Beast*, 166.

3. These paragraphs on differentiation are quoted and adapted from two of my previous books: chap. 14 of *When the Body Says No: The Cost of Hidden Stress* (Toronto: Vintage Canada, 2004) and chap. 9 of *Hold On to Your Kids: Why Parents Need to Matter More Than Peers* (Toronto: Vintage Canada, 2005).

4. M.E. Kerr and M. Bowen, *Family Evaluation: An Approach Based on Bowen Theory* (New York: W.W. Norton, 1988), chap. 4, 89–111, provides a full discussion of differentiation.

CHAPTER 22 POOR SUBSTITUTES FOR LOVE

1. A. Goodman, "Sexual Addiction: Nosology, Diagnosis, Etiology and Treatment," chap. 30 in *Substance Abuse: A Comprehensive Textbook,* ed. Joyce H. Lowinson et al. (Philadelphia: Lippincott Williams & Wilkins, 2005), 511.

2. Monique Giard, interview by author.

3. F. Champagne and M.J. Meaney, "Like Mother, Like Daughter: Evidence for Non-genomic Transmission of Parental Behavior and Stress Responsivity," *Prog Brain Res* 133 (2001): 287–302.

4. Daniel J. Siegel, *"Cognitive Neuroscience Encounters Psychotherapy"* (notes for a plenary address to the annual meeting of the American Association of Directors of Psychiatric Residency Training, 1996).

5. J.D. Coplan et al., "Persistent Elevations of Cerebrospinal Fluid Concentrations of Corticotrophin-Releasing Factor in Adult Nonhuman Primates Exposed to Early-Life Stressors: Implications for the Pathophysiology of Mood and Anxiety Disorders," *Proceedings of the National Academy of Sciences* 93 (February 1996): 1619–23.

6. K.T. Brady and S.C. Sonne, "The Role of Stress in Alcohol Use, Alcoholism Treatment, and Relapse," *Alcohol Research and Health* 23(4): 263–71.

7. Allan Schore, *Affect Regulation and the Origin of the Self: The Neurobiology of Emotional Development* (Hillsdale, NJ: Lawrence Erlbaum Associates, 1994), 378.

8. I. Lissau and T. Sørensen, "Parental Neglect During Childhood and Increased Obesity in Young Adulthood," *Lancet* 343 (1994): 324–27.

9. D.F. Willliamson et al., "Body Weight and Obesity in Adults and Self-Reported Abuse in Childhood," *International Journal of Obesity* 26 (2002): 1075–82.

10. T. Wills, "Multiple Networks and Substance Use," *Journal of Social and Clinical Psychology*, 9 (1990): 78–90.

11. Data and quotes for this section on Conrad Black are from the following books: Conrad Black, *A Life in Progress* (Toronto: Key Porter Books, 1992); James Fitzgerald, *Old Boys: The Powerful Legacy of Upper Canada College* (Toronto: Macfarlane, Walter & Ross, 1994); Jacquie McNeish and Sinclair Stewart, *Wrong Way: The Fall of Conrad Black* (Woodstock and New York: The Overlook Press, 2004); Peter C. Newman, *The Establishment Man: A Portrait of Power* (Toronto: McClelland & Stewart, 1982); Richard Siklos, *Shades of Black: Conrad Black— His Rise and Fall* (Toronto: McClelland & Stewart, 2004); George Tombs, *Lord Black: The Biography* (Toronto: BT Publishing, 2004).

12. Tombs, *Lord Black*, 38.

13. Robert Musil, *The Man Without Qualities* (New York: Vintage International, 1996), 416.

14. Primo Levi, *The Drowned and the Saved*, trans. Raymond Rosenthal (New York: Vintage International, 1989), 67.

CHAPTER 23   DISLOCATION AND THE SOCIAL ROOTS OF ADDICTION

1. Eckhart Tolle, *The Power of Now* (Novato, CA: New World Library, 1997), 18.

2. Joanna Walters, "$15 Billion Spent on Beauty," *The Guardian Weekly*, 3–9 November 2006, 7.

3. Paul Taylor, "Shop-till-You-Drop Disorder Taxes Both Sexes," *The Globe and Mail*, 6 October 2006, A13.

4. Joe Drape, "Setting Restaurant Records by Selling the Sizzle," *The New York Times*, 22 July 2007, 1 and 21.

5. "Big Tobacco Lied to Public," *The Washington Post*, 18 August 2006.

6. "Ending Our Tobacco Addiction," editorial, *The New York Times*, 30 May 2007.

7. "Narcotic Maker Guilty of Deceit over Marketing," *The New York Times*, 11 May 2007, A-1.

8. Lewis Lapham, "Time Travel," *Harper's Magazine*, May 2007, 11.

9. "Work-Life Balance? Not for One in Three," *The Globe and Mail*, 16 May 2007, C-1.

10. Tolle, *The Power of Now*, 23.

11. "Facts about Prisons and Prisoners," The Sentencing Project, October 2003, quoted in Amy Goodman, *The Exception to the Rulers* (New York: Hyperion, 2004), 129.

12. U.S. Department of Justice, Bureau of Justice Statistics homepage; www.ojp.usdoj.gov/bjs/crimoff.htm.

13. Robert L. Dupont, *The Selfish Brain: Learning from Addiction* (Center City, MN: Hazelden, 2000), 31.

14. B. Alexander, "The Roots of Addiction in Free Market Society," Canadian Centre for Policy Alternatives, Toronto, April 2001, 12; www.policyalternatives.ca/bc/rootsofaddiction.html

15. Dupont, *The Selfish Brain*, 31.

16. *Agence France Presse*, reported in *The Vancouver Sun*, 30 September 2006, A

17. Aboriginal women between the ages of 25 and 44 are five times more likely than all other women of the same age to die as a result of violence, reported a Canadian federal study in 1996, "making them the prime targets and the most vulnerable in our society" (quoted in Stevie Cameron, *The Pickton File* [Toronto: Knopf Canada, 2007], 163). In the U.S., according to Justice Department figures, "more than one in three American Indian and Alaska Native women would be raped in their lifetime, almost double the national average of 18 percent." In the vast majority of cases, the perpetrators are non-Native. ("For Indian Victims of Sexual Assault, a Tangled Legal Path," *The New York Times*, 25 April 2007, A15.)

18. Harold H. Gordon, "Early Environmental Stress and Biological Vulnerability to Drug Abuse," *Psychoneuroendocrinology* 27 (2002): 115–26.

19. Michael A. Dawes et al., "Developmental Sources of Variation in Liability to Adolescent Substance Use Disorders," *Drug and Alcohol Dependence* 61 (2000): 3–14.

CHAPTER 24   KNOW THINE ENEMY
1. Julian Sher, "Canada's Top Child-Porn Cop Is Turning In His Badge," *The Globe and Mail,* 10 June 2006, 1.

CHAPTER 25   A FAILED WAR
1. Bruce Alexander, *Peaceful Measures: Canada's Way Out of the "War on Drugs"* (Toronto: University of Toronto Press, 1990), 3.
2. Norm Stamper, *Breaking Rank: A Top Cop's Exposé of the Dark Side of American Policing* (New York: Nation Books, 2005); excerpted at http://www.alternet.org/drugreporter/22227.
3. Quoted in Judge James P. Grey, *Why Our Drug Laws Have Failed and What We Can Do About It: A Judicial Indictment of the War on Drugs* (Philadelphia: Temple University Press, 2001), 126.
4. Elizabeth Rubin, "In the Land of the Taliban," *The New York Times Magazine,* 22 October 2006.
5. "Cocaine Wars Turn Port into Colombia's Deadliest City," *The New York Times,* 22 May 2007, A-3.
6. George Povey, "The Purgatory of Prohibition," *Columbia Journal,* January 2007,
7. Alan Travis, "Revealed: How Drugs War Failed," *The Guardian,* 5 July 2005.
8. Grey, *Why Our Drug Laws Have Failed,* 50.
9. Gary Becker, *The Failure of the War on Drugs,* http://www.becker-posner-blog.com/archives/2005/03/the_failure_of.html.
10. Donald G. McNeil Jr. "Drugs Banned, World's Poor Suffer in Pain." *New York Times,* September 20, 2007, A1.
11. Grey, *Why Our Drug Laws Have Failed.*
12. Mark Stevenson, "Mexico to Decriminalize Drug Possession," *Associated Press,* 29 April 2006.
13. Peter O'Neil, "Canada Looks to U.S.A. for Drug Policy Hints," *The Vancouver Sun,* 12 December 2006, A1.
14. "Effective Drug Control: A New Legal Framework for State Regulation and Control of Psychoactive Substances as a Workable Alternative to the "War on Drugs"; http://www.kcba.org/ScriptContent/KCBA/druglaw/proposal/FAQs.pdf.

CHAPTER 26   FREEDOM OF CHOICE AND THE CHOICE OF FREEDOM
1. Jeffrey M. Schwartz and Sharon Begley, *The Mind and the Brain:*

Neuroplasticity and the Power of Mental Force (New York: ReganBooks, 2002); Jeffrey M. Schwartz, *Brain Lock: Free Yourself from Obsessive-Compulsive Behavior* (New York: ReganBooks, 1996).

2. Schwartz and Begley, *The Mind and the Brain,* 367.

3. Eckhart Tolle, *The Power of Now: A Guide to Spiritual Enlightenment* (Vancouver: Namaste Publishing, 1997), 191.

4. M.H. Teicher, "Wounds That Time Won't Heal: The Neurobiology of Child Abuse," *Cerebrum: The Dana Forum on Brain Science* 2(4) (fall 2000).

5. B. Perry and R. Pollard, "Homeostasis, Stress, Trauma and Adaptation: A Neurodevelopmental View of Childhood Trauma," *Child and Adolescent Clinics of North America* 7(1) (January 1998): 33–51.

6. The research on brain impulse and activation is cited and discussed in detail in Schwartz and Begley, "The Mind and the Brain," chap. 9, 302–7.

7. A. Hirsh, "Discharge Against Medical Advice: Perspectives of Intravenous Drug Users" (University of British Columbia Family Practice Research Day Presentation, 2 July 2002).

8. N.D. Volkow and T. K. Li, "Drug Addiction: The Neurobiology of Behaviour Gone Awry," *Neuroscience* 5 (December 2004): 963–70.

CHAPTER 27   IMAGINING AN ENLIGHTENED SOCIAL POLICY ON DRUGS

1. Anne McIlroy. "Get-tough policy on drugs doomed, experts say." *The Globe and Mail,* October 1, 2007, p. A-4.

2. Jiddu Krishnamurti, *On Relationship* (San Francisco: HarperOne, 1992).

3. Roy A. Wise, "The Neurobiology of Craving: Implications for the Understanding and Treatment of Addiction," *Journal of Abnormal Psychology* 97(2) (1988): 118–32.

4. C. Heim et al., "Pituitary-Adrenal and Autonomic Responses to Stress in Women after Sexual and Physical Abuse in Childhood," *JAMA* 284(5) (2 August 2000): 592–97.

5. D. Morgan et al., "Social Dominance in Monkeys: Dopamine D2 Receptors and Cocaine Self-administration," *Neuroscience* 5(2) (2002): 169–74; S.P. Martin et al., "Effects of Dominance Rank on *d*-Amphetamine-Induced Increases in Aggression," *Pharmacology, Biochemistry & Behavior* 37 (1990): 493–96.

6. Robert Matas, "Consider Legalizing Drug Use, Panel Says," *The Globe and Mail,* 17 November 2006), S-6.

7. http://www.csdp.org/publicservice/halsted.pdf.

8. Rod Mickleburgh and Gloria Galloway, "Storm Brews over Drug Strategy," *The Globe and Mail,* 15 January 2007.

CHAPTER 28   A NECESSARY SMALL STEP

1. Pamela Fayerman, "Unhealthy Lifestyles Cost B.C. $1.8B a Year," *The Vancouver Sun,* 5 October 2006, 1.

2. Canada, Department of Justice Canada, NewsRoom, website of the Department of Justice, 19 February 2001; http://www.justice.gc.ca/en/news/index.html.

3. Gary Mason, "Insight on Insite from Across the Pond," *The Globe and Mail,* 24 August 2006, S-1.

4. B. Fischer and J. Rehm, "The Case for a Heroin Substitution Treatment in Canada," *Canadian Journal of Public Health* 88 (1997): 367–70.

5. Jane Armstrong, "Is Free Heroin Just a Quick Fix?" *The Globe and Mail,* 31 January 2005, 1.

6. Peter McKnight, "Give the Addicts Their Drugs," *The Vancouver Sun,* 29 April 2006, C5.

7. G. Alan Marlatt, *Harm Reduction: Pragmatic Strategies for Managing High Risk Behaviors* (New York: The Guildford Press, 1998), 40.

8. A. D.-M. Uchenhagen et al., "Prescription of Narcotics for Heroin Addicts: Main Results of the Swiss National Cohort Study Zurich," Institute of Social and Preventative Medicine, University of Zurich, 1999.

9. D. Small and E. Drucker, "Policy Makers Ignoring Science and Scientists Ignoring Policy: The Medical Ethical Challenges of Heroin Treatment," *Harm Reduction Journal* 3(16) (2006).

10. "The NAOMI Project," *The Vancouver Sun,* 28 January 2005, A5.

11. Evan Wood et al., "Summary of Findings from the Evaluation of a Pilot Medically Supervised Safe Injecting Facility," *CMAJ* 175(11) (21 November 2006): 1399–1404.

12. Rod Mickleburgh, "RCMP Takes Heat over Insite," *The Globe and Mail,* 12 December 2006, S2.

13. "Harper Has a Duty to Gather All the Evidence About the Injection Site," *The Vancouver Sun,* 8 June 2006, A22.

14. Camille Bains, "Insite Expands with Onsite Detox Centre for Addicts," *The Globe and Mail,* August 27, 2007, S-1

15. Mark A. Wainberg, "The Need to Promote Public Health in the Field of Illicit Drug Use," *CMAJ* 175(11) (21 November 2006): 1395–96.

16. Allan Woods, "Ottawa Ignores Support for Injection Sites," *The Vancouver Sun,* 6 November 2006, A1–A2.

CHAPTER 29   THE POWER OF COMPASSIONATE CURIOSITY

1. Pema Chödrön, *Comfortable with Uncertainty: 108 Teachings* (Boston: Shambala, 2002), 9–10, 57–58.

2. Gabor Maté, *Scattered Minds: A New Look at the Origins and Healing of Attention Deficit Disorder* (Toronto: Vintage Canada, 2000), 4.

3. Anthony Storr, *Solitude* (London: HarperCollins, 1997), 22.

CHAPTER 30   THE INTERNAL CLIMATE

1. E.A. Maguire et al., "Navigation Expertise and the Human Hippocampus: A Structural Brain Imaging Analysis," *Hippocampus* 13(2) (2003): 250–59.

2. Antonio Damasio, *Descartes' Error: Emotion, Reason, and the Human Brain* (New York: G.P. Putnam & Sons, 1994), 112.

3. Marian Cleeves Diamond, *Enriching Heredity* (New York: The Free Press, 1988), 150.

4. Ibid., 157.

5. Ibid., 164.

6. B. Kolb and I. Q. Whishaw, "Brain Plasticity and Behavior," *Annual Review of Psychology* 49 (1998): 43–64.

7. G. Kempermann and Fred H. Gage, "New Nerve Cells for the Adult Brain," *Scientific American* (May 1999): 48–53.

8. Jeffrey M. Schwartz and Sharon Begley, *The Mind and the Brain: Neuroplasticity and the Power of Mental Force* (New York: ReganBooks, 2002), 252–53.

9. Schwartz and Begley, *The Mind and the Brain*, 289.

10. J.M. Schwartz, H.P. Stapp and M. Beauregard, "Quantum Physics in Neuroscience and Psychology: A Neurophysical Model of Mind-Brain Interaction," *Philosophical Transactions of the Royal Society B* (2005): 1309–27.

11. Walter Kaufmann, trans., *Basic Writings of Nietzsche* (New York: Modern Library, 1992), 685–86.

12. Daniel L. Schacter, *Searching for Memory: The Brain, the Mind and the Past* (New York: Basic Books, 1996), 190.

13. Wilder Penfield, *The Mystery of the Mind* (Princeton, NJ: Princeton University Press, 1975), 55, 62, 114.

14. Schwartz, Stapp and Beauregard, "Quantum Physics in Neuroscience and Psychology," 1309–27.

15. Mark Epstein, *Thoughts without a Thinker: Psychotherapy from a Buddhist Perspective* (New York: BasicBooks, 1995), 111.

16. Daniel Siegel, *The Mindful Brain: Reflection and Attunement in the Cultivation of Well-Being* (New York: W.W. Norton, 2007), 25.

CHAPTER 31   THE FOUR STEPS, PLUS ONE

1. Jeffrey M. Schwartz, *Brain Lock: Free Yourself from Obsessive-Compulsive Behavior* (New York: ReganBooks, 1996), 11.

2. M. Schwartz and Sharon Begley, *The Mind and the Brain: Neuroplasticity and the Power of Mental Force* (New York: ReganBooks, 2002), 224.

3. Schwartz, *Brain Lock*, 41.

4. Ibid., 71.

5. Ibid., 97.

CHAPTER 32   SOBRIETY AND THE EXTERNAL MILIEU

1. Kevin Griffin, *One Breath at a Time: Buddhism and the Twelve Steps* (Emmaus, PA: Rodale Inc., 2004), 92.

2. B. McEwen, "Protective and Damaging Effects of Stress Mediators," *New England Journal of Medicine* 338(3) (15 January 1998).

3. Marian Cleeves Diamond, *Enriching Heredity* (New York: The Free Press, 1988), 163.

CHAPTER 33   A WORD TO FAMILIES, FRIENDS AND CAREGIVERS

1. Edward L. Deci, *Why We Do What We Do: Understanding Self-Motivation* (New York: Penguin Books, 1995), 30.

2. Maia Szalawitz, "When the Cure Is Not Worth the Cost," *The New York Times*, 11 April 2007, A21.

3. Thomas De Quincey, *Confessions of an English Opium Eater* (Ware, Hertfordshire: Wordsworth Classics, 1995), 18–19.

4. Byron Katie, *Loving What Is: Four Questions That Can Change Your Life* (New York: Three Rivers Press, 2002), 4–5.

CHAPTER 34   THERE IS NOTHING LOST

1. Julia Kristeva, *Black Sun: Depression and Melancholia*, trans. L.S. Roudiez (New York: Columbia University Press, 1989), 5.

2. Eckhart Tolle, *The Power of Now: A Guide to Spiritual Enlightenment* (Vancouver: Namaste Publishing, 1997), 23.

3. D. Tankersley et al., "Altruism Is Associated with an Increased Neural Response to Agency," *Nature Neuroscience* 10 (2007): 150–51.

4. Victor Frankl, *Man's Search for Meaning* (New York: Washington Square Press, 1985), 164.

5. Joseph Campbell, *The Hero with a Thousand Faces* (Princeton, NJ: Princeton University Press, 1972), 285, 286.

6. A.H. Almaas, *Diamond Heart, Book One: Elements of the Real in Man* (Berkeley, CA: Diamond Books, 1987), 21.

7. Edmund Spenser, *The Faerie Queene* (New York: Penguin Books, 1987) canto v, book 2, line 39.

8. St. Augustine, *Confessions*, trans. Garry Wills (New York: Penguin Books, 2006), 41.

APPENDIX I   ADOPTION AND TWIN STUDY FALLACIES

1. J.S. Alper and M.R. Natowicz, "On Establishing the Genetic Basis of Mental Disease," *Trends in Neuroscience* 16(10) (October 1993): 387–89.

2. K. Kendler, "A Gene for . . .": The Nature of Gene Action in Psychiatric Disorders," *American Journal of Psychiatry* 162 (July 2005):1243–52.

3. Robert Plomin, *Development, Genetics, and Psychology* (Hilllsdale, NJ: Lawrence Erlbaum Associates, 1986), 9.

4. C.R. Cloninger et al., "Inheritance of Alcohol Abuse," *Archives of General Psychiatry* 38 (1981): 861–68.

5. S.R. Dube et al., "Growing Up with Parental Alcohol Abuse: Exposure to Childhood Abuse, Neglect and Household Dysfunction," *Child Abuse & Neglect* 25 (2001): 1627–40.

6. J.S. Alper and M.R. Natowicz, "On Establishing the Genetic Basis of Mental Disease," *Trends in Neuroscience* 16(10) (October 1993): 387–89.

7. K.S. Kendler et al., "A Multidimensional Twin Study of Mental Health in Women," *American Journal of Psychiatry* 157 (April 2000): 506–13.

8. M.A. Enoch and D. Goldman, "The Genetics of Alcoholism and Alcohol Abuse," *Current Psychiatry Reports* 3 (2002): 144–51.

9. L.A. Pohorecky, "Interaction of Ethanol and Stress: Research with Experimental Animals—An Update," *Alcohol & Alcoholism* 25(2/3) (1990): 263–76.

10. G. Slap et al., "Adoption as a Risk Factor for Attempted Suicide During Adolescence," *Pediatrics* 108(2) (August 2001): E30.

11. D.W. Goodwin, "Alcoholism and Heredity: A Review and Hypothesis," *Archives of General Psychiatry* 38 (1979): 57–61.

APPENDIX II   A CLOSE LINK: ATTENTION DEFICIT DISORDER AND ADDICTIONS

1. K.M. Carroll and B.J. Rousnaville, "History and Significance of Childhood Attention Deficit Disorder in Treatment-Seeking Cocaine Abusers," *Comprehensive Psychiatry* 34(2) (March-April 1993): 75–82.

2. D. Wood et al., "The Prevalence of Attention Deficit Disorder, Residual Type,

in a Population of Male Alcoholic Patients," *American Journal of Psychiatry* 140 (1983): 15–98.

3. J. Biederman et al., "Does Attention-Deficit Hyperactivity Disorder Impact the Developmental Course of Drug and Alcohol Abuse and Dependence?" *Biological Psychiatry* 44(4) (15 August 1998): 269–73.

4. Dr. Richard Rawson, Associate Director of the Integrated Substance Abuse Program, University of California at Los Angeles, Teleconference, 26 April 2006. Available from U.S. Consulate, Vancouver, BC.

5. B.R. Van den Bergh and A. Marcoen, "High Antenatal Maternal Anxiety Is Related to ADHD Symptoms, Externalizing Problems, and Anxiety in 8- and 9-year-olds," *Child Dev* 75(4) (July-August 2004): 1085–97.

6. M.H. Teicher, "Wounds That Time Won't Heal: The Neurobiology of Child Abuse," *Cerebrum: The Dana Forum on Brain Science* 2(4) (fall 2000).

7. M.J. Meaney et al., "Environmental Regulation of the Development of Mesolimbic Dopamine Systems: A Neurobiological Mechanism for Vulnerability to Drug Abuse?" *Psychoneuroendocrinology* 27 (2002): 127–38.

8. Nora D. Volkow et al., "Depressed Dopamine Activity in Caudate and Preliminary Evidence of Limbic Involvement in Adults With Attention-Deficit/Hyperactivity Disorder." *Archives of General Psychiatry*. 64 (2007): 932–940.

9. T.E. Wilens et al., "Does Stimulant Therapy of Attention-Deficit/Hyperactivity Disorder Beget Later Substance Abuse? A Meta-Analytic Review of the Literature," *Pediatrics* 111(1) (January 2003): 179–85.

10. T. Sim et al., "Cognitive Deficits Among Methamphetamine Users with Attention Deficit Hyperactivity Disorder Symptomatology," *Journal of Addictive Diseases* 21(1) (2002): 75–89.

11. Meaney et al., "Environmental Regulation."

APPENDIX III   THE PREVENTION OF ADDICTION

1. An indispensable resource to all parents and also to all professionals working with families and children is the seminal work on healthy child development by my friend, colleague and mentor Dr. Gordon Neufeld. No other authority has articulated so clearly the devastating impact of the growing tendency of children to connect to each other rather than to nurturing adults, nor the prevention and management of this phenomenon. See Gordon Neufeld and Gabor Maté, *Hold On to Your Kids: Why Parents Need to Matter More Than Peers*.

ACKNOWLEDGMENTS

My first thanks go to the men and women who have trustingly laid their lives open to me as their physician and as a writer and who agreed to tell their stories for this book. As I mentioned in the preface, their oft-stated motivation was to help others understand addiction and the experience of the addict. Working with them in the Downtown Eastside continues to be my privilege. I also thank non-patients such as Stephen Reid—and others whom I cannot name—who have shared with me and the reader their struggles with addiction.

I gratefully acknowledge the financial assistance provided by the Canada Council for the research and preparation of *Hungry Ghosts*.

The knowledge, perspectives and generous time shared by the following outstanding researchers and clinicians have greatly enhanced my understanding of addiction and the addiction process: Drs. Jaak Panksepp, Aviel Goodman, Bruce Perry, Jeffrey Schwartz and Bruce Alexander.

I owe gratitude to four editors. Diane Martin, Publisher at Knopf Canada, has a deep and compassionate interest in Vancouver's Downtown Eastside. She has encouraged *Hungry Ghosts* along from its conception and, as with all my books, her judicious editing has greatly improved the finished work. My son Daniel has served as front-line editor, reviewing and reworking each chapter as the manuscript was being written. His lyricist's gift for language and for recreating dialogue has enlivened many passages: among other felicities, the reader has Daniel to thank for Dr. Fell's "hard day at the OFC." His personal acquaintance with the author and with the Portland Hotel clientele has helped keep the work honest—as has his acute awareness of his father's tendency to sometimes lapse into overdramatization and medical-scientific prolixity. I thank Daniel, too, for his frank and insightful passages about his own experience. My wife, Rae Maté, has contributed much to the writing: her detailed, empathic yet unsentimental critique has helped shape the manuscript from beginning to end. At her Rockwood, Ontario, farmstead copyeditor Kathryn Dean laboured prodigiously against a looming deadline, cleaning up the manuscript with sympathy and a deft touch, incorporating and improving my last-minute changes with forbearance.

I am grateful to Ed McCurdy for the title suggestion, and to the friend identified in the text as "Anne" for sharing her nuanced understanding of the Twelve-Step process and for her astute comments on Part I of the manuscript.

Many other people have read and critiqued all or parts of this work during its preparation. Their insights and forthright critiques have all been most helpful—difficult as I may have found them to gracefully accept at first sight. I owe special thanks to: Margaret Gunning, Mairi Campbell, Dan Small, Kerstin Stuerzbecher and Liz Evans.

In my author's note I have already expressed my appreciation for the contribution made by the artistry of photographer extraordinaire Rod Preston. All readers of this book will, I'm sure, share my gratitude for his work.

Finally, words are inadequate to thank Rae once more for her indispensable belief in my work, her steadying influence and, above all, her loving support.

PERMISSIONS

Grateful acknowledgment is made to the following for the permission
to reprint previously published material:

Quotations on pages 31 and 223 are from "Junkie" by Stephen Reid, from *Addicted:
Notes from the Belly of the Beast*, edited by Lorna Crozier and Patrick Lane.
Published 2001, 2006 by Greystone Books, a division of Douglas & McIntyre
Ltd. Reprinted by permission of the publisher

Quotations on pages 35 and 246 are from *The Drowned and the Saved* by Primo Levi,
translated from the Italian by Raymond Rosenthal. English translation © 1988
by Simon & Schuster, Inc. Reprinted by permission of Simon & Schuster Adult
Publishing Group.

Quotations on pages 140, 260 and 261 are from *The Selfish Brain: Learning from
Addiction* by Robert L. Dupont, M.D. Copyright © 2000 by Hazelden Foundation.
Reprinted by permission of Hazelden Foundation, Centre City, MN.

Quotations on pages 168, 204, 286, 343 and 357 are from *The Mind and the Brain:
Neuroplasticity and the Power of Mental Force* by Jeffrey Schwartz and Sharon
Begley. Reprinted by permission of HarperCollins Publishers.

Quotations on pages 183, 186 and 435n are from *Human Behavior and the
Developing Brain*. Reprinted with permission of the publisher.

The quotation on page 185 is from *The Developing Mind: Toward a Neurobiology of
Interpersonal Experience*. Reprinted with permission of the publisher.

The quotation on page 213 is © Maurice Walsh, 1987, 1995. Reprinted from *The
Long Discourses of the Buddha: A Translation of the Digha Nikaya*, with permission of Wisdom Publications, 199 Elm Street, Somerville, MA 02144 U.S.A.,
www.wisdompubs.org.

The quotation on page 251 is from *Requiem for a Dream*.

Quotations on pages 255, 259, 287 and 389 are from *The Power of Now: A Guide to
Spiritual Enlightenment*, by Eckart Tolle, published by Namaste Publishing.
Reprinted with permission.

Throughout this index the abbreviation *AA* will be used to indicate references to Alcoholics Anonymous and the abbreviation *DE* will be used for references to the Downtown Eastside. Quotation marks will be used to indicate pseudonyms (for example, "Celia").

GABOR MATÉ, M.D., is the author of the bestselling books *Scattered Minds: A New Look at the Origins and Healing of Attention Deficit Disorder* and *When the Body Says No: The Cost of Hidden Stress*—published in ten languages on five continents—and co-author, with Gordon Neufeld, of *Hold On to Your Kids: Why Parents Need to Matter More than Peers*. Former medical columnist for the *Globe and Mail*, where his byline continues to be seen on issues of health and parenting, Dr. Maté has had a family practice, worked as a palliative care physician and, most recently, with the addicted men and women in the Downtown Eastside of Vancouver.